WARRIOR'S WAY:
Ben Singer Grows Strong By Learning The Strength Secrets Of Ancient Warrior Societies

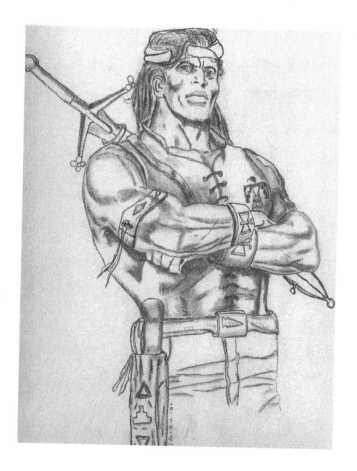

By: Jon H. Hansen, M.Ed.

Order this book online at www.trafford.com/07-0956
or email orders@trafford.com

Most Trafford titles are also available at major online book retailers.

Note for Librarians: A cataloguing record for this book is available from Library and Archives Canada at www.collectionscanada.ca/amicus/index-e.html

Printed in Victoria, BC, Canada.

ISBN: 978-1-4251-2781-7

We at Trafford believe that it is the responsibility of us all, as both individuals and corporations, to make choices that are environmentally and socially sound. You, in turn, are supporting this responsible conduct each time you purchase a Trafford book, or make use of our publishing services. To find out how you are helping, please visit www.trafford.com/responsiblepublishing.html

Our mission is to efficiently provide the world's finest, most comprehensive book publishing service, enabling every author to experience success. To find out how to publish your book, your way, and have it available worldwide, visit us online at www.trafford.com/10510

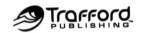

www.trafford.com

North America & international
toll-free: 1 888 232 4444 (USA & Canada)
phone: 250 383 6864 ♦ fax: 250 383 6804
email: info@trafford.com

The United Kingdom & Europe
phone: +44 (0)1865 722 113 ♦ local rate: 0845 230 9601
facsimile: +44 (0)1865 722 868 ♦ email: info.uk@trafford.com

10 9 8 7 6 5 4 3 2 1

Warrior's Way

Chapter One: Ben Singer Learns To Sing

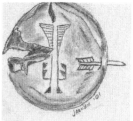

"Now let's hear you howl, Benny," Dick Sand said. "Like one a them Hollywood Indians."

Ben Singer stopped shuffling around the campfire and let the rage and shame and the bright new hate that was seething in him come up and focus in his eyes as he looked at Sand across the fire. Firelight glinted off Dick Sand's shiny uniform buttons and his big deputy sheriff's badge.

And from the eyes and off the milk white fangs of Sand's grinning Doberman police dog.

The Black Prince.

Tonight Prince looked like his namesake. He stood near Sand, haunches quivering, his red-lit eyes locked on Ben. Waiting for, aching for, the command that would launch him across the fire. Dick Sand loomed massive and powerful, the firelight glinting redly in his eyes. He didn't need any help whipping the likes of Ben Singer.

Sand smiled a broad, slow smile and stepped closer to Lester Pearson who lay near his feet puking softly, almost apologetically, into the dry dirt around the picnic table. Sand's sharp, metal-tipped Justin cowboy boots aimed at Lester's midsection like twin 44 caliber pistols, cocked and ready to fire again.

"You want to fight some more, Tubby?" Sand's grin evaporated. A darker tone colored his voice. "If you don't you best keep dancin' and start howling."

Acid contempt dripped from his words scorching Ben's mind, chilling his heart.

Sand" big hands moved down to rest on his hips and Ben saw him lean forward just a little. An icy current of fear trickled down Ben's nerves, snuffing out his anger. Dick Sand was a dangerous man.

Powerful.

And cruel.

Ben grabbed his upper arm and squeezed, trying to cut off the waves of agony that rolled up from his elbow to his neck. Was his shoulder dislocated? He worked the joint. Pain flashed up his shoulder and slammed into his head but the shoulder moved freely. Like Professor Schwartzen says in law class, cops can do that. Hurt you and still leave nothing to show the judge.

Ben felt his face flush. His heart picked up the beat of a war drum. I'll make you pay for this Sand. I'll hang you out to dry. Hound you with the law till you'll wish you could hide in Hell.

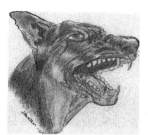

"You can't get away with this Sand .. you know this constitutes assault and battery by a police officer. I'll see you in prison for this .."

Sand kicked Lester again, hard, just under the breast bone, the steel shod tip sinking out of sight into his belly. Lester's mouth started working like a catfish out of water. Ben saw Lester hunch over and heard a keening whine come across the fire. It brought a deep-throated rumbling growl from the Black Prince, who still stared hard at Ben.

"How you getting from here to the highway Benny? Let alone go find yourself a judge. Now I said like a Hollywood Indian, Singer. And I won't tell you nice again"

Sand's face had lost all expression now and Ben's insides went watery when he saw the deadness of it. Only Sand's eyes were alive, squinted down, measuring Ben. Like an undertaker sizing up a dying man, fitting him into his grave.

Where's a cop when you need one? Right across the fire from me But the Law Ben so loved and counted on had no place around this campfire tonight. Only raw physical power. The one thing Ben Singer truly despised. Embodied tonight in Deputy Sheriff Dick Sand, the strongest man in Warren County.

Firelight glinted blood red on the metal tips of Sand's boots as he shifted his feet. Lester hunched over and a small mewing sound made it past the vomit on his mouth. Prince looked from Ben to Lester and back again, grinning in the flickering firelight.

The air turned thick, with an overtone of impending violence. Like the humid stillness just before lightening splits the sky and a booming thunderclap announces torrents of rain and hail.

Ben couldn't catch his breath.

Ben saw Lester looking at him. Misery stood out in every line on the black face reflected in the guttering firelight. A mournful face, full of shame and pain and something else.

I can't take it any more, Ben, his look said. I'm sorry, but I just can't take it any more Please? Make it stop?

Lester was his friend.

But what can I do, Lester? How can I help?

Fighting any more was out.

I tried that, Lester, Ben thought raggedly. Dick Sand's too big, too strong, too mean.

He could tell Sand he was placing him under citizen's arrest. Order him to cage his dog, take off his gun ..Stop hitting me ..Now there's a plan

If you were your father's son you could stop him. Grandpa Tsosie's voice spoke in his mind. You would tear off his arms ..That's what your father would have done to Dick Sand ..Just pull his arms off.

Ben slammed a door in his mind. Revulsion flooded through him. My father is a drunk. And a bully. He felt his face flushing hot. Nobody would want to be like my father .

Sand shifted his feet, seeming to grow impatient with Ben's hesitation. Lester flinched and moaned, but dared not move away from Sand's feet.

The depth of evil in Dick Sand scared Ben. He realized, late, so very late, how little he knew about Deputy Sheriff Dick Sand.

Ben shifted his sore body. The pain in his mind hurt worse. Shuffling around, patting his face, making comic noises Shameful ..I'm Navajo, we don't do those Plains Indian war dances in the first place .. Ben felt heat building up around his heart, a burning that rose to his eyes and made them water. What should I do? What can I do?

Nothing ..Ben was ashamed ..nothing.

Shaming. That's how Navajo's discipline children. Make them ashamed. Tease and belittle them in front of others.

He remembered how his uncles had shamed him. His whole body felt the burning, eye watering flood of feeling he felt then ..and now. Ben would rather die, here, now, than be shamed by Sand.

But he won't hurt me. He'll just kick Lester again ..And I can't stop him.

All Ben Singer, the avid student of the Law, could do now was make a fool of himself if it would help his friend.

Ben's right arm hung useless at his side but he raised his left hand and used it to make the ridiculous imitation of an Indian war cry that every child knew. The shame burned in his face as he shuffled his feet in time to the noise.

Oo-woo-woo-woo

Oo-woo-woo-woo

Ben tasted dirt in his mouth each time his hand patted his face. And he felt some black emotion wriggling in him.

Shame. In a whole new dimension.

Bigger, deeper than anything he had ever felt before. Misting out and filling up every niche and nook inside him. He looked up once, out across the valley, alight in the night. He felt like a prisoner gazing through a wire fence at another world.

A world he could never rejoin.

He felt so alone. The longing for someone to help, even to just look on in sympathy, flooded him with an ache that made his throat close in a gasping, agonizing cramp.

He saw the headlights on Sand's big Suburban, reflecting the firelight in a cold, red and silver glow. Like the dead eyes of an Aztec war god. Gazing on its next sacrificial victim. Pitiless, unheeding. Aloof and cold. Above noticing the humans suffering here tonight.

After that Ben kept his eyes on his feet. And he kept up his shuffle and his stupid Hollywood war whoop.

After a couple of minutes, long, face-burning, humiliating minutes, Sand seemed to tire of his game with Ben.

"That's better, Benny-Boy. Now come on over here. We just got to have ourselves a talk."

Ben moved cautiously around the fire. Sand's next words, spoken softly with his easy-going West Texas drawl, hit Ben like blows from his fists, hard .from a totally unexpected direction.

"Now Benny, you got to make up your mind, right here, right now, that you're going to say goodbye to that purty little gal of yours and leave Warren Valley before sunrise tomorrow."

Sand's grin was back.

Ben was stunned.

****

Chapter Two

"We need to talk, Benny," Sand had said on the phone. "I know who killed TJ."

"Killed? TJ was murdered?"

Ben had heard the shock in his voice and had felt a needle-sharp pain in his stomach.

Sharp as the needle the EMTs had found stuck fast in TJ's arm. He felt cold sweat beading on his upper lip, starting to trickle down his back.

"Terry said--"

"Don't matter what she said, Benny. You followin' me? You turned him into a snoop.

Now he's dead "

The silence hung heavy on the line. Ben rubbed his stomach.

"You told me you was turning him, putting him out on the street as a snoop. Make him like you. You said you was a snoop once too. That's how you got your fancy scholarship, you said."

"I was trying to help him get straight, get off the street, not become an undercover cop .just identify the dealers in his school. He was only 13-- "

"He ain't getting any older, Benny. Question is, what you gonna do about it?" Sand's voice was edged with impatience, ..or scorn. "I know who helped him shoot up."

Ben saw TJ's damp, mottled face framed against the pillow where he lay in the emergency room, hooked and wired like an astronaut. Only TJ wasn't headed for outer space.

Terry was there, holding the teen ager's hand. She suffered quietly for TJ, who was brain-dead and couldn't suffer for himself.

Murdered

Someone held TJ down and put raw Mexican heroin in him? Destroyed his mind? Ended his life.

A crime against all human kind, he heard his Grandpa Tsosie say in his head. Each bilaa 'ashdlaa 'i (five fingered one=human being) is unique. Each mind must be respected. No one can do such a thing and not become something evil and inhuman.

Someone who killed children. Ben had felt a little surge of fear pulse through him, like when Grandpa Tsosie used to tell spooky stories about the dine naldlooshi, the were-men who dressed in animal skins and killed a brother or sister so they could get dark power. They could run fast as a truck, it was said. As long as some evil helper stayed in the hogan and worked the magic for them. Yes, and they could yank little kids out an open truck window along some dark highway. To never be seen again. Ben felt a shiver crawl along his backbone as Sand continued.

"You best be at Tibble Fork Campground tonight. See if we can keep you outta jail on this Folks around here don't smile on people who get little kids killed tryin' to be a do-gooder.

Nine o'clock, Benny . Be there. Bring Lester with you, not Terry .or anyone else. We gotta play this close to the chest. Don't make no more mistakes. You'll get somebody else killed and don't be late ..And oh yeah. Singer .." Sand's voice dropped to a harsh whisper. "Be careful. Don't talk to anyone. You don't know who you can trust."

****

Ben was careful. Lester sounded like he had the flu when Ben called him, but he readily agreed to come. Next he broke his date with Terry: "I have a paper due tomorrow for law class and it just isn't finished." "You perfectionist", she had said, but he could hear the affection in her voice. He hated to lie to her, but she would insist on coming and if things were as dangerous as they sounded he didn't want her anywhere near Tibble Fork tonight.

They arrived at the campground on Ben's Honda Goldwing road bike just before nine.

Oh yes, Ben was careful all right ..

Big mistake number one

Nothing prepared him for what happened when Sand pulled in. This early spring night the rest of the campground was empty. The fire he and Lester built barely held back the somber darkness of the black lava rock walls around them. The air was chilly and the fire warmed them but little.

The moment Sand arrived things started getting strange. Lester backed off behind the picnic table like a small dog going to the end of its tether to escape an approaching cougar.

Because, of course, as Ben saw now, Lester knew what was going to happen.

At least he thought he did. On reflection Ben doubted that Lester would have come at all if he'd known what Sand was going to do to him.

He only knew what Sand was going to do to Ben.

But Lester is my friend .

"I'm glad you and the nigger could make it, Benny."

As he spoke Sand moved over and casually sat on the picnic table, both feet still firmly on the ground. Ben looked at Lester and saw there the hurt Sand's words caused. But he was startled when he also saw fear scrawled on Lester's face.

"There's no need for that kind of crudeness here, Dick," Ben had said.

"Oh, you got to be straight up with people, Benny. Otherwise folks don't know where they stand. And when folks don't know where they stand, they put on airs. They pretend they're something they ain't," before he could stop himself Sand automatically corrected his grammar, "aren't."

As you say, Sand. Putting on airs tonight, are we?

Proper speech was something Sand struggled with in the classes they shared at Warren Valley Community College. Ben felt a grin stretching his face.

Though huge and naturally powerful. Sand was often amusing as he bumbled along, trying to get the educated polish he seemed so hungry for.

Sand paused, realizing maybe what his grammar was saying about him, not Lester.

Without another word he'd lashed out with a powerful arm and slapped Lester hard in the chest, grabbing his shirt, and throwing him forward into the firelight. Ben opened his mouth to say something like: Heyyy! Knock it off. Sand.

But just then Sand looked at him.

Ben had never seen such malevolence in a human face. It cut off his words like someone had pulled the plug on a tape player. His mind went blank, the words stuck in his throat. And then the Black Prince moved like a ghost into the firelight, to stand looking from Ben to Sand and back again.

Ben froze in place. Lester rolled over on his back to get away from the fire, but made no move to get up.

While looking straight at Ben, his eyes glittering redly in the firelight. Sand kicked Lester in the stomach, hard, with the pointed, metal-tipped toe of his custom-made Justin cowboy boot.

Lester rolled over in agony and began to vomit, all the time clutching his stomach, but made no move to defend himself.

"You know where you stand, nigger?" Casual, almost conversational. A horrifying counterpoint to the look on his face and the violence of his actions.

Despite his fear, Ben felt outrage building quickly in him.

This was sick. This was blatantly illegal. Sand couldn't do this ..

Sand put a hand under Lester's arm pit and with one hand effortlessly lifted him completely off the ground and then dropped him. Lester instantly sat down, bent over, totally inert, offering no resistance, showing no antagonism.

"See, Benny, Lester knows where he stands. "You gonna play your part tonight, huh, Les?

Lester didn't move. He sat as though carved from the surrounding lava rock. Sand's boot-tip found his kidney in a vicious, probing kick and Lester straightened up, the twisted scream coming from his throat sounding like the word Yesss! was being wrung from the lava rock itself.

Ben had had enough. He jumped the fire, planning to use his momentum to shove Sand away from Lester.

Big mistake number two.

Ben wasn't small, he weighed a flabby 220 pounds, but he felt like he had just tried to shove the side of a sky scraper. Sand didn't budge. Ben felt his rock solid body as he was jolted by the impact. Sand was a head taller, so he couldn't see his face, but he heard Sand's gleeful laugh.

Then he was shoved violently backward, lost his balance, stumbled down into the fire pit, felt the scorching flames and danced awkwardly backward and fell sprawling in the dirt.

Ben saw Sand through a red haze as he got up and rushed back at him, swinging hard and fast. Sand batted down his arms, practically paralyzing them. Then he grabbed Ben's right arm, pivoting into him, and doing an over the shoulder throw

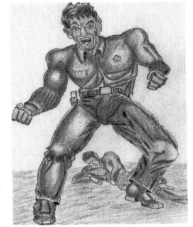

that had Ben going easily up over Sand's head and then crashing down to the ground. Sand held onto his arm and would't let it rotate and Ben felt an excruciating pain shoot through his arm and shoulder.

Ben didn't remember feeling the breath rush from his lungs, only the solid smash of his upper body on the ground and the burning in his chest as he tried to breathe.

The pain was awful. He heard a weird, unearthly sound as he rolled over onto his side. It was Lester, but it was also him, the voices combining in a strange, unharmonious, keening duet.

A non-musical tribute to pain.

And to defeat.

And to shame.

Prince whined along with them for a moment and then growled deep in his chest when Sand turned and glared at him.

Even through the pain Ben's mind screamed: Why? Why's this happening? This man has taken an oath to uphold the law He has to know I'll prosecute him for this, send him to jail ..Ice water flushed through his body ..Is he planning to kill us?

Sand moved away, looming large across the fire. He leaned casually against the picnic table his huge arms folded across his chest. His boots again within easy reach of Lester, who could not run away from Sand because of the dog.

Prince moved around the back of the table, not coming between Sand and Ben, and stood next to Sand. His tongue was hanging out now. gleaming red against the white fangs and the blackface. To Ben he was grinning , alert, tense. Like the tag team partner outside the ropes of the wrestling ring Waiting eagerly for the signal that would launch him into action.

Sand ignored him.

Ben struggled to make his pain-fogged brain work. But Deputy Sheriff Dick Sand wasn't giving Ben time to think.

"Get up, Benny," Sand said. "Let's see you dance. And howl like a Hollywood Indian."

****

Now Sand was telling him to get out?

Leave the valley? Before daylight? Quit school? Leave Terry behind? Abandon everything he was working so hard for? Ben rubbed his stomach hard. But the pain wouldn't let up. Between his belly and the pains shooting up through his shoulder he was getting dizzy, lightheaded.

Scared.

San's grin was slow and lazy, huge with enjoyment, and terrible. Sand seemed to be saying: I can keep this up all night, Singer. How about you?

Not me, Ben thought.

He couldn't look at Sand.

Or at Lester.

Ben felt his confidence shred inside him. The space it left was huge and dark and empty and lonely in a way Ben never imagined anything could be. His eyes misted and burned as the loss hit him.

You cryin', Benny-Boy?

Sand came over and took his chin and lifted it. Ben twisted his head away and kept looking at the ground, not meeting Sand's eyes any more. Trying to ignore the grin.

Suddenly Sand's hand gripped his jaw hard and twisted his face around until he had to look into Sand's eyes. He saw a great, uncaring emptyness, like the empty headlight eyes of Sand's suburban. And a glint of something Ben could not name.

But it scared him. Made his knees weak, his insides watery. Pain, shame, fear combined in him creating an anguish that dominated him, shutting down logic, creating a crawling, animal fear that fought to control his mind .

It was so awful, outrageous, so unexpected, that Ben couldn't wrap his mind around it.   He'd come tonight, Oh so innocently ..thinking he and Sand would jointly come up with a plan to revenge TJ's death. Bring the full weight of the law down on the heads of those who supplied death-dealing drugs to children. Do some good that would be a credit to them both.

Not this. Never in his darkest dreams did he envision this

Numbly he stared back at Sand. He couldn't think of a thing to say. But even through the haze of pain part of his mind saw Dick Sand in the bright orange jumpers worn by jail inmates.

He would find some way to make it happen.

Sand looked at him as he took a step back. Calculating, like he was somewhere inside Ben's mind.

"He won't testify, you know," Sand said.

He looked over at Lester who was curled into a ball under the table.

"Will you, Lester ole buddy."

Sand's voice sounded reasonable and very, very self-assured.

"No." The voice sounded like it was emerging from under a rug.

"What's that you said, Lester? Maybe Benny didn't hear you."

Lester's voice got louder, and higher, almost hysterical.

"No! I said I won't testify against you."

Sand smiled at Ben.

"So you see, Benny-Boy, you've got no case. Just your word against mine. And my word says that you and Lester were resisting arrest."

Dumbfounded, Ben blurted: "Arrest? Under arrest? What have we done? You walked up and kicked Lester for no reason at all. Then you assaulted me, harassed and humiliated us both--."

"Humiliation, Benny? You into humiliation? Well we got some here for you."

He turned to Lester, who still lay huddled under the picnic table, his arms wrapped around his head. Sand nudged him with his boot.

"You want to tell him, Les? He might rather hear it from you since you're, how do you say it ..a principal actor in this little play?"

Sand's laugh was like a cold, hollow wind.

Ben saw Lester's head shaking from side to side, but he wouldn't turn over and look in Ben's direction. He just lay there like a wounded animal that expected, even hoped, to die.

He looked as beaten, as defeated, as Ben felt.

As Sand moved toward him, Ben flinched and started to duck away.

Sand just grinned, took him roughly by his sore arm, and escorted him to the back of the big four by four suburban. It was Sand's personal vehicle, provided by him, as a service to the county, the way Michael Jordan had provided a bus for his baseball team. It had Sheriff's Department decals, and a whip antenna for the powerful radio that tied him into the state police dispatcher up in Hatch. It had a personalized license plate that no one made fun of:

LAWDOG.

Ben wondered again why a man as rich as Sand said he was wanted to play deputy sheriff in a mountainous county in Utah.

Too tired too much pain for thinking hard about anything except how much Sand was hurting him. He just wanted this to end. So he could turn Sand in, with or without Lester's help. Sand was dreaming if he thought Ben was going to give up his scholarship and Terry and his future as an attorney for his people, the Navajo.

Just because Sand said so. He felt some anger and indignation start to seep back into his blood.

Then Sand opened the back door and took out a video cassette and showed it to Ben.

"It's all on here, Benny. You want to see?"

Sand had a glittering look in is eyes.

He's relly proud of this, whatever it is....

How ridiculous was this going to get? Sand wasn't stupid, but this was making him look pretty dumb.

You can't have anything on that tape, Sand, because I haven't done anything wrong. You know it. What's this all about?"

Sand said nothing, only grinned his big, self-satisfied grin. The grin that Ben was learning to hate ..and fear. Sand just put the tape into his portable VCR/TV and watched as the machine lit up, the blue screen saying: PLAY.

Curious in spite of his anger and pain, Ben watched the flickering images that emerged from the snowy static on the screen. First he saw a campfire, then two shadowy figures on a blanket near the fire.

Disgust flushed through him. He had never watched pornography in any form, just as he'd never used drugs or alcohol. His traditional Navajo training under Grandpa Tsosie at Chinle had taught him that anything that had been artificially extracted out of the ebb and flow of human life, that became concentrated, distilled, set apart from its natural state was evil and dangerous, even deadly to the human spirit as well as to the human body.

Despite his inexperience, he became aware that what he was seeing was far more than x-rated. He was about to turn away in disgust when the camera began to zoom in. Ben recognized the campsite. It was right here in Tibble Fork Campground. The next thing that slammed into his mind was that the two figures on the blanket were men ..and in the next second a bombshell exploded in his mind.

Complex torrents of emotion ripped through him and then gathered around his heart and squeezed down until he couldn't get his breath. And a thousand rushing thoughts assailed his mind, competing for attention all at once, till his mind just went blank, like an overloaded computer, and all he could see was that the two men on the blanket looked just like Lester Pearson and .Ben Singer.

Through a haze Ben heard Sand☐s voice, calm, objective, dispassionate saying:

"What do you think, Benny-Boy? Good work, huh? Nobody will have trouble telling who it is Why shame on you Benny. Who knew?"

There was pride and satisfaction in Sand's voice. Like a man with a job well done behind him.

""Thaaa ..that's a lie!" Ben said in a stage whisper, not loud, yet harsh, unbelieving. "Where did you get something like that?"

"You mean this here evidence, Tubby? That led to you and Lester resisting arrest? That evidence that Ole Les will swear to in a court of law? That what you mean, Benny?"

Lester was listening. Ben heard him moaning and crying from his place under the picnic table.

Suddenly, as quickly as a giant Grizzly can go from innocent fun to murderous rage, Sand's mood switched from amused indifference to something ugly and dangerous. The malevolence re-emerged, choking off Ben's mind, filling him with raw fear.

"It don't matter where it came from. What matters is that I got it. What matters is that Lester's daddy is a Southern Baptist Minister down in Texas."

He turned to Lester.

"What do you think, Les. Shall we send him a copy and tell him it shows you

9

getting an award from WCCC? That he should set it up and invite in all your family and friends? What do you think? Good idea or not?" Sand's voice whipped across the space between them and lashed Lester mercilessly. "You best get out from there and start talking, Lester."

Lester crawled from under the table. He scrabbled, hands and knees, then crab-wise over to Ben and hugged him around the knees.

"Please, Ben," he said, his voice full of pain and fear. "Don't do anything to make him send it. If that was my life style I could stand up and say so, but it isn't. It would just kill my folks ..Ben .Please!"

Lester's sobs were deep and heart wrenching, and Ben suddenly had no idea what to do. Any nebulous plans floating around in his head evaporated like raindrops in a campfire.

Sand took his time about turning off the VCR and ejecting the tape. He held it in one big hand and tapped it lightly against the open palm of the other. He grinned at Ben, but the eyes were cold, calculating, measuring.

Ben stepped away and looked up at the dark sky in agony. Why's Sand doing this? He had to admit he's never liked Sand, too much like his own father .a brash bullying braggart. Rough and tumble fighter who had beaten anyone in Warren County dumb enough to take him on. But he had shut crime down in his part of the county. Like turning off a faucet of filthy water. Lawbreakers didn't prosper on Dick Sand's turf. He was the logical person to ask for help with TJ. Ben figured he could overlook the parts he didn't like about the Dick Sand he knew

But this Dick Sand? The one who had showed up at Tiibble Fork Tonight? He was like something out of Stephen King's mind. Twisted in ways Ben couldn't begin to fathom.

Then the sea of physical and emotional agony in which Ben's brain was floating froze like Arctic ice as an image flashed through his mind. He saw his grandfather watching Sand's tape. No devout Christian was ever more outraged by such activity than were traditional Navajos. Ben's hands began to sweat at the thought of his family dealing with such an accusation, backed up by such graphic evidence as the tape. Their reputations in their home communities would be ruined. Their enemies would gain great power over them. The taint of suspicion would verge on the crimes of Navajo witchcraft and would torment the whole extended family.

Try as he would, Ben's exhausted mind could find no reason for what Dick Sand was doing to him. And to Lester.

Sand's behavior was so unexpected, so far outside reasonable humanity that Ben knew he could never have anticipated it.

The phone call, the mystery in Sand's voice, the words "I know who killed TJ", the instructions to bring Lester, but not Terry.

It was all a set up.

A trap.

Like setting a snare for a cow.

What was the purpose? Ben couldn't be a threat to anyone. Pain stabbed through his shoulder, making him wince. The action caused a shudder of pain through his whole body, fogging his mind, confusing his thoughts.

"Why are you doing this, Dick?" Ben heard the wonder in is voice. "What are you trying to prove? What can you possibly have to gain that's worth committing a major crime like this? I thought we were going to work together, with TJ, to do some real good ."

Wrong thing to say. Ben knew it instantly as he saw Sand's face grow hard again, the meanness springing into his eyes.

"Why? It ain't for you to know, Benny-boy. Best you don't know .." Smile that didn't reach the eyes, broad wink, vicious elbow deliberately slamming into Ben's sore shoulder, refreshing the waves of agony rolling up his arm and into his head. " I could tell you but then I'd have to kill you ."

Sand's laugh was full of glee.

He enjoys this! He likes to hurt people ..torture them. What kind of man is this? How did he ever get to wear a badge and a gun to become the law itself in parts of Warren County. To be embraced as a brother officer by good men and women. To be trusted by the community ..

Sand pulled a clipboard from the seat of the cab.

"Let's get this done, Benny. I got lots to do yet tonight. Can't let the little stuff get in my way."

Sand's huge finger directed Ben's gaze to the papers he held in his hand. He had trouble focusing well enough to see the heading.

"This here's your letter to the dean, giving up your scholarship and withdrawing from school. You sign it and I deliver it. You leave Warren County without saying goodby to anyone ..anyone. That clear, Singer?"

Ben was growing numb as the enormity of this began to hammer him. Not even to say goodby to Terry?

"Lester and I will make your excuses. It won't matter what we say cause you won't ever come back to call us liars."

Sand's voice cut like the night wind that stirred the fire. Ben shivered. Sand reached out and grabbed his shirt front, jerking him up roughly, jolting pain lancing his body.

"Take your act somewhere else, Tubby. If you want a life, live it somewhere else. Somewhere far from here. You come back to my turf and I'll know it. Right away. Then this tape will get more replays than a bad TV movie." Sand's voice took on the force of a sledgehammer and each word reverberated through Ben like a blow, chipping away any courage or anger left in him.

Sand shook him again sharply then brought his face down close to Ben's. Ben couldn't look away. He stared stupidly into the depthless dark pools of Sand's eyes and saw there black despair.

"Do you hear me Singer? Are we communicating? Do you know where you stand? Are you going to play your part in this here little drama?"

Ben's head was rocking back and forth with each jerk like a dashboard kwepee doll. Finally he worked the words past the pain that was closing his throat.

"Yess .yes I hear you."

Sand stepped back and shoved the clipboard into Ben's gut, holding it there until Ben took it in a shaking hand. His mind had stopped working. He couldn't tie thoughts together fast enough to make a picture that made any sense. Sand wasn't giving him any time to think and he held all the cards. Sand wasn't talking legalities or right and wrong.

Only naked power.

Sand roughly broke into his scrambled thoughts.

"Now, Lester, you tell Benny-Boy here what happens if he shows his face in Warren County again. You'll tell everyone that what's on that tape is gospel. Right?"

The grizzly still spoke with Sand's voice. Lester's hands shook like leaves in a high wind. His head twisted side to side, back and forth, back and forth. Sand's boot tip just touched Lester in the rib cage and he smacked the tape sharply into the palm of his hand. The noise sounded like a shot in the quiet mountain night.

"Won't you, Les."

Lester began to shake his head up and down. He couldn't stifle a miserable whimper and Ben could see tears coursing wetly down his cheeks. Ben was amazed. There seemed to be nothing that he wouldn't do. Not even this unspeakable thing that would destroy his own family. Ben wondered what it was Sand had on him that could dismantle his humanness so completely.

"Lets hear you say it, Lester. Might as well let it all hang out while we're just here among friends."

The dead tonelessness of Sand's voice made the word friends sound like a curse.

"So that Singer here knows the score. He just might make a big mistake if we don't help him see it like it really is right off."

"Yes!", Lester said, absolute conviction ringing in his quavering voice. He slumped and stared at his hands. "Yes, I'll say it's all true if Ben comes back .."

Lester was kneeling now, his chin sunk in his chest and his eyes glued to the ground. But he sounded like he really meant it. Ben was convinced that he would do it. The heavy sense of hopelessness building in him grew into an all-consuming panic.

Twist and turn as he would in his mind, he could find no way out. Like a wild horse testing its pen with the memory of the open range still coursing hot in its veins, Ben began to feel trapped.

If only he had time, if the pain would just stop for a moment, if he could control his fear .but Sand wasn't giving him any time at all. And he couldn't let Sand arrest him and take him to jail. He had to stay free to have any chance at all of stopping Dick Sand. That's the only thing in his foggy brain that seemed clear to him. He's holding all the cards ..I have to play his game .

The beating he'd taken, the awful vision of irresistible evil Sand had shown him, Lester's vulnerability and Ben's responsibility for what might happen to him, all ate like acid at his confidence.

Sand tapped the clipboard.

"Time's up. Let's have that autograph."

The edge in Sand's voice, the movement of his shoulders, told Ben that the violence that seethed just below the surface was breaking though again.

The emotional turmoil surged and heaved like storm-driven waves of ice-cold water that settled around his heart and squeezed down on his breath and made him pant. He felt that he was shifting his weight first to one foot, then to the other, like an indecisive, terrified elephant who smells tiger, but doesn't know which way to run. He felt himself wringing his hands in an agony of doubt and horror at the choice he faced.

"Now don't whine about it, Benny. Face it like a man if you can."

Sand held out his pen.

"Terry wants it this way too, you know," Sand said. He was grinning again. "You're just in her way. I'll take good care of her for you."

The words generated pure agony in Ben's soul. But he could see no way out. Sand was invincible. And inhuman, unfeeling, and uncaring. He'd enjoy doing everything he threatened and more.

Suddenly Ben was afraid for Terry. There was no appeal to feelings of common human decency in Sand.   To him compassion, pity, must seem a weakness. Something that only made people weak and vulnerable. Ben looked once into the dead eyes looking back at him.   What he saw there was soulless, unmoved and determined. Setting as they did, above Sand's huge grin of anticipation, the eyes chilled Ben to the heart. No hope, no way out of this campground except one.

Ben took the pen and, hand shaking, eyes misty, signed away everything he cared about.

Chapter Three
Leave Home Without It

Sand dropped Lester off on a street corner to make his own way home. He watched Lester limping painfully as he walked away. Sand smiled, pulled out a scrambler radio/telephone concealed in a compartment between the seats and speed dialed a number. He hummed a little west Texas cattle song as he waited.

"Hey, Herschel. I just left Tibble."

"Went okay, did it?" Herschel said.

"It went. Pearson did his job and the tape did the rest."

"So he's pulling out."

"I'm headed to Singer's now to make sure he leaves."

"That so-"

"I'm calling Montero tonight, telling him to start his mules up the trail."

"I thought you decided to wait until this thing was finished."

Sand shifted in his seat. The grizzly came back in his voice.

"Ain't no tomorrow for us, Herschel. Can't wait no more on Singer or anybody else. Montero called. If we can't move right now he's going to pull his money .Look elsewhere. Startin' tomorrow…"

"That soon? I thought he was big on you, Dick."

"Ready or not, it's got to go now, and you got to make it go hear?"

"You want us to take him? That it?"

'No. That's not it, Herschel. Blinky and that jerk friend of his will do the dirty work. They say they want in. I'm gonna find out if they're serious. We need more grunts for the front line work. But I want you and Virgil saddled up and in the startin' gate come first light. Best you come on over into Nephi. And bring your field gear and huntin' rifles ..We got to make sure this happens. If those two fools mess up you'll need to get them and Singer."

"But not in Warren County ", Herschel said.

"That's why I pushed Singer so hard. To get him away from here, even if just for a day or two."

Sand pulled up half a block from Ben's apartment and backed the van down into the dark shadow cast by a huge pioneer poplar tree. He didn't like what he was hearing.

"Oh yeah? Sure it's getting' tight, Herschel. I aint no gypsy with a crystal ball. How was I supposed to know that Singer was setting up a snoop to come after us? Huh? Tell me that, Herschel. I nearly puked when he told me. He could have told someone else instead. I always said hangin' out at the college could pay off. And it did. Wouldn't that be fine, Singer on our case. And TJ holding us up for blood money . I tell you it was a near thing there.

"And nothing is solved yet. Not by a West Texas country mile. We can't suddenly have bodies showin' up all over Warren County. And we can't wait any longer. This has got to go, got to, hear? What ever it takes. Make sure ..just make sure you're in place come sunup ."

Sand rummaged on the seat and passed Prince a Pig☐s ear to gnaw on to keep him from getting restless. He took a long slow breath and tried to change his tone.

"When I checked Singer's record I couldn't believe that a fat, stubborn Injun kid could do so much damage. He's some kinda twisted Boy Scout. If he don't like you he gets the law after you however he can. Uses the legal system like a fighter uses his fists .. I think he might've even got Orvil busted down in Arizona ..Yeah. He's still servin' time down there in Yuma so far as I know. He don't send me no Christmas cards. Too hot down there for Christmas anyhow. That's why Singer's got to go.

"But I showed him tonight that the law's no substitute for a good right arm. Had him cryin' before it was over. ..But I'm getting better. I didn't lose it and kill him outright, though I was sure mad enough. Hey, I'm just learning to deal with my "immpulsivity issues" as they say over at the egg head factory."

Sand's gleeful laugh echoed in the night, but only the Black Prince noticed.

"You mean like since TJ you learned, Dick." Herschel looked and Virgil and rolled his eyes dramatically. "Where is he now?"

"I'm watchin' his place right now. He's in there packin' to leave even as we speak. I got a way to tie another knot in his tail before he leaves. I'm not leaving nothing to chance, Herschel. Make sure you and Virg don't either. You know what we stand to get out of this. You're my main man, big fella. I got to know I can count on you."

"Sure, Dick, you can count on us. You know that."

Sand shifted the phone to his other ear.

"Okay, then. Get crackin' guys. Keep your radio on. You will be hearing from me first thing."

The silence on the other end told him that he'd made his point.

He broke the connection and put in a call to Blinky Scopes.

"Well, you and your buddy ready to rumble? Our boy will be hitting the freeway about sunrise--

"Don't give me that. You can't be not sure this late in the game. You know way too much to turn back now, ole buddy .You wanted in, you said, Blinky. You and your evil twin. Well here's your chance to make your bones. You and Two-Step got to get set to take care of Singer first thing tomorrow, just make sure he's out of this county and it looks accidental."

"Listen. I'll make sure Singer leaves Warren Valley. You just make sure you don't lose him. You know his bike. I'll tell you which way he turns when he hits the road in the morning."

Sand listened a moment.

"This operation's already underway. You're in. You're on damage control. You 'n Two-step are the garbage men. Just make sure you take out the garbage ..in the morning."

"Just get the guy. That's all you got to do. Yeah, I guarantee he'll at least leave the county.

He don't want his girl to see the tape ..and I think he's scared for her. Yeah, he should be, alright. He don't want her to end up like TJ so he needs to keep her out of it. He won't do nothin' tonight or tomorrow to put her in danger. If he tries, I'm right here on his doorstep to stop him. I got one last little send off in store for him in the morning. All you two got to do is make sure you're ready at the freeway to follow him whichever way he goes. I'm bettin' it's south, back to the reservation. Get some rest. You'll have a busy day. With a big payoff after. You'll soon be driving that new Outlaw truck you got your eye on."'

Or you'll end up on the freeway lookin' like road kill.

Sand laughed at something he heard. "Yeah, I just might do that. I'm gong to call her right now."

Warrior's Way

Tough to get good help now days .

Sand killed the connection and then dialed again.

'Hello, Terry? Dick ..Dick Sand. Listen, I need to talk to you Terry ..There's something maybe you oughta know .Wait! ..It's about Benny and I really, really think you'll want to hear this .. "

Sand felt his grin stretching his face as he started talking quietly, confidentially, into the phone.

In Fairview, up close against where an old Ute Indian war trail led up onto Skyline Ridge where the Great Western Trail crossed the Colorado Plateau as it snaked its way from Mexico to Canada, Herschel looked at Virgil.

"I got a bad feeling about this, Virgil. Too many loose ends. And Sand's killing people again."

Virgil shrugged and turned off the VCR and TV.

They watched Terminator every so often.

For inspiration.

"He didn't kill Singer…."

"Yeah. Bragged just now he was learning to handle his impulsiveness issues. If he is, he's changed his spots just today."

"He's a frog on a hot stove, hoppin' whichever way. Liable to land anywhere anytime."

"Say, Virg, you think Sand has anyone else working for him. People maybe we don't know about, I mean."

"Could be. Yeah. Knowing him, probably—"

"I mean scary people. People with guns and a bad attitude."

"Like us, you mean."

"Yeah. Like us, only not us."

"You don't trust Sand? That it?"

Herschel looked around like he was maybe wondering if the room had been bugged and Sand was listening. He took a sideways, slant-eyed look at Virgil.

"You think Sand likes us, Virg?"

"Nope."

"Me neither. I don't mean that he hates us, or anything."

"No, you don't mean that. If he hated us we'd know right away."

"Just no human warmth there."

"What you getting' at, Herschel?"

"I don't suppose we could just not go, and say we did."

'Take his money and not get caught in his crazy plans ..''

"Or just get out altogether, maybe." Herschel ran his fingers through his buzz-cut hair.

"You really think Sand has a handle on all this, Virg? This big plan to make us all rich?"

"Nope."

"I worry, Virg. Sand gets nervous and goes off like a cheap Chinese rocket. Shootin' off the launch pad in five directions at once."

"Unpredictable .that's what you're saying. A danger to his friends and his enemies."

"He thinks, then double-thinks and then rethinks everything again. Spooky as a one-eyed steer in a cactus patch."

"He won't believe nothing you tell him."

"Yeah. You heard me try to ask him a question? You see this little rim of red around my ear? That's what you get for tryin' to give Dick Sand advice. When he decides he sees a threat—"

"Meaner than a grizzly with a busted tooth . Like with poor little TJ."

"That's why I asked if you think he likes us. Even just a little."

"No, Herschel. No, I don't think we mean anything at all to him."

"Not on a personal level."

"Yeah, that."

"So we better go on over to Nehpi, huh?"

"Yup."

"Cause, if he don't like us we better not get him mad."

" Could be somebody out there now spookier than us."

"Sand would set 'em on us in a minute. Just like he's ready to set us on the two stooges."

"In a Heartbeat."

"Yeah". Hand through the hair, "I think you're right, Virg. Could get dirty right quick cause he don't care nothing at all about us and you know, Virg .

"Sand half way liked TJ."

They moved out under the huge concrete slab that lay beneath the big mountain cabin, a walk out basement affair with half the cabin extending out on posts to create shelter for two muscle trucks and three trailers. One trailer held two beefed up Dirt Hogg ATV's with extensive racks fully packed with camp gear for a two week's stay in the mountains, one with a pair of street legal, JR655cc dirt bikes that had the full power competition package installed and tuned by Virgil, and one with two rare Polar Cap Kr-900 Icelandic competition snow mobiles, again beefed up and fine tuned by Virgil. Sand only provided the best.

They were soon lost in a technical discussion of what equipment they should take on the three hour haul across the shoulder of Mt. Nebo and down into Nephi Valley, along I-70.

About what they might need to make sure Ben Singer didn't live another day.

Chapter Four
Ben Singer Learns To Run

Ben stumbled on the Navajo rug as he drug his aching body from the kitchen into his tiny living room. The jolt sent a wave of agony racing up his arm and into his head. Three aspirin hadn't touched the pain. Not even Grampa Tsosie's favorite horse linament helped.

But the pain faded from his awareness as he sipped again from the witch's brew of emotions that boiled inside him..

This time it was red-hot rage.

He saw Sand in chains. In court. His sentence being read by the judge ..Murder in the first degree. Murder in support of criminal activity ..Mr. Sand you can, in Utah, choose death by hanging or death by firing squad You must now choose which manner of death you wish to experience ..

Ben was there, looking into Sand's eyes

There's a way some way. I always found it before .

Others had tried to shame him. In the Navajo way. At first schoolmates teased him, beat him, taunted him about his father .called him "The Navajo Hulk". "You gonna turn into the Hulk, Ben? We wouldn't like you if you got mad?" "Your dad can whip everything but a wine bottle. You're going to be just like him, huh Ben.."

Ben had fought back. Hard. But not with his fists. One or two fights convinced him that wasn't the way. There was the punishment, the loss of esteem in his mother's eyes. He'd had to find another way. So he did.

He studied school rules and later the law and learned how to make it all work for him. Then he set traps for his tormentors. Took advantage of their weaknesses. Caught them red handed and dirty. Then personally saw to it they were punished. It wan't long until Ben was left alone.

In more ways than one.

But no one tried to shame him again, not even his uncles.

The Law became a god to him. His defense and security and his religion. Easily replacing the old Navajo ways Grandpa Tsosie loved to prattle about. Ben rubbed his stomach.

I won't believe there's not a way some way.

The mantle clock softly chimed twice. Two a.m. He'd wandered the house for an hour listlessly trying to decide what he could take in the saddle bags of the bike. Wondering what to do with the rest.

He saw Terry smiling at him from his desk. The picture had been taken at Tibble Fork. Where I betrayed you tonight ..

He sipped afresh from the witch's brew. Shame burned his face. I failed you. I failed Lester He hugged himself as the pain in his belly got stronger than the ache in his shoulder.

You failed yourself, first, Ben, Granpa Tsosie said in his mind. You put your trust in the white man's way, the white man's law. There's your first mistake, right there .ever trusting the Bilagaana. Thinking they would let you be one of them ..

Ben shook his head sharply and let the pain shut Granpa up. This was a battle they'd had before. Ben was in no mood play it through his mind now.

There would be a way.

Ben would find it.

If Sand gave him time

Terry smiled sweetly up at him. Why shouldn't she? She didn't know what had happened. How poorly Ben had dealt with Dick Sand. That he had to run until he found someplace to stop. To think this through. How this will hurt you ..Everything we've planned ..You trusted me but there's nothing I can do. I have to leave to protect you. Hurt you terribly to save you .

Ben felt Sand testing him. Would he kill Terry if she suspected anything? As he must've killed TJ .The thought sent a shiver through him. Ben had never dealt with a murderer.

Those kind of men, Ben, Grandpa Tsosie whispered in his mind. They are the worst. They have crossed the river of Death. They can never cross back over or ever become what they once were. They are no longer Bila' Ashdlaa'ii. They still have five fingers like us humans. But they have no soul. Don't make the mistake of thinking you can reason with them ..None of the other Animal People ever have one among them as dangerous as a former human being who has murdered his own kind.

To Ben's tired mind helping Terry now meant leaving her in the dark .and she would imagine the worst.

With Sand's help.

Ben wouldn't be there to defend himself.

What use was the law against an outlaw cop who held all the cards?

Did I kill TJ? The same as killed him. Put him in jeopardy without a second thought. And Lester No more. I can't hurt them any more ..

The witch's brew of emotion in him turned black and cold. His head ached miserably. He was too tired to think. Time was running out. He would have to go.

Emotion flooded him. If only .. he could hear her voice one last time ..

He found his hand reaching for the phone, speed dialing Terry's number It rang three times before he heard her warm, sleepy voice in his ear. Just long enough for TJ's face, as he lay in his casket at Burgon's funeral home, to flash into his mind. She'd be dead like TJ

"Hello .Hello, who is this? Ben? Whoever you are, I can hear you breathing. Say something or get off the line .."

Suddenly bright headlights slammed into his eyes. Then dimmed so he could see parking lights. Then the inside light went on and he recognized the hulking figure of Dick Sand, sitting in the shadows in his van. Just down the block, under the big trees. Watching. Letting him know he was watching.

The phone turned red hot in his hand and he slammed it back down on the cradle. Breaking the thin thread of communication between himself and Terry. Forever?

He heard the big engine in Sand's police van start up and then rumble as it went past on the street. Going? Or only changing location

Ben had to sit down. He held out his hands, watched them shake. He was that tired .or scared. He couldn't think of one thing he could do to Sand. He felt helpless for the first time in many years. Somewhere inside him in some place of feeling and not of language Ben felt as vulnerable as a baby. He felt disarmed. Helpless unable to formulate any plan.

Except to run away ..

His eyes jerked to the clock. Fear washed through him and sent a shiver down his back. Before daylight. Gone from the county ..not much time left ..

****

Ben was ready. The saddle bags of the Honda Gold Wing held only what he needed for traveling.. He locked the door and slipped Terry's picture into the side pocket of the bike. All he could do was turn off his mind. Let habit take over now and get him started on his way to where?

It was still dark outside but on the eastern skyline the stars were fading.

He heard Sand's voice, smelled his sour breath, felt him standing close to him in the night as he had prepared to leave Tibble Fork.

He heard Sand's parting words. Get out of town before sunrise, Indian. Don't let the sun rise on you in my county. You hear me, Tubby? Ben thought he heard Sand's footsteps returning and he felt a shiver run up his back. He nodded his head and said Yes, I hear. Before sunrise. Now Ben couldn't control the sudden anxiety he felt, the need to be on the road To be going ..Somewhere

The Gold Wing's motor hummed quietly to life. Ben brought the big road bike down off the kickstand and used toe pressure from his foot to drop it into gear. Blinking lights signaling a left turn, he eased the clutch and drove down the sloping drive way and out onto fourth south. At 6 A.M. there was no traffic at all. The bike thrummed and responded to every touch of the throttle as he shifted through the gears and cruised through the lights and onto State Street. He could hit the freeway by driving straight down fourth . But he couldn't make himself do it.

Almost by itself the bike turned and headed down to 1200 south. The route that would take him to the freeway by way of the college.

The late April air was crisp but the day was clear and the sun would highlight the Eastern Wasatch Mountains in about an hour. He saw a few cars, including a police patrol car, the officer speaking on the radio, as he drove down State. Two early morning paper boys were pumping along, half asleep still. Both perked up to watch the big Honda road bike go by.

What if I turned around, chased down the cop, and told him everything .This is my fault . I can't just let this go ..Let Sand win.

The tape? Even with Sand in jail, would that save Lester from humiliation? Would Terry be safe? Would I be safe?

Ben raised and rotated his shoulder, trying to ease the steady, throbbing ache that was working up into his head, lodging just behind his eyes.

No. No one was safe from Dick Sand and whoever was helping him. Ben had to leave. Until he found a way to counter Sand's power. Babbling to the police, who would have to start from scratch. Accusing the man who single-handedly shut down crime in his part of Warren County ..By the time anyone listened to Ben Sand would know. There is no animal more dangerous than a former human being who has murdered his own kind

Ben knew just what Sand would do. Ben felt the fear misting through him again. I provoked Sand and he killed TJ. Now I have Lester and Terry's lives in my hands .

What he did could affect Lester and Terry just as disastrously as his ill-planned sting operation had affected TJ Fatally.

The WCCC campus ran up against I-15, the north-south running freeway Ben would have to take to get out of the county in time. Which way do I go? North or South? The Cheshire cat from Alice In Wonderland responded ..When you don't know where you're going it doesn't much matter which way you choose ..

Things were happening too fast. There was no place else that he wanted to be. Everything he cared about was here. If only I could see her .just one more time . In a few hours classes would take up again. But Ben wouldn't be there.

He came down the hill, around the sweeping curve that took twelfth south to the freeway and saw the college buildings off to his right. He started trembling when he saw the main building complex where he'd spent so much time studying in the library, snacking in the eatery, and hanging out with Terry in the lounges. This place was home to him.

I'm really losing this, he thought. And Terry too.

He felt the bike slow down and realized that he had let up on the throttle. Just then he saw bright lights flashing in his rear view mirror. He was too stiff and sore to turn his head and upper body. But he could see plainly enough in the mirror what it was.

What he saw were the flashing, whirling pursuit lights on top of Dick Sand's Warren County Sheriff's suburban.

Ben again drank from the witch's brew of emotions inside. Only now it was cold .all the fire gone out .

Ben felt a sick feeling stir in him. The fear and the shame from last night flushed through him stronger than ever and gathered around his heart. He realized that his body had a feral, animal fear of Dick Sand that his mind couldn't touch with reason or logic .or his old faith in the law.

He pulled over and, still not looking back, watched in the mirror as Sand pulled to the curb. He stopped back fifty feet or so. Too far, not the usual police procedure. Ben got little time to wonder about it.

Sand wasn't alone.

And it wasn't Lester. In the pre-dawn gloom the passenger was backlit by the lightening eastern sky He'd recognize her anytime, any where .

Terry.

A groan made it past his clenched teeth.

Terry riding with Sand as Sand stopped Ben just on the edge of the freeway on-ramp. Ben's insides twisted themselves into knots that would have disheartened an Eagle Scout and the pain bolted up into his chest to rival that in his shoulder and head.

Why, Sand. Why? You haven't hurt me enough? You have to twist the knife?

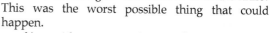

This was the worst possible thing that could happen.

You said you wanted to see her again ..well, here she is .

In a moment of blind panic Ben thought of dropping the bike into gear and running for it. Wouldn't Sand love that? Give him an excuse to run me down? Arrest me ..If I'm lucky.

Ben spread his feet to hold up the bike and took his hand off the throttle and rested it on his leg.

Unbelievable. What could Sand be thinking? Sand must have gone to considerable trouble to get her here this early. How did he know where I was? Ben saw again in his mind's eye the patrol car he'd passed on State street with the officer talking on the radio.

He could see Terry's head bobbing and arms gesturing and Ben wondered: If I do the wrong thing will he kill us both?

Ben heard the van door open. A powerful shiver wracked him, doubled the

Warrior's Way

pain in his head. He would rather be dead than be here, now. But you don't want her to die ..do you?

Terry practically bounced coming out of the truck. She started walking quickly towards him. Ben had no idea what to do. The person he loved most in the world was coming to him, her face twisted painfully by overpowering emotion. What have you done to her, Sand? What lies have you told her?

What if he'd shown her the tape

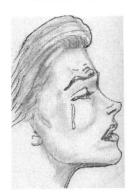

Ben felt himself gasping, his chest heaving. He didn't dare lift the visor on his helmet or risk letting Terry see his face. Shame and visceral fear struggled in him for dominance.

How he loved her! He knew if she broke down and cried or tried to hug him he would dissolve into a helpless, blubbering heap. That Sand would have to kill them both ..

But she didn't. She drew up on the curb.

"Ben," Terry said.

He could hear the tearing strain in her voice. He turned a little toward her, the hurting making him feel slow and stiff and distant and cold. He didn't trust himself to get off the bike or to say anything.

Terry was standing on the edge of the curb, hands clutched in front of her, fingers twisting and untwisting.

"Dick says you're leaving today."

The pain was there in her voice. But it was overlaid with an emotional distance, a holding back that he had never heard before. Like she was talking to him across a gulf as wide as the Grand Canyon.

"He says you're going home To be married."

His heart burst in him as he saw and heard the anguish that came out with the word 'married'.

"He said it's something your family has been planning for years. He said you knew all about it, but that you didn't want me to find out "

Sand was helping him burn his bridges .right down to bedrock.

Terry took another step toward him, almost slipped off the curb. Then she drew back, perhaps stung by his silence or the fact that she couldn't see him clearly through the visor of his riding helmet. He was too ashamed, too afraid for her, to take it off and look squarely at her. She put her arms down rigidly along her sides and raised her head in the classic pose of a movie actress bravely facing the absolute ruin of everything in her life.

"I hope you and your new wife will be very happy together, Ben."

He saw the twin tears start down her cheeks, preparing the way for what would be many more to follow. She raised a hand and brushed at them awkwardly, smiled a twisted, beautiful smile that snapped something in Ben.

He could stand no more. He cherished this woman. He'd made her a part of his plans, his life, of himself. He couldn't leave her like this.

He started to move to set the bike up on its stand so he could go and take Terry in his arms. As he turned back he caught a view of Dick Sand in the rear view mirror. He was standing outside the truck now. He was grinning his huge, self-satisfied grin as he stood big, tall, powerful. The Alpha Dog. The man. With his right hand he was tapping a video cassette on the open palm of his left hand.

The video tape.

Ben felt all his emotions wink out inside him like stars at daybreak. He sensed the emotional ashes sifting quietly downward to dust over, blacken and hide all the bright hopes that his life had held Was it only yesterday? He felt his breath gush out in a shuddering sigh. It seemed so long ago.

He looked back at Terry. He worked his mouth around until he got out his words.

"I've got to go, Terry. I'm sorry."

He saw her hands fly up to cover her face and he saw her shoulders begin to heave. But he could bear no more. No more. He was finished. Dick Sand had just ripped out the last thread. The emotional fabric of his life, every hope and dream in which he'd clothed himself, fell away. And he was naked in the world.

He fled like the coward he knew he was.

As he roared away he didn't look back. But he couldn't help seeing two figures in his rear view mirror.   Dick Sand standing big and powerful by the curb and Terry, pressed against him, hiding her face in his chest while he gently stroked her hair. Sand was looking at him over the top of Terry's head and even in the mirror, through the mist in his eyes, Ben could see his wicked grin.

Chapter Five
Ben Singer Plays Chicken

Ben Singer punched the big Gold Wing into the morning freeway traffic, the motor screaming, the RPM gauge redlining through each gear.

Don't think. Don't feel ..Drive.

At just under ninety Ben flashed over an overpass and ran up on two 18 wheelers, side by side, filling the lanes. One trying to pass, the other not giving any ground. The space between them narrow.

Very narrow.

He laughed, the sound hollow and bitter inside his helmet. He understood why Indian men played Yellow Line Chicken. Dead drunk. Roaring down the middle of the road on their bikes, forcing oncoming traffic to swerve or hit them head on. Racing till death rode with them. Blotting out their pain. They couldn't die in battle, seeking the lives of their enemies. Not any more.

So they found another way to stop the hurting .

Ben flashed between the trucks, the bike skittering and bucking in the backwash of turbulent air between them. Twice he almost hung it up on the flatbed rig and as he broke past them he reached out and slapped the fiberglass fender of the off-side Peterbilt.

Grizzly Bear Slapping, modern Indian style

Racing away he saw both truckers, reacting by instinct, swerving apart. Their air horns sounded a dopplered note, angry and shrill, then descending in pitch as he drew away.

He raised both hands as fists, high above his head and screamed a long, primal howl that boiled up from his gut. He swayed from side to side, making the big bike sway back and forth across the white lane lines. Just short of rear-ending a shining gray and black Lincoln he brought the bike upright, jerked hard enough to make the tires squeal and flew past on the edge of the road, spitting gravel, fighting for control. He reached out and kicked the car's door as hard as he could and felt the shock travel up to his knee.

I can feel ..I'm still alive Damn .

The Lincoln started a stuttering, tire-smoking stop only to see the trucks bearing down from behind. By the time the Lincoln fishtailed back up to freeway speed Ben was half a mile down the road, weaving in and out as he passed vehicle after vehicle. Horns blared, drivers swerved back and forth like week end dirt track amateurs.

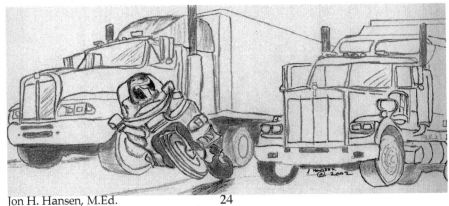

You want to know where I am, Sand? Am I out of the county yet? Just listen to the police calls. Crazy Injun on the warpath ..Headed south for the Big Res down the old Spanish Trail.

Killing himself because he can't kill you. Can't beat a white man at his own game-the law. What happens when you put your faith in the wrong things. ...

That was your first mistake, My Grandson. That's were you left the Pollen Path and started down the wrong way. Thinking you could be white even marry a white woman. Thinking the white man's laws were any good at all to us Brownskins ..

Ben howled again to drown out Grampa Tsosie. To shout down his brain. To drown out the pain that infected his mind and burned his heart. He couldn't do anything now.

It's too late.

Too late. Too late to be a white man. Too late to be a Navajo. Too late to believe in the law. Too late to do anything .but run away.

Ben sped on into the brightening day. The traffic thinned dramatically as he left Spanish Fork and headed over the shoulder of Mt. Nebo and on toward Nephi.

Why did the chicken cross the road? To snuff the guy on the other bike ..

No bikes, few cars, but there would be a speed trap near the freeway overpass down by Mona. Did he care?

Mona. His dazed and foggy brain zeroed in on Mona.

Why? Just a sleepy little farm town

What's the Word? Thunderbird! Thunderbird wine

The favorite breakfast drink of every Navajo wino in the great Southwest. Something his dad had taught him. By example. Ben felt a polyglot, acid mix of fear, resignation and recklessness.

Well .Why not?

You couldn't buy alcohol just anywhere in Utah. Only in a state liquor store.

Like the one in Mona.

Never had a drink Ben? Scared to because your dad's a drunk? Well you never got beat up and lost your girl and your scholarship all in one day before, either.

This calls for a celebration!

You're starting a whole new life here. Your dad showed you how to do it. All you have to do is follow his example. You already know how to be a failure. Plenty of Indians have blazed that trail for you.

You know exactly what to do. All you got to do is give up the struggle and let it happen.

In Mona.

You can kill yourself the old fashioned way ..one drink at a time. Betcha Sand will let you alone when he finds out ..Just so he can watch the fun.

Come see Ben Singer, the Falling Down Drunk, entertaining daily ..limited engagement. Come one, come all. And it all starts in ..

Mona.

Ben saw the sign, Mona exit one mile.

He throttled back and brought the bike down off the freeway and onto the quiet streets. Wondering just where the liquor store was. Trying to remember now what he'd never really paid attention to before when he and Terry took their Sunday drives down through the country.

Terry

He saw again in his mind's eye the picture of Sand and Terry together, Terry

Warrior's Way

sobbing softly into his chest as he gently stroked her hair. And the awful, evil and triumphant grin on Sand's face. A crashing pain radiated through him. What could Sand not do to her now that she so vulnerable?

It's hard to admit you're beat, isn't it, Indian,. . That you are leaving your friends in the hands of a monster.

Ben heard the distant rumble of thunder. This early in the day it meant a downpour for sure later. Did he care? What's the Word?

Where was that liquor store?

******

Terry fumbled for the doorknob. Rhetta. The roommate from the Dark Side. Was she home? No. Her shift at Zuka Juice started at seven. It must be later than that ..

Too late. The tears, squeezed out by the spasm of sorrow that grabbed her heart, blurred her image of the door. Too late .. Was she that dense? Ben that smooth? Those hours and hours together. Helping him study. Prepping him for his tests, helping him prepare his work, get his grades, keep his scholarship. And along the way sharing her life with him. All her secret dreams.

Trash. To him it was all just worthless trash. Oh, the help with his classes, that was valuable to him all right. Cynical? Was he that cynical? To use her. Entangle her feelings and all the while he was just using her as a study guide? Then dump her without a word, and ride off to marry someone else? How could she have missed seeing it coming? Was she really that clueless?

How on earth could she pick up and go one now .alone.

All alone.

A knot formed in her stomach and she couldn't swallow past it or get her breath around it, except in heaving gasps. She didn't want to see another soul. Just get to her room and shut herself in and cry ..and then cry some more.

She gave the door knob a vicious twist, shoved the door open with a foot, and as it banged against the wall she came .eyeball to eyeball with Rhetta. She must have been standing right there. Just waiting for Terry.

"Rhetta, what are you doing here?"

"I dogged work-"

"I can see that, Rhetta. Why?"

Rhetta moved quickly up to Terry, too close, seeing the red-rimmed eyes, the lines of sorrow that Terry couldn't control. She reached out to grab Terry's hand, but she jerked it away, raised both hands up near her shoulders in a warding gesture. She took a side step, to get around Rhetta. Rhetta moved to block her way.

"Hellooo. Like, I told you, girl ..Tried to warn you. Didn't I. About Indians . Now be honest with me, Terry. Like I tried every way I could, without coming right out and taking out a billboard ad or something."

"What are you talking-"

"About Ben dumping you, of course "

"How on earth do you know anything at all about that-"

"Dick like called me, of course told me all about it. Oh Angel, I'm like all sooo sorry-"

She almost managed to look sorry. If you ignored the feral glint in her eye. She had the juiciest gossip the campus had had all winter.

"Dick Sand called you?"

"He was like afraid for you Terry. Thought you shouldn't be alone at a time like this .."

"He told you about Ben leaving"""

"Now Angel, you just go ahead an cry if you want to. Get it out. girl."

Terry tried to step around Rhetta and get to her room.

"I don't want to talk about this right now, Rhetta."

Terry had to brush her eyes with the back of her hand. To clear the mist away before she ran into the wall.

"You like don't have to face this alone, Terry. I'm here for you, baby."

"Rhetta, please .I need to think this through. Sort out my feelings ."

Rhetta moved to block her way and put her hands on her shoulders and, pushing firmly, stopped her. Terry put her head down, but Rhetta bent down and looked up at her. Rhetta was enjoying this.

"Sure you do, girl. We'll do it together. Like set down and make a list of all the stuff I told you about. You'll be able to understand me now ."

Terry swept Rhetta aside and made it to her room. Just as she started to close and lock the door the phone rang.

"That will like be for you, Terry."

"Take a message."

"Its your dad."

Rhetta's voice was muffled by the closed door, but Terry heard her all right. She yanked the door back open.

'How do you know that Rhetta?" Terry didn't like the sound of her own voice.

"Because I called him a little while ago."

"What!?"

"You like need family around you at a time like this "

"Rhetta! You-"

"You can just thank me later, Terry dear. Sure, you like all made a big mistake. But life's not over. We can help you put something together. Make a plan. Your dad sounded pretty serious when I told him and all-"

Terry spun and ran back into her bedroom.

"I'll take it in here and Rehtta " Terry turned and gave Rhetta a look that made her take a step back, "stay off the other phone."

With no more willingness that she would have felt picking up a rattlesnake, Terry lifted the phone.

"Daddy?"

****

"You got him in sight, Blinky?

"Naw. We lost him this side of Spanish-"

"Don't say lost dirt bag. You can't lose him. I explained this all to you already ."

"Look, Sand, you got a scanner. You know what happened. He took off like a gut shot coyote, dodging between cars and trucks, weavin' around, doing more than ninety in heavy traffic. Like he wanted to die--what'd you do to him back there?"

"That's my business. I did my job. But he didn't die, did he."

"Well, we couldn't follow him. We ain't on bikes. Even the highway patrol couldn't do it."

"You see them?"

"Naw .don't worry. There's just a bunch of hopping mad citizens. We're passing Mona right now. We'll keep going fast as we dare. We can't afford to get stopped by the Bears or the County Mounties. Find him for us. We'll do the rest."

27

"Better than so far, you mean?"

"Hey, Sand, don't get yer nose outa joint. Give us something to work with here. We ain't the CIA or nothin'.'"

Sand broke the connection.

Hard to get good help now days ..

He hit the speed dial. Hershcel picked up on the first ring.

"Where you guys at?"

"Just coming outa the canyon at Nephi, still on the high ground where we can watch the freeway. And the clouds. They already got black bottoms out west of here. We're gonna get rained on pretty soon."

Sand let his breath out in a gush.

"Alright. That might help drive him to cover. You been listening to the police calls?"

"Yup, we have that. Most interesting-"

"So you seen him go by?'

'Nope."

'No? At the speed he was traveling he should've gone by fifteen minutes ago. Or else be road kill somewhere down there."

"Neither ..Uh wait .Blinky and his buddy just went by. Really tearin' up the road-"

"I just talked to them, they said he was ahead of them. You sure you're where you say you are? How long you been there?"

"Now, Dick, don't you get upset. We done just what you said and we been sitting up here since before first light. We come on over last night 'cause we got the sense that this is important to you-"

"You haven't seen Singer .But Blinky just passed you "

"Yup."

"If you guys are being straight with me that means Singer got off the road somewhere south of Spanish Fork."

'Yup. Seems so.'

"Where ..?'

'You asking me?"

'Shut up, I'm thinking ..''

"Don't let me interrupt- I gotta find him got to. I'll have to put out an all points on him, get the locals and highway patrol to find him-"

"Throw him in jail, you mean."

"No .No that would ruin everything. I got to think this through. You people stay put. Don't budge, hear? You see him you let me know right off .''

"Yup."

The line went dead. Herschel cradled the phone and turned to Virgil.

'Well, Virg, what you think? Is our Boss unhappy or what?'

'Got to be a better word than that. If he was a wolf he'd be chewin' off his leg to get out of this trap."

"Somebody's leg '

'Yeah. Not ours, though cause we're right where we're supposed to be doin' just what he wanted-"

"And your point is?"

'Ooookay .So, what you want to do? Rush down to the freeway and ask if anybody's seen a crazy guy on a big gold bike?"

"Not me."

"Or we could just stay right here, keep our backs up against this mountain here and sit lightly in the saddle .'

'In case that old Lobo chews off his leg and comes lookin' for somebody to take it out on."

"Sand don't like failure, that's sure as sunup .."

"Or thunder and lightnin' in the spring."

****

'State Dispatch? Deputy Dick Sand, Warren County. Uh, I need a "locate, report, do not detain" for points south of Warren Valley, especially along I-15. The subject is riding a hunter green over yellow Honda Gold Wing. Last seen headed south at high speed near Spanish Fork. He's wanted for questioning in the investigation of a drug-related death. Please ask the officers to contact me directly on the state-wide frequency. It's important that he not be detained, only located. Thank you will that go out immediately? Thank you again."

Sand turned his suburban through the cross over near Benjamin and headed back toward town. It was best not to get too far from Mount Nebo. Some of the local cops didn't have radios that would reach him further up the valley. And he really, really, needed to find Ben Singer.

Now.

****

"You got any Thunderbird wine?"

Ben stared around the store like Indiana Jones looking into a snake pit. His hands trembled.

Alcohol was a power among his people. A dreadful power. No good ever came from using it. It was destroying his own father. Among his people drink ruined lives everyday.

I'll bet it stops you from thinking, though.

The clerk edged toward the cash register. He's got a gun there. Ben moved his arms away from his sides and rested his hands on the counter. It occurred to him to pop up the visor on his helmet. The store clerk didn't seem reassured by what he saw.

"Down that third aisle, on the bottom shelf." He pointed with his left hand. The right one never moved. He stayed near the cash register like a goose guarding its nest egg.

Ben went back and got the wine. He half expected it to burn him as he picked it up and it nearly slipped from his shaky, sweaty hands. The bottle was smoked amber so he couldn't see the color of the wine. But he thought of it as blood-red.

What's the word? Thunderbird!

He looked carefully at the multi-colored symbol of the sacred Indian Thunderbird--bringer of rain, giver of life. It was so pretty. Like a cobra is pretty. Thunderbird wine was not the cheapest. But the symbol made it the wine of choice with many Indian alcoholics. Including Ben's father.

Ben paid for the wine and left the clerk standing by the cash register.

What's the word? Thunderbird!

Drink it all now? Then try Yellow Line Chicken one more time? Give the whites another shot?

Well, why not?

Ben heard a car and looked up in time to see an old couple going by. They

29

looked at him and at the bottle. The woman said something he couldn't hear, but the look of disgust on her face said it all. Dirty drunken Indian. Wino.

Ben felt his face burn.

How often he'd heard those words about his father. It hurt to think that now they applied to him too.

So much for the law.

How else can I get through this? Endure this.

He could raise a toast. To years of commitment and hard work. Drown it all in a single swallow of the searing, scorching heat-lightning of the Thunderbird.

The Mormons around here didn't drink at all. And, until now, neither did Ben, though not for religious reasons. Ben didn't drink because his father was alcoholic. Ben feared that he had a genetic weakness that would make him a hopeless addict if he took even one drink.

Maybe it was time for him and the Mormons to part company. Maybe it was time for Ben to stop thinking that he was better than his father. Better than his people. Maybe it was time.

Suddenly he was so tired he could hardly stand. He was out of Warren County. Sand didn't know where he was. It would be raining soon. Hard. The black clouds to the west promised that.

Here comes the real Thunderbird.

Why ride any further? Why not camp, wait out the storm and get acquainted with his new way of life?

Well, why not?

Ben gassed up the bike at Thornock's Conoco gas and go, nodded to a Burnham County deputy sheriff as they passed in the doorway, remounted the bike and followed a side road that a red-brown road sign promised would lead to: "Chateau Lake State Park and Campground-one mile".

As the bike purred smoothly down the two lane road Ben felt a looseness inside, a recklessness that he had never known before. But he immediately put it into words in his mind. What have I got left to lose? The answer echoed away again into the dark, hollow emptiness inside him. Nothing, Ben. Nothing at all left to lose. You left everything back there in Dick Sand's arms .

As he rode west he wasn't surprised to see how big the glowering purple-black cloud mass had grown, towering up over the hills, stretching as far as he could see. It was just how he felt inside.

Ben stopped at the entrance, filled out an envelope and deposited three dollars in the metal slot in a long steel tube. He took the stub with him and cruised the campground. Other campers, including another Gold Wing driver, were loosely scattered around the circle of camp sites. All of them were working quickly to put up shelters before the storm hit.

He found a place that was protected by trees and masked from the road by some oak brush. Instinctively hiding from Dick Sand. In a few minutes he had a fire started from wood supplied by the camp host. He heated spam and beans, and inflated an air mattress by blowing painful breaths from his aching chest. Not more than a minute at a time passed that he didn't think first about Terry in Dick Sand's arms and then about the Thunderbird in the side carrier. Finally he got it out, stripped off the sack and set it on the picnic table seat near his bed.

****

'Where you at, Blinky?"

"Burnin' up the road south of Nephi."

"Slow down."

"Slow down? I thought you wanted us to catch—"

"Slow down, fool. Turn off at Sidney Hollow and get your tails back up here!"

"That don't make no sense. We ain't passed him anywhere—"

"I put out a " locate but do not detain" on him."

"Yeah .So?"

"They spotted him in Mona, at the liquor store, followed him to the gas station just to make sure it was him.. It was him. He was dumb enough to use his credit card. He's checked in at the Chateau Lake campground."

"Sitting out the storm. Smart."

"Smarter'n some, for sure. Big storm coming. Should cover you nicely, if you don't mind gettin' wet."

"We ain't wimps, Sand. Like I told you. You find him, we'll do the rest."

"Well here's your big chance. Make it look like an accident .lightning strike maybe .whatever. I don't care. Just get him, you hear?"

"Oh yeah, Sand. I hear you fine. We're on our way back, runnin' into rain already. This is a big one. It'll be dark early and everyone will be indoors. Anybody else out here working for you?"

' ..No. Why do you ask?"

"Just wonderin', Sand. If we had any back up, like."

'Nope. This one's all yours. It's a simple job. Like shootin' jackrabbits. Like shootin' drunk jackrabbits most likely. Seems Benny's followin' after his old man. Only you got to shoot straight, that's all."

"Bang, bang," Blinky said and hung up.

****

"Okay, Herschel. You still in the same place?"

"Yup, pretty much."

'I got Dumb and Dumber turned around. You should see them soon."

"Best be soon, Sand. That gully washer's getting fixed to howl. It's getting dark, and the rain will screen us from seein' the freeway."

"Well, move down closer, then Herschel. You can't crouch up in them hills all day like gun-shy coyotes."

"You located him, then."

"Yeah. Chateau Lake Campground, after a stop for wine. He's down there fixin' to fall off the wagon. Should be plain easy."

"Easier'n TJ, you mean."

' I want you to backstop these jerks. Not too close in case they get themselves caught, but close enough to see what they do."

"We can do that."

'Then see that you do. This little detail is takin' way to much time. Too many resources. Getting' too public."

"Stay in touch, Dick." Herschel hung up.

Chapter Six
Ben Singer Meets His Father

Thunder rumbled to the west and gusty winds kicked up dirt and grit around him as Ben cleaned up after his sparse, hasty lunch. He pulled out the tarp he carried and made a lean-to to cover the bike with a small space left over for his ground cloth and blanket. Sleeping wet would just be one more discomfort for his tired, aching body to endure. His shoulder was swollen and tender to the touch and still sent sharp stabs of agony racing along his nerves when he reached out for something or tried to raise it above his head. He took three aspirin from his first aid supplies and saw the bottle of wine nestled among the gear on the table, lurking there like a small sand rattler hiding in a boot on a cold morning. Ready, without warning, to sink it poisonous fangs into his body.

Ben felt exactly the same fear and attraction and curiosity that he felt when he saw a snake.

Ben took his aspirin, with water. Then he stiffly lowered himself to the ground and leaned back against the bike, working around till he found body parts to rest on that only hurt a little bit. Lightning flashed a mile or so away. The thunder, when it followed, was deep, long and powerful. The storm had begun to move now, down off the hills, approaching the other side of the lake.

Ben wondered idly if there were fishermen out there in metal boats with carbon fishing rods in their hands. If there were they had better be moving to shore. Golf courses aren't the only dangerous places in a lightning storm. It occurred to Ben that he was in the trees, sitting on the ground leaning against a heavy metal bike. But it was so easy just letting the feeling float back up in him that he had as he rode away from the liquor store.

What is there left to lose Ben? Nothing. Nothing at all.

His gaze returned to the colorful Thunderbird symbol on the wine bottle. The Thunderbird, giver of rain, and it was raining in the hills. Giver of life through renewed plant growth and bounteous harvests.

And behind the sacred symbol on the bottle, alcohol. The taker of life. Worse, the destroyer of families. The harbinger of sorrows and enduring sadness and of lives vainly, poorly, sadly lived. Ben saw his mother's face in his mind's eye. She knew all about that, Ben thought. My father taught her well.

Ben felt a surging, almost warming flush of rage fill him up. Yeah, Dick Sand. My father could pull your arms off and beat you with them. If he could get the bottle out of his mouth long enough, that is.

Lightning flashed again, followed almost immediately by the boom of the thunder. Ben glanced at the approaching storm, and then looked back at the wine bottle. The clouds looked black now, turning the day dark and chill. They were malevolent, charged with electric power. The thunderbird of legend brought the powerful, slashing Male rain that filled the gullies and washed away homes, trucks, even entire herds of sheep. Not like the gentle, steady rain that went on for days and blessed the land. His people called that Female rain.

Today the male Thunderbird rode the heavens in all his destructive fury. While Ben gazed at the Thunderbird wine bottle, feeling it was even more dangerous. It had killed the love between his mother and father and made him grow up persecuted and lonely.

He'd only seen his father once. It had been enough, and more, to convince him that he didn't ever want to take a drink.

But that was before I met Dick Sand. He makes wine seem tame by comparison.

Ben eased his back and thought of Navajo Mountain and the day he saw his father.

Ben remembered that he'd felt weak and helpless that day, too. He was some where between eleven and thirteen at the time. Too small at any rate to protect his mother from the rage and violence that surrounded them that day. He was riding with his mother, bouncing over the washboard road that led to Navajo Mountain trading post.

Navajo mountain loomed larger and larger on the horizon as they approached. It was a huge mound of black rock that could be seen from many places in the northern part of the reservation. Ben remembered as he rode the stories Grandfather Tsosie and others told him about the place. And about the people who lived there.

To Navajos the land of the dead was to the north. And dark and brooding Navajo mountain marked the northern boundary of the lands of the Navajo. That association alone would have tinged the place with an aura of mystery and dread. But there was much more.

Beyond, the land fell away into spectacular deep rock canyons and extensive bad lands as the land dropped away to the San Juan and the Colorado rivers. It had been home to the 'Anaa'i Saani whose ruined cliff dwellings still dotted the canyons.

'Anaa' meant war in the Navajo language. 'Anaa'i meant "the ones which were enemies or strangers". And Saani meant the old ones. To a Navajo anyone outside of his own clan was dangerous. Strangers Navajos might seek to harm you with supernatural power that they used for evil purposes. Even other Navajos. Especially other Navajos. It was no accident that the language confused stranger and enemy. In the Navajo mind they were one and the same.

Navajo Mountain was north. It bordered on the ruined lands of a dangerous people. And the "ghosts", ch'iindii, of dangerous people was doubly, triply dangerous to the living. But Navajo Mountain Navajos could live there, apparently unharmed. That bespoke of special powers that made other Navajos nervous. A "long hair", a traditional Navajo with his hair in a bun at the back of his head who also came from Navajo Mountain was looked on with awe and dread by others.

But that wasn't all. The Naakai had come to Navajo Mountain 300 years ago, coming up from Mexico where they killed the Aztecs and took their gold. Then they killed pueblos around Santa Fe and took their land. Then they came to Navajo land and took their children to be slaves in Albuquerque. Hard men in hardened metal shells with pikes and horses and guns and a thirst for gold and glory. And at Navajo Mountain they had found silver.

All the Indians in America had learned to dread it when the Spaniards found precious metals. For all Spaniards considered themselves Caballeros, and gentlemen don't soil their hands with common labor. That's why God had made the Indians. More than one tribe was exterminated, worked to death in the mines and in the fields of the Spanish gentlemen. When they could the Indians slaughtered them and then covered mines and guarded them to see that they were not rediscovered. A man named Hashke Neihnii from around Monument Valley was said to guard the Navajo Mountain silver mines. His name meant something like "Warrior's Rage" and he simply killed anyone who came around looking for them.

Navajo Mountain was a dangerous place.

Warrior's Way

In Warren county there were countless stories and lots of real evidence that the Spanish had mined for gold in Utah. Why not then in Northern Arizona. And what better place than at Navajo Mountain where the ch'iindii of the Navajo slaves worked to death in the mines could join those of the 'Anaa'i Saani and mix their malevolence together. It took a special power, according to Grandpa Tsosie, to be able to live at Navajo Mountain. Powers that good people didn't want to fool around with.

Navajo Mountain was a melting pot. Paiutes lived nearby and intermarried with the more purely Asiatic stock of the original Navajo. And Spaniard warriors mixed their genes freely with the native stock. Until, when Dominquez and Escalante visited them in 1776, they said the Piautes, who had beards like Europeans, looked more like themselves than any other tribe they had ever seen. Thus, some Navajo Mountain people participated in the Navajo culture. But they were not Navajo people in their genes.

Ben's father was a Navajo Mountain Navajo.

Ben knew much of this before he saw his father. The day he saw him Ben discovered what that really meant. Seeing Navajo Mountain growing larger on the horizon as they approached only added to the queasy feeling in his stomach that had been there since his mother had announced that they were coming here so that Ben could meet his father.

"You don't remember ever seeing him, do you" she said as they were driving the last mile up the wash boarded dirt road that lead to the Navajo Mountain Trading Post.

Ben only shook his head.

"Well it's high time you did. You're very much like him in many ways. You need to know your roots."

Ben's mood got darker. His mother thought of him as different from her family, more like his father. He looked down at what he could see of his body. His bones were large, his feet outsized for his height. He was not pudgy Pueblo nor was he tall and angular traditional Asiatic Navajo. He was broader and heavier than any other boy he knew his age. Was Ben a Navajo Mountain Navajo too?

He felt like someone who might test positive for AIDS as he thought about how this could affect his standing in his mother's family. Especially with his grandfather Tsosie. Grandpa Tsosie, and his whole family, and especially his daughter, Ben's mother, were traditional, genetic Navajo. It was like having family who came over on the Mayflower was to Anglos. Either you did or you didn't. Either you were or you weren't. Ben began to worry seriously that he wasn't.

Navajo Mountain Trading Post appeared through the trees. It fit the locale. Built to be defended, with rifle ports, thick walls and a dirt roof. Far from any town, from any source of help. Ben wondered when the traders had last had to shut it up and defend it.

When he saw the fight going on in the parking lot he remembered glancing at the doors and windows to see if they were forted up in there today. Ben wondered if his dad was inside, preparing to defend the door.

Alone by his bike, in the gathering storm, Ben smiled at the irony. He hadn't known, hadn't been told, but he had assumed that his father worked in the store.

In the parking area the local crop of alcoholics were shouting and shoving like ravens deciding who gets the eyes and the guts of the dead rabbit on the highway.

Ben looked at his mother's face for a clue to what was happening. He saw her looking at a beat-up red Ford pickup with Arizona plates. The look on his mother's face told him that this was the local bootlegger. Ben couldn't see what was going on but the look on his mother's face scared him. She looked like a doe looks when she spots a mountain lion creeping up on her fawn. Like she was seeing something crawl from under a rock. Something poisonous that kills its own kind.

Then Ben saw a wino holding something under his coat, a ragged gray suit coat too big for his emaciated body, one pocket torn and hanging by the bottom part, the cloth grease-stained and filthy. Grass, weeds and dirt sticking out from it here and there made him look like an alcoholic Indian version of the straw man from Wizard of Oz. He and the others had slept under the trees, waiting for daylight. They had probably pooled their coins or pawned their shoes or something for the money to buy wine.

But the drunk wasn't playing fair. With an elaborate, almost clownish look of craftiness the drunk backed around a truck and began running across the parking area. Ben heard angry voices raised in howls of protest and anguish. He saw three or four drunks rushing like inebriated linebackers after a halfback as they tried to follow the wine thief's trail through the trucks parked around the trading post. From the front steps an old man and woman stood together watching the spectacle, shaking their heads sadly.

The wino halfback made it safely to a decrepit old Chevy sedan that had one flat tire and looked like it couldn't make it from the store to the highway. Ben had seen such mobile wrecks, filled with both men and women, headed here, there, and nowhere all his life. Too often they became a tangled coffin on some lonesome stretch of road or became a hurtling, aimless missile that ended the hopes and dreams of helpless, innocent people who's only mistake was to be on the road at the wrong place and at the wrong time. The reservation highways were dotted with crosses put there by grieving families to mark the sites of fatal accidents. Most of them related to alcohol abuse.

Inspired by the wine and the threats of his fellows, the O J Simpson of Navajo Mountain made it to the Chevy, clambered in and shut and locked the doors. His face peered out briefly at his frustrated pursuers. Ben could see him clearly across the way, a look of comic triumph, not just on his face, but exuding from every part of him. A man in Paradise who had everything he'd ever dreamed about. He was Adam, in the Garden of Eden, and he had it all to himself. He settled back and ignored the pounding and the shouts of those lesser people who were excluded from heaven and who howled the gut wrenching howls of lost souls in darkness. He grinned foolishly and began to work at the cap seal of a bottle of Thunderbird wine.

The noise of the men gathering around the car became raging, almost hysterical in volume and tone. Navajos do not have profanity in their language because it carries no tradition of a Christian God for people to degrade. But within that limitation, they were telling the thief what his fate would be in terms that made Ben shudder.

Then, suddenly, there was a silence so sudden and so profound that Ben looked around fully expecting to see a Navajo police van pulling up. But it wasn't the Navajo Police. Instead Ben saw another of the drunks coming through the parking lot. He saw his mother suddenly go tense and he looked from her face to the man and back again several times. What he saw there told him without words that this was his father.

Ben's feelings, fear, shame, self-pity, hit him so hard that he was soon looking out through a misting of tears. As he watched the thought kept pounding through his brain. Why show me this? What does this prove, what am I supposed to be learning? That my father is a drunk? How will that help me to live a happy life in harmony with my world, as Grandpa would want. I see my roots, and my roots are rotten.

Still, Ben looked, for curiosity is among the strongest of the traits that make bilaa' ashdlaa'i (the five fingered ones) human. Ben saw first the head and shoulders of a man who must be six feet tall or more. Tall for a Navajo. And thick. A squarish head and shoulders that seemed to extend twice as far as they should from the man's neck to their tips. There was nothing here of the tall, slim, Asiatic body type of the original Navajo/Apache racial stock. Many Navajo who had sheltered the Pueblo during the great revolt against the Spanish in the 1600's had the short, stocky, sometimes potbellied body that showed the Navajo/Pueblo cross breeding that took place then through mixed marriages.

This man showed none of that. This man was a Navajo Mountain Navajo. As he

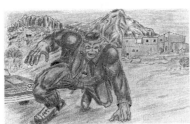

passed the gaps between trucks Ben saw that his belly was totally flat and his waist was wide, not tapering in white man's fashion. And he had a peculiar almost foot slinging gait that moved his body along so smoothly that Ben could only think of the tigers he'd seen in the Albuquerque zoo pacing in their cages. Every movement was controlled and cushioned by muscles that contracted and relaxed in turn as he moved. His movements were at once smooth and powerful.

And menacing.

He had lantern ears, large, and one had a leather thong strung though it with a piece of blue turquoise on it. His back was straight in that way characteristic of ballerinas and marines. What people called a military bearing. His neck was thick and brown as a cedar fence post. His features were not thick, as Ben would have thought, but startling in their refinement and sensitivity. Though ravaged and weather-beaten, Ben saw that he could almost pass as handsome by European standards, if he cleaned himself up.

He looked at his mother again. This intelligent, educated, refined Navajo lady. And he caught a glimmer of what must have happened a decade or more ago to bring this man into her life long enough to conceive Ben. A faint smile touched her mouth but a great watery sadness seemed to radiate from her eyes. The result was a misty eyed look that softened her face in a way Ben seldom saw. The crisp and efficient executive secretary was gone. In her place Ben saw what he now knew was a woman with a woman's passions, and fantasies, and brutal realities. His mother had lived. She had a past.

As Ben stared at this memory, slumped against his bike in the campground, he knew that many of his insights were current, not those of an eleven year old. But he felt the old amazement again that children feel when they learn that their parents are much more than nurturing grown ups assigned to them to torment and to love them.

As the man came closer Ben heard his mother say softly:

"His name is Frank, Ben."

Ben's full name was Benjamin Franklin Singer. He saw the connection right away. Ben also saw that he was going to pass right in front of their truck. In a moment Ben gazed into unfocused, red rimmed, angry eyes and saw a scowl that would have frozen the blood of the Medusa. Ben saw the dirt and the stained clothing like that the other drunks wore. And Frank reached up and pulled his coat closed as he moved past. Ben saw that his hands were large, his wrists heavy boned. Something about him made Ben think of King Kong or Mighty Joe Young. But then Ben was young at the time, and what happened next probably affected his memory of his feelings.

The man in the car looked up from his efforts to uncork the bottle when he heard the silence around him. He saw Frank coming up on his side of the car. He stopped working on the cap for a moment and then his movements became jerky, almost frantic, Ben thought. Frank moved faster, his hands working into fists, clenching and unclenching in blind rage as he moved toward the car. Ben saw again the mask of rage his father's face wore as he went past the truck and could see why the man in the car was scared. But scared or not, it seemed his thirst drove him to empty the bottle into his stomach even if it was the last act of his life.

When he got to the car Frank kicked out at the door and it crumpled like an aluminum pop can did when Ben squeezed it. The car rocked on the springs, but the flat tire held it in place. The sound was solid and loud and the man inside stopped opening the bottle and looked out at Ben's father. Ben hear a low, almost rumbling noise and realized that it was coming from his father. Frank Singer bent in the legs, his back still perfectly stiff and straight and placed his hands against the car at the top of the windows. With one heave, one intense burst of muscular energy, Frank tipped the car up.   His shirt and coat ripped at the back with the massive effort and Ben had a glimpse of the huge cords of muscle that contorted and bunched into knots with the effort he was making. He shifted his hands one at a time to the under side of the car and heaved it over on its side. Ben was looking head on at the car and could see the man inside fall to the bottom of the car, struggle, get to his feet and fling the door open.

Frank was gathering himself to push the car the rest of the way over when the door popped up, held by a desperate man who was standing on the steering column and holding out an unopened bottle. By now the oil was beginning to drip down the motor and the smell of gas drifted across the parking lot.

Frank took the bottle and listened briefly to one of his companions who was pulling on his sleeve and gesturing at the car. He must have been the owner. Frank nodded, walked around to the other side and put the bottle in his coat pocket before heaving the car over again on its wheels. Ben couldn't see the man inside. He was on the seat or the floor. Ben didn't know if he was hurt or hiding. Ben's father didn't give the car a second glance but walked away through the trees with the other drunks in tow. In a moment they were passing the bottle around among them.

That struck Ben as strange at the time. If his father was so dominating why did he bother to share at all? He glanced at his mother and saw her looking at him with a face like the Mona Lisa, full of feelings that were hard to read. But hope and pride were mixed in there among them, he was sure.

"Why didn't he just keep the wine for himself?" Ben said.

"Because he's a warrior, Ben."

Ben felt his face wrinkle as he puzzled over that. His mother must have seen that he knew little about the world of men, let alone the world of warriors.

"He's a warrior without a war. A natural leader of men because he has great strength and intelligence, yet considers others his equal. He does not need others to serve him or bow to him to make him feel good about himself. He shares what he has

Warrior's Way

with his comrades, whoever, or whatever they are."

"What good can he see in drunks," Ben heard the wonder in his voice.

"Alcoholism is their condition, Ben. But human beings is what they are. Just as slavery was the condition of the blacks, not what they were. They were human beings in servitude. They were not slaves. Can you see that Ben?" Her voice said that this was important. But Ben could not make the connection.

"They're so dirty." was all that he could think to say. His mother looked at him like she used to when he carelessly broke something.

Suddenly she reached down and started the engine and put the truck in gear. Ben started to feel relief flooding into him. They were going home.

Then he was horror-struck when he saw that his mother was going after his father. She caught up quickly to the group as they passed among some cedar trees beside the road. She beeped once as she pulled up. Ben felt his insides turning watery as he saw several pairs of alcoholic eyes leering at his mother and at the new truck. Lopsided smiles broke out on every face as they saw that she was a woman and almost alone. In his mind Ben heard the warning screech of the blue jay rising suddenly to a crescendo: Look out, Ben ..Look out!

Ben searched inside himself and found only the sickening knowledge that he couldn't do the least thing to help his mother if these men decided to hurt her.

As Ben sat alone in the wind driven cave next to his bike, watching the storm lash the lake with wind and rain and vicious strokes of lightning, his feelings of the past for his mother and his feelings of today about Terry and Lester and Sand mixed and exploded and burned through him like a white-hot fire. He gazed into a blackening sky and felt helplessness, hopelessness, frustration and outrage filling him till it gushed out of his eyes as tears and emerged as a moan from this lips.

That a man like Sand could drive him away from everything dear to him. What Sand had done, gleefully inflicting pain and humiliation on others, rubbed Ben's mind raw and tortured his nerves like salt in a wound. Ben saw clearly now that Sand was everything he hated. Everything that he wanted to strike out against in life.

But Sand operated on a level Ben couldn't match Couldn't hope to match. Somehow these emotions and the one's surging in him the day he met his father seemed to meld together and drain away every ounce of energy and every spark of hope in his soul until he was as dark inside as the skies above him.

In his mind he saw his father as clearly as he had the day he looked at him through the truck window. Ben's father gazed steadily at the truck, not really seeing the occupants, perhaps trying to focus his attention through his alcoholic haze. To make his brain realize what was happening. Another man started for the truck and Ben's heart started beating like a small bird's in the grip of a cat. Ben's mother leaned out a little and said:

"Frank?"

Ben's father jerked as though he'd been hit and Ben watched him struggle as he focused on his mother's face. Suddenly he moved, not shoving the others aside, just going through them as though they weren't there. They weaved and rocked like bowling pins brushed by a rocketing ball.

"Da' Desbah?" he said as he got closer. He was peering like he was looking through heavy fog.

"Yes, Frank, it's me." she said.

Ben saw surprise in his father. His whole face became almost round, clownish, ridiculous looking. Then the thoughts must have flashed through his alcohol-soaked brain like bullets from a machine gun. Ben saw joy, curiosity, hope, self-consciousness and abject shame play across his father's face in a matter of seconds. He saw him pull his coat together in front and brush his fingers quickly through his hair and then try to hide his filthy hands with their cracked and dirty fingernails.

By then Ben was aware of the other men, the leers, the filthy things they were saying, the kidding his father was taking.

One said: "Who is it this time, Frank? She looks a lot richer than the others that come looking for you."

Ben saw color coming up into his mother's face. Was she embarrassed by what they were saying or upset that other women came after his father? Ben never found out.

But his father must have seen her reaction. His face changed in an instant as the mouth pulled down like the mask of a Greek tragedy and he turned and looked at his brothers of the bottle. The laughter and the jeering stopped instantly. They looked like they wished they were anywhere on earth than here with an angry Frank Singer.

"She'esdzaa nt'ee' " he said. Softly the sibilants and the glottal stops coming out rapid fire, not to be misunderstood.

This was my wife.

None of the men failed to get the message behind the words. They backed away and moved off among the trees. No one seemed to care that Ben's father still had the wine in his pocket.

Frank Singer moved closer and peered into the truck. Ben marveled again at the presence his father had, even drunk. He looked like ancient kings were supposed to look. Except for the dirt and the ragged clothes and the awful stink of sour wine and an unwashed body and the ravaged, hollow, haunted look in his eyes.

Ben saw the pain there in a way he'd never seen pain before. It hurt him so bad he had to look away. Now, thanks to Dick Sand, he was feeling that same pain again, deep inside himself.

"Who's this with you here?" his father said.

Ben noticed that his English was accent less and wondered where his father had gone to school to learn the language so well. The voice was deep, full timbered and well modulated. Almost soothing to Ben, who was seething in a cauldron of competing emotions.

"Benny, I named him Ben after you."

Ben couldn't bring himself to look up at his father. He wiped his damp hands on his levis and studied his shoes.

"Da' t'aash 'anii? Shiye'. His father's voice was almost reverent.

'Yes, Frank it's true. Ben is your son."

Ben found himself looking up, into his father's eyes. He saw there red blood veins, dirt, a broad sober face .and something glinting deep within them.

Now, being older, Ben knew what it was. Pride and love and a bottomless sadness that almost sucked Ben down.

His father turned and called to the other men.

"My son is here," he said. 'This is my son and his mother brought him to see me."

From a safe distance some of the men waved and saluted Frank Singer for his good fortune. Like a ragged band of the French Foreign Legion, about to disappear forever into the desert, but waving bravely nonetheless.

Then, for a moment, in the strength of the emotions he felt, Ben's father forgot the years and all that had and had not passed between them. He looked a Ben's mother, hope a raw mask on his face.

"Can you come home with me?"

His eyes dropped immediately as the truth tore into him. Ben saw his mother stir slightly on the seat, as though she wanted to get out of the truck and hug his father, to just go away with him. Then she glanced at Ben, the look of anguish carefully, but not fully screened from him, then back at his father.

"I mean," he added hastily, "just for a while, to show Ben to my mother?'

To prove that I'm not a complete failure as a son his tone said.

"No, Frank. We can't do that. We have to get back to Chinle and your son must go to school. He's a good student. The best in his class.."

Ben saw her eyes going soft and misty again.

'You can be proud of him', she said sadly.

But we can't be proud of you, Ben thought.

"Thank you," Frank Singer said. 'For bringing him for me to see. I'll remember him now."

Ben saw the heartache again. The melancholy cloud settled back on his father's shoulder. Frank slumped a little and seemed to withdraw back into himself.

"He asks about you and I wanted him to know you. "

'Yes, well ..now he knows me. Who I am ..What I am.'

He gazed after the other men, seeming to gather his emotions together, getting ready to move on down the destination-less road he walked.

"Goodbye, Frank."

"Good bye, Desbah. Tell my son to do well in school ..to grow and be something good He could do that for me ..for us. I'd better go now. Thank you again." He glanced back at her. Their eyes locked, held, then his slid away. He pulled his ragged coat around him and strode away with his peculiar, powerful gait, his shoulders no longer so straight and stiff. The emotional burden he carried was pulling him down now, as no physical burden could ever do.

"We'll go home now, Ben ."

Her voice held a lifetime of soft regrets. She started the truck. Ben's father moved back, off the road. As they drove away he stood looking after them till they became lost in the dust the truck was making. Ben knew this because he looked back until he could no longer see his father standing in the road. As he turned around and settled in for the long trip home Ben suddenly realized that he hadn't said a single word to his father. Not a word. His father had never heard his voice.

His mother pulled over less than a mile down the road. Ben saw her taking great, gulping breaths and her voice was shaky when she spoke to him.

"I don't mean to defend him to you Ben. I wanted you to meet him and talk to him and to let him know you. But it just didn't work that way. You'll have to come to your own peace about this, now that you know.

"Try to understand, Ben. He's a warrior without a war. A warrior, a fighter, by nature. But he doesn't have the weapons to fight today's battles. He's a man who's answers don't fit the questions of life. The questions asked of us by a modern society."

Ben was beginning to feel that his mother should have put this off until he was older. The ideas meant little to him. He looked down at his feet, enduring, polite. He loved his mother, but she often puzzled him. She seemed to want to talk to him about the things grownups found interesting. He supposed that single parents did that sometimes. They wanted someone to talk with and their kids were always handy. He loved her and he could do that for her.

But he couldn't see anything great about having a truculent, overbearing drunk for a father.

"Can we go now Mom?" Ben asked quietly, trying not to let anything show in his voice. But his mother wasn't through yet. Perhaps she was really talking to herself, to explain again why she lived alone and was still in love with such an unlovely man.

"He's also responsible, Ben. Always remember that. He could have ruled his nature and channeled his strength and his ability to lead others. He could have lived at peace with his world." The sadness in her caused her to slump and to seem older.

Ben sensed something of the years, the happiness, and the memories that would never be because of his father and the choices he'd made.

Then a thought struck him that took his breath away.

She thinks I'm like him in many ways.

Ben felt fear working in him. Am I a Navajo Mountain Navajo? Am I like my father? He longed to see his body grow tall and slim and willowy. Not like Frank Singer.

She took his arm, and Ben could still feel the painful pressure of her grip and the direct look straight into his eyes. Ben could still feel his amazement at this for Navajos considered a direct gaze to be rude and watched the lips of the person they were visiting with. This gave them an air of suspicion to whites, shifty-eyed was the phrase he'd heard. It was enough that day, that direct gaze and the surprise of it, to burn it into Ben's memory, deep and long. He also could remember the misty sad-eyed look he saw there and caught a vision of the lonely soul that lived in his mother's body.

"Don't make his mistake, Ben. Don't give in to the temptation to use your mind and your skill to hurt yourself and those around you. If you don't discipline yourself your strength and skills will be used for evil purposes by others. Or you will waste you life's energy without ever becoming the best that's in you. Take the best that I have given you and the best that your father has given you and give it the best that you have brought with you.

"You're like him, Ben, in so very many ways. Now you know why you're bigger than all the other boys. And why you don't look like the old time Navajo like your Grandpa does. And why you don't look like a pueblo Navajo. You're a Navajo Mountain Navajo. There's a lot of mixed blood up here because of the Utes and the Paiute and others. And you know that grownups who know about Frank look at you a little strangely. Be what you are, Ben. Be the best person you can be."

The best I can be is a Navajo Mountain Navajo and an alcoholic like my father, Ben thought.

Ben took this to heart in his own way. He vowed never to touch alcohol. And never to act tough. He vowed to be a traditional Navajo, almost shy and unassuming. To go even to extreme measures to live in harmony with those around him. To make no waves. To be practically invisible. To use his mind and not his body to get what he wanted.

Then the persecution started.

Then he became a warrior of sorts, a soldier of the Law.

I succeeded too well, he thought. His eyes refocused on the bottle of Thunderbird. Dick Sand beat me down. And when I wanted, really wanted to fight back, I was too soft and he was too strong. And here I am. With nothing left to lose.

Why wasn't I more like my father. The picture of Sand and Terry together floated up into his mind. He felt a mixture of rage and anguish that made his stomach cramp. His father would have stuffed Dick Sand and his dog under the suburban.

I wonder where my father is right now. Probably sitting in jail somewhere.

Ben's mind was tired and his body hurt and nothing made sense. He felt his hair rise on the back of his neck. A sure sign of an impending lightening strike. Here I am, he thought. Come and enlighten me. Burn everything out inside me and let me rest. But it didn't happen.

With a thunderous crash lightning hit somewhere out in the lake, backlighting the curtain of dark, fierce, male rain that was just reaching the shore. In a moment the rain lashed at him and drove him into the hole he'd prepared for himself. The rain splashed on him, wet his face as he lay in misery and pain on the ground. He could have told himself that the wetness on his face was just rain if it hadn't been for the salty taste in his mouth that mocked him.

He heard Dick Sand's voice in his mind, insulting, belittling:

You crying, Benny?

Yes, Ben said.

Yes, I guess I am.

But there was no one to hear.

Chapter Seven
Ben Burns

Dick Sand sat alone in his suburban near the top of Mount Nebo, on the loop road near the nature trail where he could see into the Nephi-Warren Valley area to the west and into the Fairview Canyon area to the east. Nebo was the biggest mountain around and a great place to monitor radio traffic and to use his powerful radio-telephone to call southern Arizona.

Outside Prince roamed the cedars and aspens, ambushing mice and pot guts and marking his territory. If anyone was dumb enough to try to get close, Sand would know ..instantly.

He punched a hidden latch, allowing the passenger seat to tilt back and reveal a compartment containing the telephone handset and a Browning .338 Winchester Magnum scope-sighted rifle. He couldn't resist stroking stock. The reddish-brown, checkered maple was sensual to him and he felt his face pulling up into a grin. No chance to use it on Singer though ..Too bad.

He saw Ben Singer in his mind, a small hole in his chest, half his lungs blown out his back, trying to take one last breath. Yeah, this rifle would do it all right ..Too bad he'd have to pass. The machinery was operating and shortly Singer would just be an ugly memory

Sand turned on his telephone and settled back to wait till nightfall. To the west Chateau Lake lay up against the eastern foothills of the Sheeprocks. In the declining light the lake water looked leaden and cold as it disappeared into the mist and clouds of the approaching storm. When he couldn't see the lake any more he started the big suburban, whistled up Prince, and headed back down the loop road toward the Interstate, fifteen miles down the mountain. He was grinning his big self-satisfied grin all the way.

He was thinking ahead .what he did best, he thought .Now he was seeing himself gently embracing Terry, helping her accept the news that Ben Singer was dead.

Oh yeah, that will be fun ..for a while.

He whistled a tuneless cattle drover's ditty as he drove through the gathering storm.

****

Ben Singer jerked awake to the sound of sirens entering the campground. Their pulsating screech scorched his nerves like liquid fire. Lightening flashed lighting up the area in strobe-like brilliance that only made the following darkness more inky-black. The thunder's concussive pounding followed instantly. The smell of ozone filled his nose and static electricity made the hair on his neck stand on end.

Static electricity or stark terror.

In his mind the sirens were heading straight at him. His sleep-sodden brain heard them as the hounds of Hell, racing over the ground, sniffing out the spoor of a doomed soul, lunging against their leashes, dragging their awful masters forward through the crashing darkness.

Fear beyond reason surged in him making him so weak he could barely lift his head.

Sand's found me. He's coming for me. If I'm caught everyone will know about the tape ..

Shame burned his face, shortened his breath and mixed with the terror to make a stink rise from his body that made his stomach cramp. He turned on his side and retched dryly. An awful pain seated itself in his shoulder and sent succeeding waves of agony down his arm. He felt his fingers growing numb and cold.

He rolled on his back, wearily giving himself up as lost, buried like a drowning man, deep in an icy sea of sorrow and regret.

Then, his tired brain finally managed to tell him that the sirens were winding steeply down, stopping. But not here, at his campsite. On the other side, perhaps a hundred yards away. Could they have mistaken the other biker for him?

Like a man on death row gazing at a reprieve, Ben felt a small flutter of hope gusting into his mind, fragile as butterflies. In but a moment they lay dead at his feet.

How long was it going to take Sand to see, even in the pouring rain, that he had the wrong man? How long would it take him to move along the circle of campsites and find Ben? Even as the thought hit him, as the hope died, he heard sounds of a truck motor rumbling toward him through the night.

He pulled himself out of the shelter, into the frigid downpour, stiffly pulling his poncho over his head, paying a terrible price in pain for trying to move so fast after laying on the cold ground. Running away in the dark would hurt even more, but maybe he should at least try

Then it was too late. Ben saw two orange-yellow parking lights showing dimly through the rain and the brush that concealed his campsite, coming at him through the rain. Before he could react a large four-by four truck with oversized wheels and a rack of running lights on a bar across the top went rumbling past, accelerating and heading the wrong way around the campground loop road.

Ben jerked back so fast he slipped on the muddy ground and almost fell. New waves of pain raced down his arm. The thought cut through the fog in his mind, riding a shot of adrenaline that coursed through him like an icy wind.

Sand's suburban! Sand's out looking for me right now. He knows I'm here

Ben's empty stomach cramped hard enough to cancel the pain in his arm. Even as his eyes showed his tired brain that the truck wasn't Sand's and that it wasn't stopping ..And it was avoiding the flashing lights over at the other campground.

Another brilliant stroke of lightening arrowed through the night, illuminating the black clouds above him and seeming to release extra torrents of rain. He also felt a distinct slap on the top of his head from the electricity released by the storm. Close ..way too close. The center of the storm must be right overhead ..

Sand's a witch ..maybe it'll hit him ..

He peered into the darkness as if he could see the next bolt before it shot out of the murky clouds scudding just above the trees. Lightening was the great enemy of the Navajo who often traveled over flat open spaces where they and their horse were the highest things around. They believed that lightening hunted witches. Any lightening-caused death was troubling to a Navajo family .

Too much to hope for ..not something to count on now I've got to save myself.

The lighted dial on his Timex Marathon told him he'd slept four and a half hours. This storm was not the one that was approaching when he fell into his exhausted sleep. These storms don't last four and a half hours. This had to be another storm, perhaps bigger and more intense than the first ..

As he struggled into the rest of his rain gear his mind finally got through again

..something out there in the night wasn't right The darkness didn't have the right look about it There was an unnatural source of light somewhere behind the curtain of rain.

Then a gust of wind lifted the downpour just long enough to show Ben a huge bonfire burning on the other side of the campground. It took several seconds for his exhausted mind to grasp that no normal fire could be burning in the steady downpour ..He peered around the brush screening his campsite and saw the glow like lamplight through thick glass .That's where the sirens stopped .

Hope made him giddy.   What if they don't know I'm here? What if some accident had brought them here? What if Sand wasn't even around not lurking out there somewhere in the dark?

Could he still get away under cover of the storm? How much longer would it last? At the rate it was coming down ..not long. A few minutes at best. The glow across the campground seemed to be getting brighter by the second

He broke camp as fast as he could working faster ..thinking of Sand--out there in the dark somewhere ..He had to put more miles between himself and Warren County. He couldn't let Dick Sand accidentally find him here, or even learn he'd stopped here .Terry's life might depend on it.

The rain started slacking off as he finished packing up and struggled to get the big bike turned around. The glow from the other side of the campground was plain now. It was huge, ugly black, oily smoke billowed up into the black clouds above. It was not a simple wood fire. It was more like what you saw when a car caught fire.

One thing Ben had plenty of experience with on a reservation where there were no fire stations. Where if a car or home caught fire you saved what you could and watched the rest burn. He began to wonder if it was an explosion that woke him up-- not a thunderclap.

Near as he could tell through the heavy rain, the fire was near the camp site of the other biker. He wondered if lightening had set the other bike afire. Hope the guys alright ..If not he'd read about it in the paper ..that is if Sand didn't catch him sneaking out of the campground.

The rain was definitely slacking off, the lightening strokes getting fewer and further away. Ben's stomach started burning like it was filled with battery acid the last thing he packed was the Thunderbird wine bottle. It glinted softly in the semi-darkness. Like the barrel of a big pistol. Ben shuddered and started up the Gold Wing and listened as it purred quietly in the drizzling rain.

Then, riding the wind, he heard what he'd been dreading. More sirens. Rapidly getting closer. He could see the bizarre colors of the swirling red and blue lights diffused through the mist. He eyes followed them as they came into the campground and stopped almost opposite him, not a full hundred yards away. Close--much too close. Maybe one of these was Dick Sand hearing the news rushing to see if by lucky chance Ben Singer was dead ..

He had to get out of here .now. Ben kicked the bike into gear and started down the loop road, headed the wrong way, like the truck he's seen earlier. There was a booming thunderclap and the rain increased again to a torrent. Good for hiding in, but hard to see the road .And any moment more vehicles could be arriving .Ambulances, sightseers .deputy sheriffs .Only one of them had to take the loop road backwards and he'd be caught ..

Three hundred yards along the road he came to a farm road that turned south. It was paved and with luck, it would take him south of town and let him cut back to the freeway or get on the state road system. A few miles south of Nephi the state roads began dividing off in all directions like veins in an old wino's face. Heading off across the state, even up through the national forests. There was an east bound freeway leading to Green River .even to Denver.

Ben would have a dozen ways he could head south if he could just get out of the box he was in...

In the distance, through the thinning rainfall, he saw two more sets of flashing lights headed down the road he'd just left. The fire would draw all the lawmen for miles ..not so bad. Fewer for him to dodge. Less chance someone will tell Sand where he was .

After a quarter mile he turned on his parking lights and the yellow glow helped him stay centered in the road in the blinding downpour. He didn't need much light as he slowly drove away. He was easing his way down the road, widening the gap, but not running in blind panic.

A jolt ran through him as he realized what he was doing, without conscious thought, just as second nature to him. He was falling back on the instructions Grandpa Tsosie, despite Ben's best efforts, had pounded into his rebellious young mind. Ben had determined never to take up warrior ways. Not after seeing his father.

But you can't overcome your upbringing. You just seemed to absorb things out of thin air. You just can't get away from the way you're raised. It pops up when you least expect it.

When you most need it, he heard his grandfather say.

Ben could even recall the Navajo story that Grandpa used to teach what he was doing.

Watch the big deer, he had said once when they were hunting up in the Carrizizo east and north of Chinle. You learn from them what to do when your enemy has the poisoned hand and you are foolish enough to let yourself be defenseless.

Ben felt himself smiling a little in the night as he thought of his grandfather. He felt a great desire to see him, talk with him. Suddenly it seemed clear to him. If he could he would go home and see his grandfather.

The poisoned hand was the Indian way of saying that if your enemy could see you and touch you then you would die because what he had in his hand could kill you and you were unarmed, and therefore could not fight back, only hide and run away.

Sometimes it was long range poison that could reach across the distance if you were careless and place a red hot piece of lead in your body, just as a Navajo witch can shoot a piece of corpse bone into you that kills you with ghost sickness if your shield is down inside your breast. Other times it would be short range death--war club, knife, pistol. The Hopi name for Navajos was "head pounder" because in the old times they favored cracking skulls with a stone war club.

The big deer, Grandpa Tsosie said, were big and old because they had learned the trick. They never ran straight away from you if they could help it. They'd run just a little way to cover and then circle to hide and to find you and watch you. Knowing where you were was important so that you couldn't surprise them. Time and again Ben had seen the big deer with the heavy horns circle out around hunters on a distant mountainside. Keeping the hunters in sight, ghosting away softly without ever being seen themselves.

"It's an old Apache trick", Grandpa would say with a grin.

It was a private joke among the Navajo. Few white men knew that the Navajo and the Apache were the same people. They spoke the same language and their ancestors came from the same place up in Canada. The Apache had the big reputation in war. But the Navajo were living exactly where they wanted to be, on their own land between the four sacred mountains. The whites had never taken it. Apparently never realizing how craftily the Navajo had dealt with them. That Navajo got what they wanted without ever being backed into an outright war with the Anglos. The round-up of many Navajo by Kit Carson during the Civil War, the Long Walk to Fort Sumner, had taught them to use their heads, not their hands

against the whites. Grandfather Tsosie's parents had escaped the round up and remained on their land. They were also among the most gifted politicians and bureaucrats on the reservation. Ben had tried hard to be like them.

But, when push came to shove, they were Apache at heart. Scratch a Navajo, the saying went, and he would bleed Apache blood.

So Ben knew, almost instinctively, where his danger was. It was behind him. But he had to avoid being even accidentally caught in the headlights of a police car. If he left unseen no casual word could get back to Dick Sand through lawmen gossiping on the radio net.

He drifted on down the road, looking back often. Leaving his helmet off despite the rain so he could hear better. He passed on west of Mona and jumped the freeway near Levan, went on to Gunnision, then Salina on the old state highway system. In each sleeping community he paused, watching, seeking cover behind an old building here, skimming quietly along a residential street there, watching always for the local police. Few towns had enough officers, or, given that, enough crime to mount a night shift.

He stayed on back roads as much as possible to dodge sheriff's patrols. When he came to the junction of eastbound I-70 it was still very dark and raining in a slow drizzle that seemed to have washed everyone off the streets and into shelter. Only truckers were using the freeway and most of them stopped at Salina.

Fitting into a long gap in traffic he blasted East down the freeway for five minutes and turned off on Highway 24. This was the ☐Navajo Trail☐ that was used by many of his people coming and going from the Navajo Reservation to the south in Arizona. It was a narrow state highway that crossed some low passes, went past the ☐Big Rock Candy Mountain☐, divided at Loa and went east to Hanksville and on to Lake Powell, passing through Capital Reef National Monument on the way. This was the famous hiding place of Butch Cassidy and the Sundance Kid. Long, lonesome empty stretches of bitter and barren land. The rain had been left far to the north. The sky was clear here, the stars brilliant and plentiful so far from the city lights. The Milky Way, the spirit path, was particularly plain tonight. The sight of it made Ben wonder if he'd walk it one day soon.

After crossing the Colorado River at Hite the road continued on then into territory occupied mostly by Navajos and their arch enemies of the old days, the Utes.

After leaving the freeway Ben put the big bike in overdrive and reached Capitol Reef well before daylight. In time to pull into another secluded campground near Natural Bridges. It was still closed for the winter, but he found a spot back in the trees, well screened by brush and trees. He was so hungry he was shaking and the benefits of the little sleep he'd gotten had long since worn off. His mind was floating in a gray fog of fatigue and despair that absorbed his energy and will like a black hole and made every thought an effort.

He prepared his bed under the tarp again, ate a can of pork and beans and took some aspirin. He soaked his arm down with Absorbine Jr. and sank down wearily. He was too tired to wake up to anything less than the noise of a freight train. He was still taking a chance-stopping here. But his exhausted and injured body could carry him no further.

Like a wounded buck he hunkered down in the brush hoping no one would stumble across him. He felt a grim satisfaction. He was half a state away from Warren County now and quite sure no one had seen him. No one had touched him with a poisoned hand. The irony of it hit him as he drifted into a fitful sleep. The only thing he could do right was run and hide.

A great skill for a warrior, his mind said in Grandpa Tsosie's voice.

If warriors were rabbits.

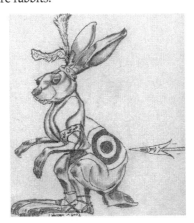

Chapter 8
Ben Singer Discovers He's Dead

Crushing weariness wasn't enough to overcome the ache in his arm. He slept fitfully never deeply. Each time a truck went by out on the highway he jerked wake, sending waves of agony through his shoulder. Light glinting on the red-rock canyon walls, at first, looked like blinking emergency lights on a police car. His sleep-fogged brain, suddenly awash in fear-fueled adrenaline, screamed that Sand had found him. But his exhausted body couldn't carry him any further. The fear couldn't drive him on.

But it wouldn't let him rest.

The headlight beams danced on the canyon walls like bonfires at a Squaw Dance. The echoing sound of tires on the asphalt boomed and echoed like enemy war drums. Each time Ben held his breath, strained to hear if it showed signs of slowing down, turning into the campground.

He couldn't reason his way out of it. Sand had done something to him, put a fear in him, that was immune to logic. An unreasoning, animal fear that made him sweat even in the early morning cold.

Sometime in the night Ben snapped awake as the singing of tires slowed, and a vehicle turned off the highway. Suddenly the darkness was pierced by the white-hot beam of a searchlight as a police cruiser with Loa City Law Enforcement decals on the side drove slowly through the campground.

Ben felt beads of cold sweat forming on his lip. He ducked down, pulled back into the brush that screened him, biting off a groan as his shoulder sent fresh waves of agony down his arm. Panting with pain and fear he leaned against the bike behind the screening brush and watched the patrol car.

When it reached the end of the first loop of the campground it turned around and crept past each campsite, the searchlight spearing the darkness. Ben was sure they would spot the Goldwing hidden in the brush. Suddenly the cruiser stopped and Ben's heart stopped with it. Ben peered cautiously through the brush and saw that the   patrolmen had 3 or 4 deer, including two magnificent bucks pinned in the spotlight.   The deer's eyes shined eerily in the night like the ghost lights Ben heard about in spooky stories Grandpa told at midnight around the fire in the hogan at Chinle.

Finally the spotlight winked out and the comforting darkness returned as the police car moved slowly back to the highway, sped up, and was gone. Wearily Ben lay back down. Nothing the policemen did indicated they were searching for him, or anyone else. Just bored, spotlighting some big deer. Planning a fall hunt that was still months away. Maybe Sand wasn't trying to track him after all. And, if he was, like the big deer circling the hunters, the safest place for Ben to hide was where they had already searched.

The night air had turned chill. Ben took some aspirin, crawled back into his blanket and fell into an exhausted sleep.

****

"You hear about the fire dance, Dick?" Herschel said. "Down in the Chateau Lake Campground. Some biker, I hear. They're saying on the police band, took a lightening bolt, gas tank blew."

"You don't say. That's tough. Real sad. Where you at?" Dick sounded like

49

Warrior's Way

someone had just told him a hilarious joke, like he was about to giggle right out loud.

"Sittin' up on Nebo by the road home, watching the smoke signals comin' up from the lake shore as we speak."

"You seen Blinky and Scopes?'

"Nope. I'll say that for them. The rain shut down visibility to nothin' and less than five minutes later this huge fireball lights up the whole valley. Then the place filled up with cops and EMT units. It was raining too bad to see anything that wasn't flashing red and white."

"Good, good." Sand tried to keep the relief out of his voice. "Well, you guys go on back over the mountain, but keep your phones on. Call me when you get back to base so I know right where you are. In case "

"In case?"

"Just don't go off the clock. I'm up on Nebo, high enough to call Mexico. They'll be glad to hear we got our end under control."

"While you're feelin' so good, Dick, how about dropping some cash into our piggy bank? We're running on empty.."

"Yeah, yeah. First thing tomorrow. Then when I get the next installment from our friends south of the border we'll all get a big payday. Meantime, stay close.'

"Yessir, we'll do that. See you."

****

"Hey, Blinky" Sand said. "Heard you did okay. Where you at?"

"Yeah, like I said, you find him, we can do the rest. We're south of Nebo headed for Scipio. We'll camp there tonight to stay out of the way of all them cops up at Mona."

'Good. Do that. I got some things to do. I'll call you tomorrow and set up a meeting. Get you paid for this night's work. Ill probably have some more work for you guys. Looks now like things are really gonna start hummin'."

"Little steady work, you think Sand? This part time stuff stinks. Means hungry times all around. Scopes and me, we got big appetites .."

And small brains ... "Yeah. Plenty for everybody. Tell you more about it tomorrow. Get some rest, but leave your phones on. I like havin' my people close .."

"Yeah, Yeah Dick, we'll just do that. Sleep with one eye open and a phone under our pillow .."

"Works for me. See you manyana."

Dick hung up. Now he could call Montero and tell him everything was set. The Mules could be on their way by daylight. All the holes were plugged, the loose ends tied up. With Singer gone By golly, I got to go tell Terry her man didn't make his wedding ..Give her another hug and lots of sympathy ..No tellin' how this might work out ..

After his call to Mexico Sand pushed the big suburban with the LawDog plates down the road to the Heber turn off. He was humming his tuneless cow puncher's ditty and smiling broadly to himself.

****

Terry lay awake in her room, Rhetta at last quiet, no longer knocking on the door, insisting that she and Terry "gotta talk. Can't let this fester, got to get it out in the open and thrash through it "

Terry shifted to her left side, trying to loosen up and relax. Nothing worked. She heard her father's voice again. Syrupy-sweet with sympathy.

"Is it true, dear, what Rhetta said?"

Try to keep the relief out of you voice, Daddy.

"Ben left this morning to go home."

"To be married, Rhetta said. He's gone to marry a reservation girl."

Indian, why can't you ever just say Indian?

'That's what Dick Sand said. Ben just said he had to leave and drove off.'

It took all her strength to keep her voice from cracking as the picture of Ben roaring off on his bike floated up in front of her as she listened to her father filling her mother in on the details.

"Just like that? Just left you standing by the road?"

She heard the undertone in his voice. I told you so. Tried to warn you. You should have listened to me.

She'd told him once the reason he objected to Ben was his fear that some of his grandchildren would be brown. Well, you don't have to worry about that now, do you Daddy.

"I can't talk about it right now Daddy. I'll call in a few days."

'Now wait a minute, Terry. We've got to talk about this ..''

"Do you want me to put Rhetta on the phone? She'd love to talk to you about this."

"Terry, don't take that tone with me. Your mother and I are worried about you. We'll drive up tomorrow if you want us to ."

"If I don't will you come anyway?"

'Terry ..''

"Or will you respect my wishes if not my feelings?"

"I, I .we.."

"Good night, Daddy.'

She'd hung up, but not before hearing a click on the line. Rhetta. Dear Rhetta.

Terry felt her nails digging into the palms of her hands. She washed out her anger by letting the warm tears start flowing down her cheeks. Ben, how could you do this. You gave me no warning. Turned my whole life upside down. Destroying every dream. Squashing every hope. Right out of the blue, like a bolt of lightening from a clear sky.

But of course, Ben wasn't here to answer those kinds of questions. He'd just gone. Leaving her to face their friends, to handle the messy, painful details all alone.

Then the tears became a flood and the sobbing, stifled in her pillow lest Rhetta hear, became an awful, anguished moan of loss and regret.

Later, lying awake in the early morning hours, all cried out, bleakness like winter inside her, Terry passed the empty time by beginning an intense, emotional rehashing of her life, her decisions, her apparent shortcomings in reading human nature (especially in men) and in trying desperately to find some way to face her classmates on campus after dear sweet Rhetta, crying crocodile tears all the way, spread the news.

Ben Singer had gone home. To marry someone else ..

****

Ben awoke to see the legs of a doe near him. She was grazing the new spring grass, carefully keeping him in sight. Ben worked his shoulder and arm and groaned. The doe pricked up her ears, turned and stotted away in that stiff-legged jump that alerted every deer for 500 yards.

Traffic was picking up out on the highway. Someone could turn into the campground at any moment. Maybe the sheriff or the highway patrol ..Was he far

51

enough away from Sand? From Warren County? From Terry? To protect her? No, in his own mind, he wasn't. He was still in Utah.

He rolled over, got up and packed the bike, ignoring as best he could the bruises and stiff muscles that made him awkward. Terry floated in the back of his mind and emotions dark and powerful washed through him. He'd never see her again. Was that possible?

What was she doing right then? Should he call her, try to talk to her? What could I say that wouldn't put her in danger? Would she even listen?

Ben moaned again, but not with physical pain. His whole soul ached for the comfort Terry's presence could give him now. If he only dared to seek it ..

But he didn't. Couldn't. Not put Terry and Lester in any more danger than they were. If only there were a way some way ..But there was none. The dark and bitter wind that had blown through his mind all night still blocked his thinking. Derailed the rational processes of his mind. Animal fear was all he had left. And he want far enough away yet.

As he started up the bike and moved toward the highway Ben realized that sometime in the night he had decided where he was going. Home. To Chinle. To talk to his grandfather. He owed it to his mother's family to tell them what had happened. They'd put up a lot of family money to help him in school. Expecting big returns when he was a reservation lawyer, probably a politician. Not a criminal on the run from the law, no matter what the truth of that really was.

He needed someplace where he could rest and think and get some advice. In his mind he saw the Tsosie camp that overlooked the thousand foot deep red rock canyon at Chinle where his people had found refuge for three hundred years. Where he had been a child, loved, a little spoiled perhaps, but accepted despite who his father was. Yes. Ben was going home.

Ben put the Honda in drive and scarcely noticed the magnificent white and red rock pinnacles of the capital reef monument and park. He rolled down through the canyons and out into the sun-baked, trackless flats that led to the outlaw country of Butch Cassidy and the Sundance Kid. He stopped for gas and milk and donuts at Hanksville, a junction where two highways met, leading to Lake Powell's recreation areas.

Leaving the Hole In The Rock Store he stopped dead when he saw a Wayne County sheriff's patrol van sitting just across the highway. The big 4x4 all cops favored in the back country had a power winch, running lights, several antennas and two deputies wearing dark glasses that reflected like mirrors. The van starting moving immediately and Ben saw spare gas cans in racks on the back and at least three radio antennas. Ben felt the fear crawling up his backbone again. He spun on his heel, walking steadily, resisting the urge to run, straight to the bike. He'd never feared policemen before. But he started the bike before he even mounted and was prepared to run for it if he could.

Anything was better than being given over to Dick Sand on some trumped up charge or other.

Anything.

As he bent over to pack the groceries in the bike's saddle bags he heard the big van moving toward him, cutting in behind him and stopping about twenty yards away. When he glanced up he saw two pairs of eyes shining in the dim interior, looking right at him. Checking the plate. The shotgun rider picked up the mike and was talking to someone. Ben jumped on the bike as smoothly as any ninety-year old with terminal arthritis and immediately pulled out, snaking through the crowded parking lot and back on the highway to Lake Powel. He watched his mirrors as he quickly brought the bike up to speed. If they were going to chase him he might as well know now. They'd never run him down between here and the muley point drop off. He knew every inch of the road and the big bike was made for running the road. Once he was on the gravel road's ungraded hairpin turns.....well they'd just have to see.....

The mirror stayed empty. Looking back Ben saw the van moving north on the highway to I-70 and Castledale and Price. Away from him. He heaved a sigh that hurt his arm, but he barely noticed. Relief flooded him until he recalled the cop on the radio. He could picture Sand getting the report. Knowing right where Ben was, where he was going. It was over 150 miles to the next junction that didn't just end in a trap at Bull Frog marina or Hall's crossing. Sand could stop him anywhere along there if he wanted to. Ben wouldn't be safe till he crossed the Colorado at Hite and, fifty miles later, turned south, down the thousand foot high cut at Muley Point where so many uranium trucks had gone over the edge, sliding off the narrow gravel road that snaked down the high plateau into Monument Valley. There he could cross into Arizona at Mexican Water and be on the Big Reservation. Navajoland. The size of New England, empty, often desolate. But home to him. Where he had friends and family and a place to be. Where he knew every inch of his home turf. There he'd have a chance.

He set the bike into overdrive and pressed the speed limit, leaning far over around the curves, fighting to keep the bike from crossing the solid yellow line. Dropping down quickly into the spectacular red rock canyons that drained into the Colorado River. To his right, South, he could see the black bulk of the Henry Mountains. Home to buffalo and desert bighorn sheep.

Soon enough he came to the high suspension bridge near Hite that crossed the big river just above the little fishing and resort village of Hite. Ben slowed on the bridge and looked down, down into the red-stained water. He saw the confluence of the Dirty Devil and the Colorado, the Devil dumping roiling red water into the relatively clear water of the Colorado.

Red and swift and cold. When he was eight a section of the bridge across the Chinle wash near his home had been washed away in a flash flood one stormy August night. Six or seven cars drove off into the smashing, churning water before someone discovered what was happening. His mother was stopped less than a hundred feet from the gap. They'd walked over and peered into the dark, churning water and Ben could still feel the vibration of the concrete piles supporting the rest of the bridge, fearing at any moment he would be plunged to an awful death.

In dry country, to a desert people who believed that their previous world had been destroyed in a flood, drowning was among the worst of all possible deaths. Growing up around arroyos that were dry one moment and running twenty feet deep from bank the bank the next, Ben had a caution about water in anything larger than a swimming pool. So he didn't linger now. He punched the bike back up to speed and climbed up the far side back onto the Fry Canyon plateau and on to Natural Bridges and the turn down to Muley Point. By then hunger and pain and relief that he had turned South at last prompted him to pull off along a wood gathering road and stop for lunch behind a screen of cedars that had been drug down and stacked in piles by huge cables drawn between twin pairs of bulldozers by cattlemen who wanted to plant crested wheat grass for the cattle, but that wouldn't grow in the shade of trees.

He was still tired. He couldn't make Chinle today no matter what and traveling at night would be that much safer. He turned on the bike's radio while he opened beans and spam and saltine crackers for lunch. It was when the Blanding station got around to state and local news that Ben learned he really had nothing to hurry or worry about.

Because he was already dead.

He picked up the tag end of a newscast from KUTA in Blanding stating that a Benjamin Franklin Singer had died in a campground accident in Mona. It was a lightening induced explosion and fire. A real tragedy since Mr. Singer was so young.

Too young to die.

Especially if only the good die young........

****

Dick Sand strolled through the parking lot at Warren County Community College, headed over toward his suburban after his class on social disorders, which he shared with Terry. He fought to suppress a big grin but inside he basked in a warm rush of triumph. In his mind's eye he saw the empty seat in class where Ben usually sat. He heard people asking where Ben was. Heard himself again telling everyone that he had left school to go home and get married. He had to practically bite his tongue to keep from blurting out that Ben was dead, killed in a tragic accident on the way home. He wanted Terry to find out from someone else. He was fitting himself for the role of White Knight in her life. He'd be a comforting big brother at first. Later? You just never know. The sky's the limit here.

He'd caught the wondering looks when Terry dragged into class, darkness in her eyes, her clothes and hair a mess. Best of all, shed bypassed her regular seat to come and set down by him like a little girl seeking comfort and safety. Oh, that made 'em sit up and take notice. A glance from him then stopped all the wagging tongues.

Sand knew he had a tough reputation. He'd personally whipped every football player or wrestler in the valley dumb enough to take him on. In the gym or on the streets. He had the reputation as the strongest man in the county. And to some as the meanest. Fortunately Terry didn't hang out with that group. So, though shed never been more than polite toward him when Ben was around, she had no reason to fear or distrust him.

He'd see to it it stayed that way. He could depend on Rhetta to keep him right up to date on everything in Terry's life.

And by now the school was buzzing, the stories flying, with Rhetta passing on inside information and having the time of her life doing it. What an ending it would be when everyone learned that Singer was dead and gone. Sand had to fight down the grin that welled up from the merry feelings that warmed his insides. He loved his power plays. Too often nobody but him ever knew about them. But not this time. This time everybody knew, only they didn't know a thing. Not really. That made it perfect.

Now if he could use Terry's feelings when she found out Singer was dead and gone for good .. That there was not the remotest hope that he might return .If he moved just right, at just the right time Rhetta would tell him when that was, without even knowing what she was doing.

This time he couldn't stop the grin. It just came. He saw it reflected from the window of his suburban as he reached out to unlock the door. Sand you ole cuss. You're good. Yessir, you're really good. Too bad your daddy can't see you now.

As the door swung open he saw the red light on the radio shining brightly. He had a call waiting from the Salt Lake dispatcher. Here's where they tell me poor old Ben has gone to the happy hunting grounds.

He punched the mike button.

"Deputy Sand here. You have a message for me?"

"Uhh, yes Deputy. Here it is. It's on that call you put in on Ben Singer."

"Yes. My request to locate him. I heard he was in an accident down by Nephi." Here it comes. Now the good news.

"Uhh ..I don't know anything about that. Perhaps you have newer information than I do. If he was northbound from Hanksville he might have been in an accident when he got to Nephi. I'm sorry deputy Sand "

'Hankesville? What's that you say about Hankesville" Sand tried to keep his voice from rising, from taking on the cutting edge he used with people who worked for him.

"That's right. Two Wayne county deputies confirmed seeing the Honda Gold Wing with a plate registered to Ben Singer at about 8 A.M. this morning and reported seeing a Native American get on the bike and travel East toward Lake Powel. I just don't see how he could have had an accident near Nephi."

"No ma'm. Neither do I. I guess I was given false information about that." Sand felt himself biting off each word like Prince took the legs off a rabbit. "Thank you ma'm. I appreciate the help. I'll take it from here."

Dick slammed the phone down, looked up to see some startled students staring at him.

Sand felt raw adrenaline powered by equal measures of rage and fear pumping through him like red hot lava. It hunched him over the steering wheel like he'd been kicked in the stomach.

He can't be there. He's dead. I told Montero that everything was set. Things are moving. Can't be stopped .

Abruptly he shut off the emotion. Resumed the icy control that he'd given up so much to achieve. That had brought him so far from a West Texas cow farm. He released his death grip on the wheel and pumped his fingers to work off the pain. Singer was the smallest part of his plans. A mere detail. Sand specialized in details. At looking at every part of an operation, from every angle. Over and over. Leaving nothing to chance. Like TJ. Like Singer.

He worked to eliminate small complications, with overwhelming force when needed, before they could become problems. That's what got him here, doing what he was doing. On the verge of raking in millions millions.

Blinkey's voice spoke up in his mind. We ain't the CIA. You find him, we'll do the rest.

"But you didn't, did you." Prince, roaming the back of the van, pricked up his ears and whined. Looked around to see if there was a threat .hearing that in Sand's voice.

Sand felt an intense flash of murderous rage--aimed straight at Ben Singer. You think you can mess this up for me, do you Injun? Blunder around out there somewhere. Put two and two together? My mules got to pass right through your land down there in Arizona. You never should have set TJ up.

"Well, Benny boy, you just got lucky, that's all. The idea was to get you before your got wise. We'll just do it a little further down the road. Maybe take out some of your family if we have to ..You'll still wish you had died .."

****

Sand almost broke the phone punching in Blinkey's cell phone number. Blinky picked up on the fourth ring and sounded sleepy, maybe hung over. From celebrating last night ..

"He's alive. He was seen in Hanksville less than an hour ago.'

He paused only seconds and then cut back in, his voice rising despite his effort to stay in control.

"I don't care about the body. You got the wrong guy!"

Sand listened a moment, then cut in.

"I'm not interested in reasons. I don't care who it is. It wasn't him, that's all. I told you fools there was no excuses on this one. Not for me, and not for you.'

He felt his teeth clenching and his face was getting hot as he imagined explaining this to Montero.

"I gave them the go ahead down south. The mules are on their way by now."

He fought down an urge to shout into the phone. Blinky wasn't sounding so sleepy now.

"They can't be reached and stopped. That's the whole idea. That's why the plan is foolproof. Except maybe you're the fools who can wreck it. No, you listen to me and listen good. He's headed for home, down on the reservation. Most likely hell go down Muley Point to Mexican Water. You better be heading for you truck right now. One of you start readin' the map. Head to I-70. Jump off by Richfield, go down past Big Rock Candy Mountain and hit the road at Loa that goes to Hanksville and on to Powell. Fifty miles or so from Hite Marina, near Natural Bridges, a gravel uranium hauling road turns south, drops a thousand feet down Muley Point to the floor of Monument Valley. Up at Bluff he can cut across the San Juan to Mexican Water and pick up the road to Chinle from there."

Sand listened as Blinky huffed and puffed, heard a truck door slam, the sounds of a high speed whine revving up through a powerful engine.

"You best hope he stops to rest. I'll get reports on him and let you know where he is. See if you can help him make it down off Muley Point in record time. You hear?"

Sand listened, then cut in his voice a hiss, intense, the rage that boiled in him leaking out like acid down the phone line.

"You won't be around to help if we have to go in down there on the reservation to clean this up. You got that, Blinky? You two stooges won't be part of it. I'll have to give you up to the big man to save my own neck. And I will. In a heartbeat. Now stop jawin' and move."

Sand resisted slamming the phone down. A broken radio phone was the last thing he needed at this point.

****

"Listen, Herschel. While we're talking you and Virgil mount up. High speed travel, no extra equipment. You movin' yet?" Dick's voice had the whiplash edge to it that he seldom used, at least not with Herschel and Virgil.

"Yep, out the door as we speak.' Herschel opened and shut the door, then kicked Virgil's foot, putting finger to lips to shush him as he sat straight up in bed. Herschel made the motions of a wolf biting at his leg and pointed to the phone. He used the patrol sign for saddle up. "What's up, Dick?'

"Dumb and Dumber got the wrong guy. Singer was spotted in Hanksville headed East about two hours ago."

"Two hours? It took the dispatcher two hours to call you?"

" I was away from the radio. That don't matter. I just kicked them where it will do the most good and sent them down through Candy Mountain to head him off."

"Oookay. What you want us to do?"

Herschel motioned frantically at Virgil who was sitting, slumped and round shouldered on the edge of the bed. He signed for rifles, food, the standard survival kits and warm clothes. 3 days stay. He missed and spun half around when he leveled a sharp kick at Virgil's shin. Proving Virgil was now awake.

"I don't hear no motor noise, Herschel. Why don't I hear motor noise? You just sittin' there listening to me over breakfast?"

"Naw, Dick. Virgil's gone to get the extra gas cans throwed in. I got to run back and get the CB's and we're out of here. Which way you want us to go, what you want us to do when we get there? ..Who we after .Singer or Blinky and Scopes?"

He made an ugly grimace at Virgil, who was now moving rapidly and efficiently. Getting dressed as he eased open the door, hopped on one foot getting his boot on, and disappeared behind the snow machines to get the gas.

Herschel reached through the open window and fired up the truck.

'Your choice, up Fairview and across the top to Castle Dale or over Soldier Summit. Either way you can hit the cut off down through outlaw country to Hankesville and get there almost as fast as Blinky can. Study your map. Watch for Natural Bridges Monument. The road turns south there for Mexican Hat, Bluff, and across the river to Chinle."

"Been through there once, but not recently. Big country, Dick. Plenty empty ."

"I know that. Don't you think I know that? We got one chance to keep this polecat in the bag. We don't get him, I got to call my people down south. Think about what that could mean."

"Yeah. Definitely not good. We don't want to have to chase him onto the Big Rez either. His turf, too many unfriendly eyes ."

"Stop telling me what I already know. Just get in position. I should get more reports and I'll update you as the patrol officers spot him. Chances are good hell stop and rest. I guarantee you he's not feelin' too good."

"I'll bet. That West Texas massage you gave him has got him tender all over today."

"Next thing " Herschel heard the ice tinging Sand's voice. Not the first time he'd heard it, and it always meant somebody was going to get seriously, probably terminally, hurt. Despite the warmth of the morning he felt the hair rising on his neck and a shiver started down between his shoulder blades. "You get the least chance, I don't want the two stooges on the team. We don't send people back to the minor leagues. We take them out of the game. They don't get a chance to learn from their mistakes. You take my meaning? You hear what I'm saying over this secure, untappable phone of ours?"

"We get you, Dick."

"Don't be dainty. This ain't dainty work. Don't matter if they get Singer or not, you hear? I already took steps to make sure Singer don't get no welcome home party if he makes it all the way to Chinle. So get rid of those two. No matter what. Make an example of them I can use later. If we miss Singer we ain't quite dead yet, but we sure ain't got no wiggle room."

"Gotcha, Dick. We understand perfectly."

"Where you at?"

Herschel rolled his eyes at Virgil, who was driving fast, the racing driver in him

Warrior's Way

fully charged and working. But they were only a mile out of Fairfield. Forty -five miles from the highway in Spanish Fork Canyon.

"We're better than half-way to Spanish Fork Canyon. Virg figures he can pick up more time dodging traffic on the big road than dodging elk in the back country."

"Keep your phone on, I'll be in touch."

"Yep, we'll do just that, Dick. We'll be right here in this truck just waiting for your call."

Herschel looked over at Virgil, mock pain and disappointment obvious in his face.

"He hung up on me, Virg. Didn't wait for me to say goodbye."

"Sand's a busy man today, Herschel. No time for the usual niceties."[

"I fear 'ole Dick's impulsivity issues are getting out of hand again."

"Seems he regrets not killing Singer outright while he had the chance."

"Yeah, he was so proud of himself. He didn't have to twist the knife before he let Singer go, either."

"That scene just before Singer hit the freeway....that musta been something."

"Singer all but killed himself on the way to Mona."

"Singer's probably really, really mad, now he's runnin' around loose. Making a fool of Sand. So far though, Sand's just blaming Blinky and company."

"He don't want Blinky and Milliken on the team anymore. Said he wants us to hand them their pink slips first chance we get."

"Uh oh. They musta done something to make him mad."

"Them and Singer. In the same boat now. They got on Depitty Dick's bad side."

"The old Lobo's on the prowl for sure, Herschel. Best we go to Devcon Four or whatever that is."

"Step up our alert from yellow to red."

"Keep a sharp eye on our own back trail."

"Case Sand decides he needs a whole new team."

"A fresh start."

"Can't mix friendship and business. That's what old Dick always says.

"No use tryin' to change his mind. Nor count on him to cut us any slack."

"We're on our own, Virg. You and me are the two Musketeers of the Old Spanish Trail."

"Both for one and one for both."

"Till we see a Lobo on our back trail."

"Then it's gotta be every Musketeer for himself."

"Words to live by, Virgil. Words to live by."

Chapter Nine
Deadfall

Sand hurried back through Warren Valley, out the other side up the canyon to Heber and up Daniel's Canyon and by a back road up onto Strawberry Ridge. He stopped when he crested out, deep in the pines where he could see out south, in the blue misted distance, the Soldier Summit area. From here, at this elevation, his radio phone had near perfect reception from all points of the compass. It was close to one of his 'Mexican Mule' stopover points, hidden down on the reverse slope from Strawberry Valley.

Best of all, from here dirt track roads led south to the Spanish Fork Canyon road Herschel was on, east to Colorado and the back door to Denver, north to Salt Lake City or Wyoming. It was seldom visited. A few deer hunters in the fall, maybe a pair of snow mobilers in the winter. Right now he had it all to himself. He let Prince out to roam and act as a moving early warning screen around his suburban.

He monitored the police band as he waited to hear from the dispatcher or police patrols, or Blinky or Herschel. As he waited his mind paced through the situation like a lion paces it's cage. Ceaselessly, restlessly. Searching for a way out. Following lines of thought, threads of feeling. Looking for weaknesses and flaws in his overall plan. Details, details, the devil's in the details. Was there anyone he could trust to get things right?

He grinned a little to himself. Best you never learn to depend on anybody, he heard his daddy saying as he whipped Sand with a rawhide quirt most men only used on onery horses. You lean on anyone, it only makes you weak. You got no control Somebody else is deciding what's gonna happen to you ..

You taught me a lot, old man. More than you ever knew. Not bad for a man who worked for other people his whole life. Sand felt a little tingle of relief pulsing through his mind, grateful again that he'd left nothing to chance with Singer. Made sure, if he made it home, he'd get a bad reception, find it hard to stay. That's what got Sand where he was. Some people would call it overkill. But it wasn't. It was just covering your bases.

You map out the turf, identify the people who can think, who can lead, the do-gooders that might tumble to what you're doing. Then you eliminate them. Quickly, quietly. Like Singer. Just a detail. Small potatoes. He should have died with no fuss or bother. You strike all at once, with overwhelming force, never giving them time to think nor to learn. Like the little street rat, TJ. With his little picture book of cheap prints made with a dime store camera. Showing Sand meeting with known pushers and dealers. Jacking Sand up for money, playing both ends of the game, threatening to give Sand up to Singer. What happened to TJ was just typical of Sand's careful approach to business. Singer.....well....

Singer was a classic example. Sand had done everything right.

He slapped his palms on the steering wheel so hard Prince came back to investigate.

It should have worked perfectly. Except Bonehead Blinky and his partner killed the wrong guy. Chances were fifty-fifty they'd miss him again. Maybe Singer would actually make it home. But if he did he'd find old Dick had been there first. That's what planning was all about.

You can run like a jack rabbit, Singer. But you can't hide from my hawks. But just for insurance I plugged up your burrow for you too.

Sand drummed his fingers on the side of the suburban and looked every few seconds at the radio-pone. Wondering. Should he call Herschel or Blinky? No use. Only upset them. He knew Herschel would have mounted magnetic decals and a flashing light bar and would be running full out looking like a local lawman's rig. They could do ninety to a hundred a lot of the way, especially with Virgil behind the wheel. No, best let them do their job. They'd never failed him .yet.

****

Ben listened to KUTA in Blanding to get the noon news. Sandwiched between appeals to shop Utah, support Utah merchants, not Cortez Colorado businessmen who don't pay Utah taxes, and the scores of the latest Monticello Blanding showdown on the high school basketball court Ben heard his name again.

He'd died in Mona in a freak accident. Lightening had stuck his camp, exploding the gas tank on his Honda. Burning him to death.

Terry will think I'm dead. How will Sand use that? They must have notified my mom. The word would be going out to the extended family to come home to Chinle for the four days of ritual mourning. His mother worked as a legal secretary clear down in Flagstaff Arizona and would have to take time off. His uncles and aunts would also have to leave their jobs. It was a major problem for them. Especially when they'd discover Ben wasn't dead.

How inconvenient. Perhaps I should do something about that ..

There were no phones near most of them. He couldn't call his Grandfather Tsosie. He might not even know yet that Ben was supposed to be dead. The nearest phone was at Mexican Water and he could be home almost faster than he could call.

But he'd have to take the Goosenecks drop off down Muley Point rather than go the long way around through Blanding. The road dropped over a thousand feet in just three miles. This plateau was as high as the monuments in Monument Valley and the road dropped down into the broad, desert valley of the San Juan River.

Should he let the police know he was alive? Terry has heard the news by now. Will it really matter to her now? Should I call her? What can I tell her? That I'm alive but still on my way home and that I still can't talk to her about why? What can I tell her that won't set Sand off and that will help her understand?

Nothing. Not a thing.

Sand thought I was dead. Now he knows I'm not. What'll he do?

A sudden thought slammed into his mind. Was that an accident or was it supposed to be me? Were the deputies in Hanksville looking for him or just checking on a stranger? Does Sand know or not? Does it matter?

Pain and fatigue made his mind as thick as motor oil in January. Too many bad choices. No good ones. There was no excuse to go back or call Terry. Or do any of the things he ached to do.

His mind went to the wine in the side pocket of the bike. Nested there like a scorpion. You can kill yourself one drink at a time. In the meantime you don't think so much. It was just waiting there to blot out his pain, dull his thoughts. Who would it hurt?

The reckless feeling of nothing to lose came back. He pictured himself at 100 miles an hour rocketing off into space at Muley Point. Then his family, at least, wouldn't be called home for nothing. If he drank the wine first they'd know he'd followed his father. It would be hard for Terry and Lester would still be living in Sand's version of Hell. But hey, there were no golden answers here. Any choice he made was going to hurt someone. Maybe himself most of all.

Ben wiped his sweaty hands on his levis.   The wine whispered to him. Well why not?

Then he suddenly saw his mother, looking at him, directly in the eyes, and gripping his arm so hard Ben thought he could feel it.

Don't be like him, Ben. Don't hurt me like your father hurt me. I'm counting on you Ben. Please don't let me down ..

"I won't, mother" he heard himself say. He was surprised at the sound of his own voice. He hadn't spoken for two days and he sounded like a bull frog trying to swallow a sparrow.

Among the Navajo fathers came and went. But mothers were always mothers. You were born into you mother's clan. She loved you unconditionally. Whatever he did, he couldn't shame his mother. Most especially not by being like his father. She'd been his friend his whole life. Bringing misery and pain upon her was something he just couldn't do.

What will you tell her about Dick Sand? About the tape? About leaving school?

He shut off his tired mind. Enough. He'd go see Grandpa Tsosie. Let them know he was alive. Then he'd decide what to do. But he wouldn't go home a drunk. He took the bottle out, tore off the cap, and poured the wine into the dirt. The sweet smell only made him want to vomit. He'd smelled it all his life on the breath of people he knew, people he'd watched destroy their own lives and the hopes and happiness of others.

He turned and threw the bottle left handed as far as he could out into the trees. It fell out there somewhere without a sound. Straining to hear it made him aware of the sound of a high speed engine howling down the road out beyond the screen of junipers. Between gaps in the branches he saw a large 4 by 4 truck with running lights flash past. It was the same type he'd seen in the dark at the campground in Mona. But there were so many like it around he thought no more of it. But as he was repacking the bike he heard faintly in the distance a siren, dopplering quickly closer. In a minute or so a police unit flashed by doing nearly a hundred, if he was any judge. Far too fast given that less than a mile down the road the asphalt gave way to gravel and two miles further dropped off the side of Muley Point down a twisting, often single lane road with a step rock wall on one side and a thousand foot drop on the other.

The first guys must have been pot hunters. The canyons abounded with Ansazi cliff dweller ruins. One of their thousand year old pots could be worth ten thousand dollars on the black market. Reason enough to hunt them. Reason enough for the local cops to chase them.

Then it was time to go. As he settled into the seat and started the engine the dark despair settled again into his soul. He pictured Terry in Dick Sand's arms and saw again Sand's wicked, wicked grin of triumph. Nothing had changed. Now he was going home and for the first time in his life that was an unhappy prospect. Nothing he was doing was solving his basic problem. Nothing was going to take him back to Warren Valley, back to Terry. Against that fact nothing else mattered much at all.

He put the bike in low and pulled carefully back out on the road. In a few miles he checked the brakes and started slowly down the grade in the deepening twilight. As he started down into the first turn, where there was a narrow turn out to pause and enjoy the view of Monument Valley spread out below, he was concentrating so hard on the bumpy road that he didn't see the fresh scrape and drag marks leading over the edge and down into a 700 foot deep declivity. Even if he'd paused to look over the edge he probably wouldn't have seen the various truck parts scattered down the cliff. Nor the bodies wedged in among the wrecks of uranium trucks and other wreckage that had accumulated over the years like dead ships in the Sargasso Sea. It might be days before anyone noticed there was a new wreck down there now.

What Ben did see, far out across the valley, was the flashing lights of the police unit, still moving fast and approaching now the intersection with the highway that led to Bluff one way and Mexican Hat the other. As he cleared the next curve he saw the flashing lights turn left, eastward. Toward Bluff. That cut him off from the Mexican Water road and he decided to travel down to Kayenta, in Arizona and back along the Shiprock Highway 160 to the turn off to Round Rock and Chinle.

He put the bike into low, checked his brakes for the fifth time and started down the next steep section. Night was coming on. There was no moon and this was no place to be after dark.

****

"Sand, how you doin'?"

"You tell me, Herschel. How am I doing? Where you guys at?'

"On the road to Bluff, just turned off the Goosenecks access road that connects to the Muley Point freeway. Man, that is some drop off."

"Don't tell me what I already know, Herschel. Tell me what I don't know. What about the Dumbo twins? How'd they come out?"

"Well, they musta dropped their feather along the way. They took off down the hill, but they didn't fly much. Mostly just crash and burn."

"You found them at the overlook?"

'Yup, we did that. And then we gave them a hearty boost and off they went, kicking and screaming. They sure didn't much want to leave our fine organization. But we gave them their pink slips and sent them into retirement."

"You haven't seen our Indian friend though ."

"Not so far. We're doing near a hundred along here. But it don't seem like he should still be ahead of us. Just too many ways from here for us to cover them all. What you want us to do?"

"For starters quit impersonating police officers and slow down to the speed limit. Stay in the area so you can respond if I get a report on him. He's still on the net and something might turn up."

"If not?"

"If not I got another plan, but I want to see this one through first."

"Okay, Dick. It's your call. You feel pretty sure he's headed home to Chinle?"

'Yeah. I've already made sure he won't get no welcome home party. If I have to I can get a chopper to do a flyover down there."

"We don't want to go in unless we have too. How important is this guy anyhow?"

"Herschel, you and Virgil done good. But that don't earn you no seat on the board of directors. You know I like to keep my options open, make decisions as the situation develops."

"Yeah, Dick we know you're flexible, spontaneous and totally unpredictable." Herschel grabbed Vigil's leg and pinched. He got a yelp and a slap for his trouble. Virgil made no noise but turned his face up like he was howling at the moon.

"You got that straight. Park yourselves at the bridge at Bluff. You can cross the San Juan River there and cut across the reservation to Mexican Water right quick and be at the Chinle turn off if I get word he went down through Monument Valley and Kayenta. Just get comfortable and leave your phones on."

"Yessir, Mr. Sand, sir. We'll be here if you need us."

"Keep your eyes open, he could come past you at any time. If he does, get him any way you can and let me know right off."

"Gotcha", Herschel said and hung up.

Herschel looked over at Virgil and heaved a huge, melodramatic sigh.

"Get him any way you can, Sand said."

"He means no matter what the cost, Herschel."

"He means 20 years to life for us, but not for him, is what he means."

"I hate it when he gets like this. He's mean, just downright mean."

"He is that.. Say Virg, is there another level above red on that alert scale? What happens if them nuclear warriors go above Devcon four?"

"I don't know for sure, Hersch, but I think its called nuclear winter."

"I swear I'm starting to feel the chill, Virgil, I purely am....."

****

Ben pulled up onto the ridge that looked down into the Tsosie camp at first light. Exhausted, hungry, road weary, sick at heart. He'd spent he night with the ghosts of his life flickering about him, just out of reach of the racing headlight of his bike. Night was always scary to traditional Navajos. A time when the ghosts of the dead wandered the land working mischief and causing soul sickness. Ben felt it in him today.

Even the site of magnificent Canyon De Chelly stretching out before him, a thousand feet deep, beautiful red rock ..home, could not lift his spirits. He worked his shoulder, cramped from hours of driving and it rewarded him with a bright stabbing shot of pain.

With a groan part physical and part spiritual he started down the ridge on a journey he'd have given anything not to have to make. Fifty miles away in the clear air he could see round rock. He'd passed it in the night with scarcely a glance. Now it stood out against the horizon, the major landmark to the east. West of him stretched massive, brooding Black Mesa. Home of Hopis and witches and to the northwest lay the dark hump of Navajo Mountain. Still in the black of night, still ominous, still the homeland of his father's clan.

His vision narrowed, darkness making a tunnel through which he peered and an emotional lump formed in his chest and burned his throat. Another day was starting in Warren Valley. Terry was beginning another day alone, as he was alone. Separated from someone he loved more than he had ever realized. Now she'd think he was dead. Her dreams would be ashes, as were his. Sand, Dick Sand, like the snake in the garden, was there.

Ben was not.

Thinking of Sand as a witch, Navajo fashion, he glanced again at Black Mesa. The old-time Navajo thought of the Hopis as powerful witches who could kill enemies by magic, even at a distance. He saw Dick Sand's grinning face, his eyes glinting redly in the firelight, superimposed on the red-dawn before him.

He's doing just that to me, Ben thought. Killing me from a distance. Just like a witch. Ben shuddered despite the warm morning air that was trying to penetrate the chill that he'd felt creeping through him all night. A chill that was vastly more than physical cold. It gathered around his heart and he felt his breathing grow short and raspy.

You cryin', Benny? Sand's mocking voice rang through the hollow emptiness of his mind.

He drug his mind back to the present. To the problems of today. He'd tried a dozen different approaches to telling Grandfather Tsosie what had happened. As he looked down at the camp the last of them vanished like the morning mists disappeared in the desert as the sun rose. At that moment he would have given anything, life itself, not to have to go down there and talk to Grandpa. Only the thought of his mother forced him on.

Just then he saw Grandpa Tsosie in the doorway of his hogan, greeting the sun and the new day. A pinch of corn pollen and a song would welcome another day of life for the old man. How many days in 75 years had he done this? It was the ritual of the conservative, traditional, old time Navajos, of the old warriors.

Ben's face burned hot now as he remembered how stubbornly he'd resisted his grandfather's attempts to teach him the old warrior ways of his people after he saw his father at Navajo Mountain. The old man had finally given up in disgust. Ben knew that in the old days, in other tribes, he would have had to dress in women's clothes and do women's work the rest of his life for rebelling against the warrior code of his people.

Grandpa had tried to get him to do several things.

Warriors, both men and women, run a race everyday, he would say. They run up the hill and back down, early in the morning. You never sit down to eat. You just

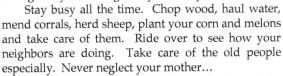

hunker down into a crouch. That makes your legs strong and you don't get lazy that way.

Stay busy all the time. Chop wood, haul water, mend corrals, herd sheep, plant your corn and melons and take care of them. Ride over to see how your neighbors are doing. Take care of the old people especially. Never neglect your mother...

Work to learn the songs and sandpaintings of the Beautyway. So you can bless yourself and your family. So you can turn evil back on the evil doers. So you can fight in the real world and in the world of spirits. That's what makes a warrior

Ben Singer, Warrior Wimp ..at your service, grandpa.

I could have used some of that at Tibble Fork Lake that night..... I would have turned Sand's evil back on his own head.....he felt the load of loss settle down harder between his shoulder blades, making it hard to steer the bike the last few hundred yards to the camp. What good were books and laws and ideals in a world that also contained Dick Sand?

He stared down into the canyon at the finger-like protrusion of sandstone that rose up 300 feet from the canyon floor. Navajo warriors had forted up there as a last resort when Spaniards or Mexicans or Kit Carson and the U.S. Army showed up and hounded them till their backs were against the wall.

They couldn't dial 911 or call in the national guard. They had instead a final place of refuge where they could sell their lives dearly or extract such a high toll of enemy dead that they would give up and go away.

Make a bow and arrows, learn to shoot and hunt, Grandpa said. Help your relatives. Especially your mothers and your sisters. In Navajo your aunt was your "little mother" so almost everybody had more than one mother.

That's what good men do. When it comes time to fight they are strong outside and strong inside with ceremonial knowledge and real power. Be a man, Ben, a true warrior. Not a killer or a butcher. A good man. That's what a warrior is, Ben. Strong in this world and powerful in the unseen world. A man that does the hard thing when it needs to be done, even if all that is is to get up and go to work every day.....

But Ben had gone another way ..The white man's way. Schooling was where Ben had power. Sifting through the categories of knowledge white men loved to create. He was powerful in the things of the mind. Or he had been. Until Dick Sand decided to introduce him to the world of brute force and the pitiless use of power.

Then Ben's big mistake caught up with him. When the chips were down he was nothing. In either the white or the Navajo world. So now he was like his father, he'd just taken a different road to get there. That was all. The end result was the same. He was caught up with the pitiful "people between" who existed but were not comfortable in either world.....

What will Grandpa think when he finds out what Sand has accused me of being? Refusing to be trained in the skills of warrior hood, bad as that was, was nothing compared to being thought of as a homosexual Navajo. One was a preference, a lifestyle choice. But in the Navajo mind homosexuality was tinged with witchcraft, incest, and evil. It spoke of a people who had left the true Dine and who had taken up with brother and sister killing witches. Such a person was more dangerous to the members of his own family than he was to strangers. Even a rumor without any evidence to back it up could ruin a person's life. Destroy a whole extended family.

No way Sand could understand what he's done.

No way Ben could have refused to leave Warren Valley.....

Throughout the long ,weary night Ben had struggled for some way to tell Grandpa the truth. He was here. The time was now. His mind was blank. He could only feel how thin the ice was that he was on. He wasn't a Tsosie. He was a Singer. From Navajo Mountain. Many of the Singers were good people. Everyone knew that. But Ben's father was a black sheep. Everyone knew that too. That they were not the true blood Navajo, the pure Athapascan Dine who first came down from Canada. Many Navajo Mountain Dine had Ute and even the blood of the Spanish Conquistadores in them.

Ben had never heard his grandfather comment one way or another about whether one Navajo was better than another. But now, in Ben's mind, the difference was as enormous, as deep as the canyon he faced.

A Navajo who went his own was considered selfish. The richness of meaning in that word to the Dine was not lost on Ben. They behave like they have no relatives, he heard grandpa say. Like Ben Singer.

Witches had to kill a brother or sister to join, to gain the evil power they used. Ben, if he wasn't careful what he did and said about Sand and the tape, could, in a very real way, be a witch to his own family.

The burning acid in his stomach strengthened by the moment. He felt his hands trembling and the pain started pounding again behind his eyes, like the steady beat of a water drum. It took everything he had in him to keep moving toward the camp and

Warrior's Way

Grandpa Tsosie's hogan.

He saw smoke rising from the chimney of the main house, where his grandfather had gone. Someone was heating the coffee. But there would be no breakfast. Traditional Navajos believed it was what you ate before noon that made you fat. And Grandpa Tsosie was a most traditional Navajo man.

It would be very rude to surprise anyone in the house. A beep on the horn, or singing a traditional visiting song was called for so that people didn't answer a knock on the door and find no one there. That would mean that ghosts were about. An evil omen indeed. Ben's shame and sorrow and smoldering rage were dangerous enough to bring home. If his grandfather had been told he was dead there would be some momentary confusion about whether he was a ghost or was real. Ben gunned the motor of the bike before he shut it down and climbed stiffly off.

Ben saw the fence was sagging around Grandpa's satellite dish and he wondered if the goats had eaten the wiring again. Hosteen Tsosie was a strange mixture of Navajo and Anglo ways. There would be no breakfast because he wasn't going to get fat. On the other hand he would watch news broadcasts from New York, nature programs from Florida, game shows from Hollywood and Farm Bureau programs from Kansas. Pragmatic was the only way to describe his philosophy about choosing what to use from the world around him. Whatever worked. So long as it worked in harmony with the Navajo Way.

The pounding in his head grew to a thunderous crescendo as he stepped in the door. He had no business being here, and he knew it. So did his grandfather. There was a stillness and tension in the room despite the sunlit beauty of the cedar wood walls and ceiling and the comfortable arrangement of the rooms.

"You're home, Shony," Grandpa said. And not in school where you should be, his tone said. Shony was short for nizhoni, pretty. A name applied to two year olds.

"Ya'at'eeh, Shichei." Ben heard the tension in his voice.

"Hello yourself, Ben. I told them I knew that you wasn't dead. Nobody called your mother. They wanted to be sure first."

Grandpa Tsosie chose to speak English to him. Without being rude Ben could not speak Navajo back. Ben felt a chill. But he didn't question his grandfather's ability to know he wasn't dead. Old time Navajos were often that way, knowing things without being told.

The hair on Ben's neck rose and he shivered. Maybe Grandpa knew everything. Would know if Ben didn't tell him everything.

Ben's mind promptly went blank. All the Navajo phrases, the diplomatic working up to things wouldn't work. Beginning with the creation of the world and working gradually down from there, in a leisurely way, until they arrived at the point. He hadn't prepared any other way to talk to his grandfather. What he needed to say was so delicate, so potentially scandalous, that Ben felt he needed to feel out his grandfather as he went along.

But this situation made him hurt inside. This was getting down to business at once in the best Anglo tradition. Grandpa was a business manager asking: What's the bottom line on this? Why aren't you in school like you're supposed to be....

The silence stretched between them while Grandpa warmed up the T.V. set and powered up the satellite dish outside. In a moment he was watching the Albuquerque weatherman, the one that drew pictures as he explained why the last forecast was wrong.

Silence was not an enemy to Navajos. If you had nothing to say it was okay not to say it. Not like Anglos who had to fill the air with noise even when they really had nothing to say. But this situation was not set in the Indian world. White values were at play here. This stung Ben, he felt like an orphan. Like he was a stepchild. Why is Grandpa treating me like a white man or a stranger Navajo?

Ben felt a mental earthquake shake him. His mind had shifted dramatically like he had fallen off a cliff and was experiencing fee fall and the fear of hitting the ground. He saw things in a new way. Saw himself in a new position within his family. His worst fears were being realized .

Is that it? The thought hit him hard. Has Grandpa always looked down on me because I'm not blue blooded Chinle Navajo? Not traditional, not off the Mayflower? He thought of his father. Navajo mountain. Mixed blood? Bad blood? Was Ben seen as a bad seed? That he might take after his father and not follow the Tsosie's way? Had his mother mongrelized the Tsosie line by bearing Ben? Was he following his father now? His empty stomach began to hurt again and he rubbed it softly.

Ben knew that you'd never felt discrimination until an Indian did it to you. Strange reversal, since Indians were almost universally looked down on by the `dominant culture' (read northern European). Almost every tribe he knew anything about had a name for themselves, not what the European invaders called them, their own name from the distant past. Like the Navajo, the Dine. It meant The People. Meaning the most important, the most favored, the best of creation. Those who followed the true path of the Creator. Something like that.

Ben was feeling unclean and unworthy. It only made it harder to talk. But Ben couldn't stand the silence, the coolness, any longer.

"I guess you're wondering why I'm here." His voice sounded like a little boy asking for a hug.

"No, not really. Why should we?" He sounded like someone had just decided to explaining how the Japanese stock market works.

Grandpa started switching channels slowly, looking for a moment at each program, like a shopper selecting vegetables in a big supermarket.

"We share profits from the family business with you so you can go to school and be a smart lawyer and look after the Tsosies around here. You get a big time scholarship to boot. Then you show up a month before school's out looking like you've been fighting with a freight train. Why should we wonder?"

Was his grandfather telling him the family thought he had been going off on his own, trying to be a big shot, a selfish loner?

This was going to be harder than Ben had imagined. Grandpa wasn't going to pat him on the head and welcome him home. The family expected things from Ben, as he did from them. Mutual dependence, everyone contributing what they could for the good of the group and getting acceptance and support in return. That had been drilled into the Navajo by thousands of years of marginal existence. The effort and cooperation of every member of the group was required just so they could survive. One person making waves, acting independent (read: being `selfish'—behaving as if they had no relatives.....) could kill the whole group. Ben wasn't pulling his own weight. His fierce independence had backfired on him, as some in his family had predicted. That's what people said about witches.

Ben was not where he was supposed to be, doing what he was expected to do to contribute to his family. It was not Grandpa who was acting cold and unfriendly. It was Ben, just by being there. He was threatening his whole family. Not with starvation, certainly. But the old ways died hard, or not at all. Ben was walking a

Warrior's Way

fine line. A wrong move, that is, another wrong move, and he'd be an outcast. The thought flushed his body like ice water. He felt a little bead of sweat form on his upper lip. He tried to keep a quaver from his voice. He had to say the right things. Grandpa might be handling this in an emotionally reserved, Anglo way. But he would listen and judge like a Dine.

"I'm sorry, Grandpa. I had to quit school. I gave up the scholarship."

Grandpa didn't turn away from the screen to look at Ben. Now he was looking at a farm bureau program from Kansas. Pig farming was being profiled. Maybe Grandpa was wishing he raised hogs, not sheep and grandchildren.

"You quit, huh?" he said.

Are you a quitter, Ben? his tone asked. Are you turning out to be like your dad? Ben heard in his mind.

"Who'd you fight?"

"A deputy sheriff. They say he's the strongest man in Warren County. He was beating a black man, my friend."

Ben's weak smile hurt his face, but Grandpa wasn't looking at him. Not looking at people was the Navajo way of telling you bad things about yourself. When they turned their backs and pretended that you didn't exist anymore, then you were on your own. Like the shunning among the Amish people. In the old days you went out and just died because nobody would feed you or help you. Ben started to feel like he was fading away a little at a time like Michael J. Fox in Back To The Future.

"Guess you lost then, huh?"

"Yes. I lost."

Ben found himself staring at the floor by his feet. He felt his face burning again with the shame he'd felt that night. The old familiar ache of loss, of aloneness, welled up again. But the anger, the outrage, were gone. They had quietly died when Ben saw Sand standing by his Suburban with the tape in his hand, when he had left Terry standing in the street, seeking comfort from Sand as he rode away. When Ben gave up his manhood and ran away.

You did it to yourself, he thought. You caused your own problem. You thought you were different, that you could live in two worlds.

You can't live in either one.

Self loathing filled up his soul.

"And you didn't try none of those lawyer tricks you talked so much about? The kind we see on Perry Mason at night around here? Instead you butt heads with a billy goat?"

Ben was stung. Grandpas and uncles taught lessons by telling stories. One of the best stories about stupidity told of a boy who tried butting heads with a billy goat to convince the goat to go the way he wanted him to go. The story was hilarious, the point unforgettable. Never come at someone from their strong side. Billy goats were designed to butt heads, men were not. Men were given brains and expected to use them. But Ben didn't feel like laughing now. He felt shamed. His grandfather had just rebuked him about as harshly as any Navajo ever rebuked a child. Scornfully questioning Ben's wisdom and even his manhood since Navajos and their cousin Apaches did not let an enemy do to them what Sand had done to Ben.

Not without revenge.

The lesson was that you never approached an enemy from his strong side. You always found the weakness and used it to your advantage. Navajos were quietly proud of the fact that they were the only Native Americans who had survived the onslaught of the European Americans and were still in control of their land. A piece of ground the size of New England.

But Ben Singer wasn't like them. Ben Singer insisted on using loser's methods. Meet things head on. Lose your temper. Then lose everything else that matters, even the good opinion of your grandfather.

Ben wanted to tell the whole story. He'd been prepared to do that when he arrived. Grandpa's coolness, the use of English, the insinuation in his voice all made Ben reluctant. Would Grandpa believe him? Ben wasn't sure anymore. His thoughts of his father kept filtering up into his mind. Is this how Dr. Jekyll felt when he at last learned that there was a Mr. Hyde in him who wanted to take control? Am I losing it? Am I going to follow after my father now? A sinking feeling inside said yes. I've lost my manhood and my woman to Dick Sand and I can't get them back from him. What's left for me now? The answer floated up from the blackness in his mind: To lose your family, too.

When the allegations about homosexuality came up it might be more than Grandpa could take. It went against one of the deepest taboos Navajos had. That and incest. Close living had bred that in them. Sharing one room shelters. Ben felt that he might be making that second mistake if he said anything. But without that fact Grandpa would not understand why he left school. Should he tell him everything? Would Grandpa only twist it to make it seem like Ben's bad side was coming out at last? How can I feel this way about a man I've loved all my life? I've never doubted his love. Why can't I rely on it now?

Can Grandpa rely on me to do what I'm supposed to do? Hardly. Grandpa hasn't withdrawn from me. I've left him. And the family. I've let them down. But there's nothing I can do to make it up. No way I can explain myself.

The answer came clear: You aren't worthy of his love. You've betrayed his trust and wasted precious family resources. And you look like your father. Now you've made them afraid that you're going bad like him. And what can you say?

The darkness strengthened in him, bringing with it a cold listless, enervating feeling that made his mind numb. Then another thought settled into his mind like a vulture alighting on his shoulder, to be his constant companion while they both waited for the inevitable end.

How do I know that I'm not becoming like him? There's no other way left for me to go. I can't stay here and I can't go back so what's left? To live alone? Maybe it was only hunger, but Ben felt like he was getting sick.

Ben had vowed after he saw his father that he would never commit suicide one drink at a time, as alcoholics did. But peering out through the blackness in his mind, he began to think of the bottle he had emptied. It was easy enough to get another.... Why not? And search as he would in the nether nooks and crannies of his mind, he could not find a reason why not.

He stood up. He hugged himself lightly, like it was cold in the hogan.

"I've got to be going, Grandpa."

Even he could hear the finality in his voice. Navajos never said goodbye unless they were standing over your grave. It was always So Long, till we meet again. Ben was saying goodbye, and they both knew it.

Grandpa turned then and looked at Ben. Not in the eyes, which was rude, but the way a good Navajo would.

"I guess you could stay, Ben. We don't feed Navajo style around here except on

69   Warrior's Way

weekends, when everybody can get home from work. We'll butcher on Friday. Saturday everyone from Gallup this way will be here. You could tell them about what happened."

Sure I could, Ben thought. I could tell them. Then I could leave. That way I'd never have to bother coming back. He had the picture of himself hanging around camp while everyone looked at him and talked behind his back about how he was letting them down. About how much like his father he was when the chips were down.

What if his mother came? What would he say? If she tried to believe him, tried to help, it would drive a wedge between her and them. Ben thought again of the sadness he'd seen in his mother's face as she gazed after his father. Don't hurt me Ben. Don't do what your father did to me.

If he'd had anything on his stomach he would have thrown up. That would be a sure sign to his grandfather that he'd been "witched" by the white man who beat him. A final nail in the coffin holding Ben's former life with his family.

I can't do that, Ben thought. I'm not that important. She must have suffered enough over my father. I can't hurt her anymore now. Her family is the only support she has. I can't risk taking it away.

"Maybe I'll come back Saturday, Grandpa. I have a lot of things to work out right now. I think I'll just keep moving. Do you know where I could find my father?"

Grandpa jerked visibly and the T.V. screen erupted into MTV's treatment of Madonna's latest hit. In a moment he moved on, settling on the morning news on CNN. Bangaldesh was reeling under the blow of a Cyclone. One hundred thousand fishermen were missing at sea. U.S. troops were pulling out of Iraq. Ted Kennedy's nephew was accused of a crime that Navajo considered unspeakable. Ben's father was dead.

But that news came from Grandpa, not from the T.V.

"You're father's dead, he died two or three years ago in prison down in New Mexico somewhere. They say he killed a Mexican in Gallup." Grandpa changed to a morning exercise program. Then to a cooking show. Ben was feeling the slick-sick, hungry feeling again.

"Funny he should die for it. We've been killing them and they've been killing us for three hundred years, ever since they started stealing our kids for slaves and we started stealing their sheep and bringing the sheepherders along to take care of them. Nothing to die over. But he died of the inside sickness. Us Navajos can't be inside too much. We have to be free to come and go, like coyote."

I shouldn't have asked, Ben thought. Now I've really planted the seed. They'll think for sure I'm going to be like him. It hurt Ben's heart to see Grandpa turn back to the T.V. and begin flipping slowly through the channels. Navajos never speak the name of a dead person for fear of calling back his ghost.

"Goodbye, my daughter's son," he said. His shoulders seemed more rounded now, his head tipped forward and his chest sunken.

"I guess you won't be needing the money from the sheep shearing this month. We'll find a use for it here."

"Grandpa, I ." Just at that moment Ben saw the blinking red light on the VCR that sat atop the TV. The light that indicated there was a tape in it. THE TAPE?!? his mind screamed at him. It couldn't be. But he dared not ask. What if it was? Would Sand do that even after Ben had agreed to leave? Ben fought to search for answers but his mind was empty, cold, and dark.

He turned and walked out, heedless of the blinding sunrise that turned into multi-hued rainbows as it struck through the mist in his eyes. Feeling the awful agony of emptiness a non-person must feel. Grandpa had not called him by name, referred to him as one dead or one whose ghost he didn't want to attract.

Non-persons were treated exactly like that.

Grandpa had turned his back, a shunning gesture, signifying that Ben no longer existed.

Non-persons were treated exactly like that.

Now Ben felt himself truly one of the □people between□. Those poor souls who had no place anywhere. A stranger to all societies. Sand was white, Terry was white, Law was a Whiteman's creation. Sand had shown him how little place he had there. He was arrogant thinking he not only belonged in that world, but excelled there.

His family had questioned his actions and beliefs but had gone along with him. Not any more. Without Grandpa's direct support the rest of the family would not help him, and his mother would be powerless to intervene. If he wasn't careful how he handled this she could become a non-person too. His own death was the simplest way to clean up the mess he was in.....

He fumbled at the bike, started it and moved back along the road to Chinle.

Face it. Your arrogance killed TJ, just as surely as if you'd injected him yourself. You've put Terry and Lester in terrible danger. Now, here at home, you have your big chance to destroy your mother's life too ..

"Don't hurt me, Ben. Not like he did ..Please." He heard his mother's voice echoing again through the hollow emptiness in his mind.

Whatever he did, he had to be very careful. He needed someplace where he could stop and try to think this through. He was a mile down the road toward Chile before he realized that he had absolutely no place to go.

****

Back at the camp Hosteen Tsosie got up slowly, like he was suddenly very old. He pushed the Eject button on the VCR, took the tape it offered, and walked slowly to the stove where the morning coffee was baking to black syrup. He lifted the lid above the fire and dropped the tape into the flames. It seemed to take all his strength to walk back and sit down in front of the TV. He flipped slowly through the channels but nothing seemed to catch his interest anymore.

Chapter 10
Ben Singer Learns to Die

The day was bright and mild and the Honda Gold Wing skimmed along so smoothly that Ben began to fall asleep. A little milk and a donut, eaten as he gassed up in Chinle, appeased his hunger. The aches in his body had been dulled by three aspirin and the gloom in him, along with the fatigue, pressed down on his body, and pushed him back into the soft seat of the bike.

He gazed about thinking of the old saying that for a person with no place to go, any direction of travel would do. He sensed Sand was testing him. Seeing what he would do. Sand would get reports as soon as Ben cleared the Reservation. Then he'd decide. Whether he'd hurt Terry or not was something Ben couldn't chance finding out. He'd killed TJ with his arrogance and ambition.

Ben couldn't bring this on his family, either. Every way he turned he was blocked. His weary body was crying for rest. His mind was losing its normal edge of vitality and clarity, taking on a blue-tinged, melancholy spirit that further sapped his strength.

Hopeless. Utterly futile. No course of action seemed reasonable or effective.

I'm beat. Physically, mentally, spiritually. There must be solutions, but I can't see a one. If I flail around trying things Lester and Terry and my mother will pay for it. Perhaps with their lives ..so where do I go from here?

At Round Rock, for no particular reason, he headed north, up the plateau, toward the reservation's northern boundary. Actually, in the general direction of Navajo Mountain. The gloom inside him was growing blacker by the mile as he brooded on his losses. To lose so much in so short a time. The weariness, the dull pain and soreness slowed his reflexes. And a great, uncaring sorrow slowed his reactions, made him dangerous to himself and to others. He couldn't find it in himself to care.

But, finally, a blaring horn jolted him awake in time to see a blue Chevy pickup swerving to the borrow pit, kicking up clouds of gray dust, to avoid smashing him head on. Fear and fatigue and the shot of adrenaline he got as he jerked the bike back over the yellow line combined to make him nauseous. He felt like pulling over and throwing up. Maybe if he did it could be like it was in a curing ceremony. The patients took emetics to throw up the evil in them before the ceremony began to restore them to the pollen path, the right way to travel through life.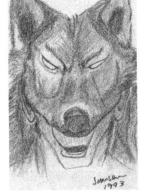

But even as the thought came he knew that he could not throw out the evil Sand had brought into his life. He saw Terry again, brave, tearful, heartbroken standing in the street by WCCC. Sand smirking in the background, tapping the VCR tape against his thigh. No, the evil had gone deep, to the bone, into the marrow of his being. Like a dark leukemia it was killing everything in him that supported life. No one could throw up hard enough to drive out something as pervasive as that. No Navajo curing ceremony could restore his former life to him.

He smiled ironically as a truth, taught in childhood, was hammered home to him again. The white man brought disease of body and mind with him to America that no

Indian medicine could cure. Avoid them, Grandpa had advised. Live as close to the old way as you can. Let the Bilagaanas go their own way until they finally fry themselves to cinders with their unholy belligerence and their blue-white nuclear fire that should have stayed on the sun where it belongs.

But not me, Ben thought, feeling the bitterness of regret like a sharp knife near his heart, twisting, torturing, tormenting mind and body without relief, without mercy or compassion.   No, not me. I had to play with fire. And I got an overdose of radiation from a white man. Now I'm turning to ashes and cinders, inside. Now there's no way to put out the radiation fire. It's too late, for me. Maybe my father went through something like this too.   That's why he killed himself with drink. He was only acting out the damage that had been done to him inside by the whites.

Ben heard a keening, almost sobbing sound fill his helmet, bounce from his visor. The dry desert air was suddenly rainbow colored as he peered through the gathering mist in his eyes. He couldn't pay attention to his driving. A big part of his mind was wallowing feebly in the center of a vast swamp of misery,   disappointment and despair. He saw the highway through a misty I haze. He couldn't swallow around the painful knot that had formed in his throat He couldn't think. It was as though his mind was a small, frightened animal that hid from him somewhere in the darkness within him. Refusing to emerge to face the ruin that was now Ben's life.

Without it he couldn't sort through the hard facts of his situation to find a way back out of the heartless maze into which Dick Sand had plunged him.

But the other emotion was still there, underneath the misery raged a boiling, nameless emotion like red hot magma, seeking some way to burst out. He was angry with a mindless rage that transcended all reason.

Am I insane? he thought? He touched the raging hate with just the bare edges of his mind, like you would gingerly test the water of a boiling hot spring. What he saw/felt there scared him. Most of all when he sensed that it was turning inward, upon him, becoming directed toward him. It was awe inspiring, like seeing the maw of a giant cannon grow rounder as it was being turned to aim directly at you. Ben felt a sudden hushed stillness in him. The moment before the awful clangor of battle begins, before the first crashing bolt of white hot lightening sears its way from the blackened sky to sizzle-burn its way through living flesh.

"It's all your fault, Ben. No one else. Just yours." He heard Grandpa's voice in his mind. Soft, sibilant, infinitely sad, speaking in Navajo the terrible condemnation.

"Jo, Ni t'eiya, shichei."

Firing the cannon of hate straight at Ben, blowing away the last vestiges of his manhood. He felt the hate inside, turned firmly inward, centered on him. I did it to myself, he thought . And with the thought the hate became self-hate and the rage shook him and multiplied the gloom, the loss, until Ben felt crowded into a small corner of himself, with the rest of him taken over by raw, surging, burning emotion.

Ben felt a grimace of distaste streak his face. You were selfish in every way. You went your own way, made everything a confrontation where you used your mind to compete. There were winners and losers and you were a winner.

You were a fool. He felt the bitter new twinge that the self-hate added to the words in his mind. You should have known better. Indians can't make it out there. Not in the Anglo world. Not against the Dick Sands who make their own rules. He felt deeply now the irony of the old saying: "When the Indian learns the rules, then the white man changes them."

Strangely, Ben could only remember now intellectually, not emotionally, the pleasure that learning and education and the anticipation of a lifetime spent serving his people had given him. He was content then with America, and his place in it. Proud to be a Native American. Now his feelings were hard-bitten, cynical, and twisted by the awful heat of the hate he felt burning him up inside, leaving only the ashes of feelings he'd once cherished as much as he'd loved Terry.

Ben felt agony in his hands. He looked down to see that he was clutching the handgrips so hard that his knuckles were white. He looked around to see where he was.

Don't make someone put a cross on the road where you killed somebody. Go somewhere so that if you die you hurt no one but yourself.

And finally, then, he knew where he was going, as though a part of his mind, a part without words, had known all along because the big bike was already on the way there.

He saw in his mind's eye the picture of a steep sandstone canyon with cottonwood trees growing along a sandy wash in the bottom. There was a spring that flowed year around. And up on the side of the canyon a shelter marked by a shield that looked like the Union Pacific Railroad emblem pecked into the rock. And rock writing everywhere. Sheltered, isolated, unvisited. Whitehouse Canyon, a tributary of the San Juan River. In the heart of the lands of the 'Anaa'i Sani. Ben felt a cold shiver move up his spine and raise the hair on the back of his neck. Only their ghosts lived there now.

He would go and see if he had power to live there among their ghosts. He most certainly had no power nor will to stay among the living.

He could find refuge there among the ruins of a people long dead and rest while he tried to plan how to live. And if no plan emerged?

Well then he could find refuge there while he died.

****

A half mile west of Mexican Water Ben stopped at the Kayenta to Shiprock highway that led through four comers to Shiprock, New Mexico. He could go north from Mexican Water, past the Rabbit Ears that more or less marked the Utah-Arizona Border, down to Mexican Hat, and into Monument Valley through Utah.

As he sat on the bike at the intersection he gazed north toward dzil ditloi, Blue Mountain and shash bijaa' the Bears Ears, two buttes up on Elk Ridge that looked like the ears of a mountain-sized grizzly bear about to look over the horizon, straight at him.

Ben felt uneasy. In the old days bear sickness was greatly feared among the Navajo. Back then Elk Ridge was a refuge for the Bronco Utes, bitter enemies of the Navajo. .The San Juan River, near the border, marked the end of Navajo territory, the last safe place to the north. There had been many good reasons in those days not to travel north. Bears and Utes and the 'Anaa'i Sani ruins made it a dangerous place to go alone.

Today Utah was Dick Sand's territory. For Ben it was just as dangerous as it had ever been. The big radio in Sand's suburban was tied into the state police network. He would know everything that went on up there, in his land. He was more dangerous than bears, or even enemy Utes. If Ben got even a traffic ticket Sand would know. He certainly knew by now that Ben was still alive.

Ben sighed and the movement sent a dull ache through his chest and down his arm. For Lester's sake, for his mothers sake, most especially for Terry, he couldn't take a chance, so he turned west toward Kayenta, driving carefully and looking in the mirror often, watching for patrol cars or Navajo Police vans.

At Kayenta he turned north, up into the southern part of Monument Valley, but still on the reservation, away from Sand's hawks.. The place where cars fell out of the sky for T.V. commercials or were perched on the high, red rock monuments and photographed from helicopters.

He turned west again toward the Goulding trading post where John Wayne and Henry Fonda and John Ford made the films like "She Wore A Yellow ribbon" and "Fort Apache". Around the back of the huge crimson-colored rock monument he passed 'Oljee' Toh, Moon Springs. The trading post there was now a national monument, filled with Navajo artifacts.

Because of his mood he saw it as if surrounded by a deep blue nuclear haze. The personal belongings of so many dead Navajo, collected in one spot. perhaps reeking of their Ch'iindii, made it as dangerous as atomic radioactivity.

Ben was fully aware that he had regressed in his thinking back to the basis from which a traditional Navajo reasoned. He had abandoned the Anglo portion of his mind. The critical, analytical part of him was gone. He didn't need that part for what lay ahead. He floated along on a burning cushion of emotion. He was dealing now with things beyond human ken. And of them all, death was the most mysterious. His Navajo mind was good enough to guide him now. He felt the darkness still spreading through him to match the brooding, darkening landscape. He could not find a ray of light or of hope anywhere inside now. His list of the things he would have to give up to go on and make a life for himself now included living without the support of his family. Trying to exist as a pitiful non-person.

In despair he moved on, thinking little, feeling much.

Then, as Navajo Mountain loomed even larger, even darker on the horizon, he angled north along a dirt road that soon became an un-traveled dirt track so sandy that getting the heavy bike through took all of his skill. No one had traveled this road in a long time, and as he passed Ben saw in his mirror a whirlwind working to erase his tracks, as though he had never come. There would be no sign on the road that he had passed this way. Whirlwinds were caused, in Navajo Mythology, by the mischievous, often dangerous, Hard Flint Boys. Some Navajos held, however, that whirlwinds were full of Ch'iindii and to be caught in one made one especially vulnerable to witches.

He felt the chill pass from the base of his spine clear up and over his scalp and he almost lost the bike. Navajos also took whirlwinds to be definite evidence of the presence of ghosts. He kept moving trying to be sure it didn't overtake him. But of course, perversely, it did. Filling his nose and eyes with fine grit, leaving a dirty red-brown film over him and the bike. Well, why not? Along with everything else, why not that, too?

A sense of dread filled his mind and turned his limbs to lead until every movement was an effort

That's when the road changed to more a wagon track, two ruts for wheels and a high center in the middle. The ground dropped off faster now, as he neared Whitehouse Canyon, and Ben fought the bike in the loose blow sand in the rut to keep it from dumping him. With his arm and shoulder like they were he doubted that he could pick up the heavy bike if it fell over. Just the strain of steering over the bumpy road was making his aching body scream at him.

The surroundings, with Navajo Mountain brooding in the near distance, a towering black dome rising out of a red and crimson landscape like a boil erupting on

Warrior's Way

the skin of Mother Earth, made him think of the Navajo description of the land of the dead. That land was underground, down a steep trail, with a sand pile at the bottom. Down there waited the dead. The fearful Ch'iindii, waiting to apply the tests to be sure you were really dead before they let you go on.

He came over a small rise and stopped, struggling to keep the bike upright, his legs shaking with fatigue. The road fell away steeply down from here into Whitehouse Canyon. The rock walls were fiery red in the twilight. They seemed to Ben to pulse slightly, as though heated red hot by the luminous fires of Hell itself.

Ben noticed the profusion of the vision weed plants. They seemed to grow everywhere around here. Perhaps the powerful witches among the 'Anaa'i Sani had planted them. Their leaves were a dark, oily green and the white flower, just now coming out, looked like the white faces of ghosts peeking out from the leaves. Malevolent ghosts because it was well known that the plant could give you visions. But it could also make you crazy or kill you outright. Strong medicine. Not for the weak to use. Things like that had to be handled by people with great personal power.

Ben felt like the single most powerless man on earth. He had no use for the weed. He had his vision. It hung before his eyes every moment. He saw his life dragging on, unending. Unendingly lonely, filled with shame and dishonor. No he didn't need help from a weed to see his future. He could already see it much too clearly. He needed, rather, to find away to forget. He regretted having dumped the wine. Suddenly Ben saw why some must turn to alcohol. To blot out the awful vision of a featureless future, even if only for a time. Ben thought again of his father, but this time with a new feeling of, almost, brotherhood. We're the same kind, you and I Frank Singer. The same kind of loser.

He paused before starting the steep, sandy descent down into the canyon, the hurt strong in him, as he left his world behind. What will they decide down there? Am I dead enough for them? Or will they send me back to Dick Sand for further processing.

At this point he didn't really care, one way or the other.

But no one was waiting for him when he finally slithered down to the bottom. More lonely than ever he started down the canyon toward the rock shelter.

Ben fought the bike along the canyon floor for less than a quarter mile where he came to the first bend in the canyon. He had to stop and get off the bike and stretch his cramping legs. He took three aspirin, drinking from a clean, clear spring-fed stream that flowed from a box canyon to his left. A miracle of sorts in a country where water was usually alkaline and bitter. A major reason why the Anasazi had lived there.

The place brought back memories. He'd made a field trip here once with his high school history teacher, Mr. Hawks, from New Jersey or somewhere. He knew nothing at all about Navajo religion. Ben remembered his enthusiasm. A small man, almost sparking with suppressed energy. Everywhere at once, glorying in each new discovery, each bend in the canyon as they hiked along.

He was having so much fun he didn't seem to notice Ben and his classmates staying in the center of the open space, clustering together like a group of nervous 5th graders passing a graveyard on Halloween. They were trying to look in every direction at once, some were almost sick with the agonizing thought that they could be walking on ground saturated with Ch'iindii. Mr. Hawkes was the only one who enjoyed himself that day. He was probably amazed at how fast Ben and his classmates got out of the canyon when it was time to go.

Ben felt his body trembling a little as he looked up along the canyon walls. This was a strange place, even by non-Indian standards. In the area near the canyon the Anaa'i Sani had built their rock houses in every sheltering cliff overhang and flat protected place on the canyon floors.

But not in Whitehouse Canyon. As far as archaeologists could determine not a single cliff dwelling, granary, or cornfield ever existed anywhere in the fifteen mile long canyon. It took its name, not from a ruin, but from a large rock-panel pictograph about two miles down the canyon. In the right light the picture of a large, white pueblo style housing complex seemed to float in the air above the canyon floor, above the tops of the cottonwood trees. The tiers, perfectly balanced on each side, looking like stair steps, also represented the Hopi symbols for eternity.

Mormons said it was a Lamanite (American Indian) version of Zion, the city taken up into heaven just before the flood and destined to return when men built a society made up of people worthy to associate with its inhabitants.

Ben wondered what they'd make of Dick Sand in Whitehouse City. Would they let him in?

Could they keep him out?

He restarted the bike and moved on down the canyon. The 'Anaa'i Sani seemed to have dedicated the canyon to some special religious function. The walls of the canyon were decorated with elaborate petroglyphs, pictures mostly of large, wedge-bodied figures dressed in elaborate costumes, head gear, and necklaces. No one knew for sure who the figures represented. Navajos didn't care. They just stayed out of the place-respectful of the powerful magic of the ancient ones.

Ben puzzled again over the rock pictures showing warriors with helmets, round shields with a bulls eye on them and upraised swords in their hands. Real, European-looking swords, not sticks edged with obsidian knives like the Aztecs used.

He felt like he was making his way slowly through the Egyptian Valley of the Dead. There was a hushed, almost church-like atmosphere in the canyon. Or graveyard-like. But that was the other peculiarity of Whitehouse Canyon, he recalled. No grave sites had ever been uncovered here.

As he got closer to the turn that would reveal the huge Whitehouse petrogylph, Ben noticed that the pictographs were becoming more numerous. When he turned the comer he saw the white pueblo floating above the trees in the twilight, framed by the dark red sandstone around it, it stood out somehow, luminescent, stark, powerful, and yet serene.

Ben saw it as cold, distant, foreign, and supremely unaware of him and his petty human troubles. Like eternal Monument Valley it had been here for a thousand thousand lifetimes. It would still be here long after Ben's miserable life was over. It had no other meaning for him. But he felt it's beauty and admired the skillful hands that had made it and even more so. the minds that had conceived it

Across from it on the opposite wall, a ten foot high petroglyph that looked like the shield on a Union Pacific Railroad station stood above a shaded cavern-like shelter. In the bottom of the canyon the stream burbled quietly over its rocky bed. Cottonwood trees, massive and old, stood along the stream banks. Tamarisk and rabbit brush and vision weed grew profusely, for the desert at least. Ben noticed that there were no birds chattering, none to be seen. There were no animal tracks along the creek. There seemed to be a spell on this land that took it outside of nature, outside of time.

Ben was embarrassed to even be here in all this timeless serenity, filled as he was with pain and rage and self loathing and hopelessness. Like a murderer in church. Out of place, out of harmony with his surroundings.

"I have no other place to go", he heard his voice, child-like, tiny in the vastness of the canyon, swallowed up instantly by the massive canyon walls. Please, let me stay here...

Struggling, he pulled the heavy bike up on its stand in the shade of a big cottonwood tree and shut down the engine. The silence washed over him with an almost physical impact. He stepped off the machine and felt he was breaking a major contact with life as he had known it. He didn't want to be here. He wanted to be back in Warren Valley, in his old life. With Terry. He looked up at the massive canyon walls and felt them sucking the life force out of him. He was so small here. So alone. So much alone ..

For reasons he wouldn't let himself examine he just left the key in the ignition.

He unpacked his gear and took his bedroll and canteen and struggled up the twenty yards of near vertical rock to the shelter. Carefully placing each foot in the hollowed out step carved by some hand that lived a thousand years ago. Alert, because he had heard stories from the old Navajos about the right-hand left foot traps that the Ancient Ones built into their steps, leaving an enemy perched high on the rock with the wrong hand or the wrong foot reaching for the next secure grip. When there was none, leaving an enemy an easy target for an arrow from the cliff dwelling above.

When he got to the top he peered inside, thinking of the entrance to the land of the dead.

He was scared in bone deep ways that he'd only felt before when Grandpa Tsosie told his ghost stories when Ben was little. He realized that he was breaking enormously important Navajo taboos. He would need a serious cleansing ceremony even if all he did now was turn around and walk away. If he stayed here the danger and the evil filth that would accumulate in him would make him as dangerous to his people as unshielded nuclear radiation was to Anglos. Only the most powerful ceremonies might help. Some singers (medicine men) held that no Navajo ceremonies were fully effective against the ancient and mysterious powers of 'Anaa'i Sani.

So?

Ben counteracted the fear he felt so easily that it impressed him. He only reviewed his shop worn list of what he would have to give up to go on living. His emotions turned off. He didn't want to think any more. He made a comfortable bed inside where there was a generous flat, open space.

As it grew dark the clear atmosphere and the brilliant stars lit the open spaces in the canyon making the dark shadows deep and spooky.

He'd rejected the idea of drinking. Following after his father, killing himself slowly, one drink at a time, would take years. That only meant that Ben's suffering would go on and on. That he would live with the loss and the pain. It would be there waiting for him each time he awoke from an alcoholic slumber. He would be like a zombie, undead, yet unable to live. Maybe Ghost Sickness is quicker.

Ben pressed his hand over his tired eyes.. The pain of his loneliness stabbed him again, making his heart ache. There was no way out of his dilemma. Non-persons had only their own resources to use to fight the battles of life. The old joke about the battle of wits and only being half prepared twisted his mouth into an ironic sneer. That's me. Just a half-wit up against an evil genius named Dick Sand.

He drank a little water and turned over to sleep. His back was toward the entrance, toward the mysterious white house that floated in the air outside, toward life.

If anything came through the entrance in the night he just didn't want to see it.

****

Ben was now into his fourth day without food and his third without water. He couldn't remember when he decided not to go back down to the bike. He had simply awakened some time in the stillness of a desert canyon night to find the decision had already been taken, almost without his knowledge or agreement. It was just an accepted fact of his life from that point on.

He lay very quietly now. After so many days without eating he felt his mind was disconnected from his body. Emotions resident in his body and brain, that he had felt so deeply before, could not reach him. The late morning sun was already gone from the cave entrance and the shade and the quiet coolness felt good. Ben saw himself now as a wounded animal that had crawled away to hide from the predators and scavengers.

I haven't seen an animal or heard a bird since I've been here. My body will last a thousand years here.

Your soul will be trapped here, in Hell, among these ghosts forever, he heard Grandpa Tsosie say. The voice was so distinct he peered around, thinking for a moment that his grandfather had come for him. But of course he was still all alone.

To divert himself from the pain of that realization he turned to thinking about what he was feeling. He had fasted for a day at a time before, participating in a healing ceremony or sing. But this was a whole new experience. At times he felt himself floating above his body, as though the connection had broken between it and his mind. He felt suspended above the blackness. The surging emotional storm he'd endured since the night Sand beat him might still be raging inside him somewhere, but he couldn't feel it anymore. He had no desire to search for it.

Except, occasionally, like high tides from an unseen storm, he'd find himself awash in an overwhelming impulse to cry. His throat would close, cutting off his breath, making his lungs burn, dimming his vision and sometimes he thought he heard someone sobbing. Perhaps is was a lonesome, long-dead Anaa'i Sani hanging around the shelter.

The soreness of his body, the strained joints, the bruises and aches all seemed further away now. No longer a part of him, belonging to some past Me he could barely recall.

He seemed to exist somewhere outside of time and space. He felt revolted by the idea that he might have to reconnect with his body, with the shambles that he had made of his life. To wallow again in the hopelessness and the endless cycle of searching only to prove over and over again that he was powerless, that there was no way out

Because there was a way out.

He could see it clearly now that he was no longer wrapped up with his physical self. It was so simple and so easy. It was right up his alley. Finally he'd found something that he could do and get it right. He smiled at the thought.

All he had to do was do nothing at all.

A solution so simple that it was beautiful. In a short time the world would just fade away and leave him alone.

He had spent hours the first two days searching desperately for a solution, trying to find a way to get back what he'd lost. The tormenting vision of Sand's tape

79

and what it could do to his mother and his family kept coming into his mind. And the vision of Terry with Sand. And Grandpa's subtle rejection and rebuke.

Ben could find no way to take on Dick Sand. The more he thought about it the more he knew that Sand was only the tip of an iceberg Sand was acting with the support of some kind of powerful organization. One that could have video tapes counterfeited perfectly. Ben couldn't help but feel amazed that anyone would consider him enough of a threat to anything to go to so much trouble and expense.

He felt like a mouse who had wandered into the elephant house at the zoo. His ignorant, innocent actions seemed to be creating pandemonium. Ben couldn't dredge up a single clue to why Dick Sand should hate and fear him so.

He did a great job on me, though, Ben had thought. Very detailed and it had worked perfectly.

But now he had no feelings at all. He had no sensation of heat or cold, he was just comfortable and simply content to sit leaning back comfortably, his body hardly saying anything to him now that he was beyond feeling hunger. Today he would not go down to the spring for water. Four days without food had weakened him a lot.

He knew he could not live three more days without water. He was on his way out of life, feeling no pain, and content to see it all end. Now just a matter of hours, he thought. Two more nights at the most and he would step out of this life and find out about what lay beyond.

I wonder who's right? The Christians? Heaven and Hell? Would he go to Hell for killing himself? Probably not, he thought. They'll meet me at the Pearly Gates and St. Peter will give me an award of some kind for doing everybody down here a big favor and getting out of their way.

Especially out of Dick Sand's way.

The thought came unbidden, unwelcome, like a drop of mud into a glass of milk. But he didn't follow the thought. Or the rage that propelled it into his mind. He just basked quietly in the total lack of emotion he felt

Maybe the Atheists were right. Nothing afterward. Just oblivion, total non-existence. Or would the Navajos be right. If you died at birth without taking a breath or lived to be very old you died without leaving Ch'iindii behind. Ch'iindii was held by the singers, the medicine men, to be the distilled essence of every evil thought and act of a human life. It was left behind at death. It contaminated the dead body and all of that person's personal possessions.

And it could make you very sick, give you Ghost Sickness as the whites translated it, though there is little connection between the Navajo concept of Ch'iindii and the Anglo conception of ghost. Ben smiled when he thought of himself coming back as the Pillsbury Dough Boy in Ghost Busters. Not quite. Something was definitely lost in the translation.

A deep up welling of emotion shook him. So intense is surprised him. He'd thought he was safety beyond feeling. Some part of him was stilt struggling, outraged at what he was doing. Somewhere inside him life was still precious and the red-hot magma that was his outrage still boiled deep inside somewhere.

He felt the impact of a string of emotion laded images in his mind and put them into words. Is this really what I want to do, is this the best way to handle things? Isn't there something else I can do? Do I really want to die? Or do I just want the hurting to stop?

"If there is, Benny boy, you won't be around to figure it out. You're on your way out"

Ben's voice was harsh, roughened by the lack of water and grating with hard bitten feeling. Something inside him stirred and rebelled at the words and then weakened and subsided.

I hope the atheists are right. Ben felt his chest lift and fill involuntarily, in big and sudden intake of breath that escaped as an audible sigh. Too weak to turn over on his side, he turned his head away from the entrance and looked at the bleak black rock wall at the back of the shelter.

Then he must have dozed in the quiet, even temperatured day because when he first heard the voice he thought he was dreaming and when he opened his eyes he saw that the sun had moved and that it was late afternoon.

He also saw that he was no longer alone. In fact, in the twilight he could see that the shelter was full. Some of the people were Earth Surface people. Others obviously were not. He was startled to see Coyote sitting erect near his feet, his eyes red spots like red hot metal, burning in the semi-darkness of the cavern. He saw Big Fly too. The messenger of the gods who too often brought bad news.

Before Ben could study the others, Coyote cocked his head sideways, wondering, perhaps considering Ben's situation. Ben heard Coyote's voice in his mind:

His shield is down. his heart is unprotected. Even a poor witch. could kill him with one shot now that he's that way.

Ben felt a darkness where his heart should be. He felt it begin to beat in his ears and behind his eyes in a steady, doleful rhythm like the beating of the drums in the death march.

He gave a start when Terry came forward, her hair girdled by a band of trade cloth, red with white flowers. As she drew nearer he saw that they were the flowers of the vision plant .   The look on her face was mysterious. Old beyond years. Her eyes held the glint of power held in check by an effort of implacable will. She had the manner of the Hand Trembler, the person who could tell you what was wrong with you. So you could get the right ceremony to restore you to harmony and make you well.

Her hand began to pass over him from head to foot. On the second pass it began to tremble violently when it passed over his chest.

"It's to late, " she said, her manner and tone cool, professional, uncaring.

"He's been attacked by 'Adilgashi'ii. His death's in him now. We can't get it back out. "

Ben bit his lip to keep from crying out and dissolving into tears. He felt so sorry for himself that the ache settled in his chest and made his heart hurt. His breath was squeezed out in little panting cries that burned in his throat like fire.

He couldn't speak Terry's name past the lump in his throat. He had to watch her turn and move away, too weak to take her in his arms and tell her everything.

Through the pain he saw Big Fly shake his head sadly and move out of the cavern. He's gone to tell Ye'ii Bichei that I'm beyond help, Ben thought That meant that even the grandfather of the gods could not help Ben now.

Coyote cocked his head and his eyes burned into Ben again.

" This is not Navajo magic", he said, nodding his head wisely. "I have seen it before in my travels.

" This is white man's sickness. Ben stayed too long with the whites. He thought he could be one of them. He lost his Dine power, or gave it away. Then he found out he had no white man's power either. "

Coyote stood up and moved back into the circle, further away from Ben as if he was afraid he might catch something.

" Now he's caught between the worlds. He floats between Heaven and earth and is nothing. Let him die. His life is useless now anyway. "

Ben wanted to shout, to protest, to plead for mercy. But Coyote's words were exactly right and the truth flamed into his brain. It hammered him into guilty silence. He had no answer for them that was not a lie. He fell back, weakness flooded through him in a dark tide. He began to slide into it's depths, drowning in guilt and self loathing and sorrow.

Coyote and the others, all but one, stood and began to move away. Terry was one of the first to leave, without even a glance in his direction. Ben felt his heart burst as he watched her leave him.

"Let the witch have him," Coyote said as he walked out. "He's no good for anything anyway."

Then he was all alone.

But not alone.

Ben felt his skin prickling, goose flesh standing out on his arms and chest and legs. A sure sign to a Navajo of impending disaster. Only one figure was left.

As the others withdrew Ben felt a shift in the psychic forces around him. There was a power vacuum when they left. An absence of the power for good. Into that 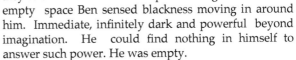 empty space Ben sensed blackness moving in around him. Immediate, infinitely dark and powerful beyond imagination. He could find nothing in himself to answer such power. He was empty.

A chilling wind howled through him and he felt anguish and regret ripping at him with claws of ice-cold steel. He was a vacuum inside. He knew that the foul, evil Ch'iindii could now fill him up completely. From head to toe, from heart to mind, forever.

He was amazed to find Indian religion and Christianity met at this point for he realized he was suffering the pains of the damned.

The shadowy figure across from him stirred and the air seemed to thicken around it. Ben saw the figure of a man topped by the head of a wolf and the chill in him froze him solid in one shattering instant of awful insight.

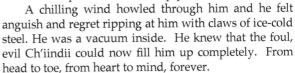

This was a dine naaldloshi, a man who had given himself to evil to get unholy power to kill his enemies, to cause lingering illness, to wreak terrible vengeance for the slightest insult.

The figure stepped forward into the little light left coming into the cavern from the early evening twilight. Ben saw the animal skin belt and from it was hanging the dreaded pouch that Navajo Wolves used to carry their corpse poison. Ground up flesh and bone of the dead.

The most fearful substance on earth.

Ben felt the dread building to a scream in him, but he could not move, not even to turn his head away from the awful sight of the man/wolf reaching into the pouch. The somber figure lifted his other hand slowly and pulled up the wolf mask so that Ben could see his face.

First Ben saw an insolent grin, broad and full of pleasure. Then the mask rose higher and in a blinding moment of horror and agony Ben saw the face emerge.

Dick Sand.

Dick Sand was the bringer of unthinkably horrible death to Ben. Ben's insides crawled in an attempt to distance his body from the hand emerging from the pouch as Sand crouched down near Ben's waist. In mind numbing horror Ben watched as Sand slowly, and cheerfully raised his hand and began to sprinkle the gray powder. He began at Ben's belt and moved slowly upwards towards his face.

At the first touch of the powder Ben felt unquenchable fire begin to scorch him. He wanted to twist, to scream out in agony. He could only lay and watch Sand's hand move along his chest, spreading the fiery pain as he went.

Then Sand looked kindly into Ben's eyes, the grin almost merry when he saw Ben's agony, like a nightmare Santa Claus about to deliver his favorite present

"So long, Benny," Ben heard him say.

Then a putrid gray film of powder filtered down and started landing on his face. On his lips. into his nose and eyes.

Instantly Ben felt his tongue swell to close his throat . He sucked violently, trying to get air past his cramping throat muscles and into his lungs. He succeeded a little, only to find he had sucked the corpse poison into himself and set his lungs on fire. The heat burned his heart and it began to race and flutter like that of a rabbit that has run too hard to escape the coyote and has burst its heart in the process.

In agony, Ben's vision started to fade and Sand's face became a distorted blur against the blackness that was closing in on him. Just before the blackness enveloped him Ben heard and at the same time felt in his throat the awful sound of the snorting, whistling noise in his windpipe. The ultimate sound of disaster, of impending ruin, of imminent death.

Then Ben gave himself up and felt like a leaf drifting down and down into the hollow blackness that had waited so long inside him.

Then, in one last sparking act of thought in a brain flickering feebly in the vast darkness, Ben Singer gave himself up to death.

Warrior's Way

Chapter 11
Ben Singer Meets His Mentor

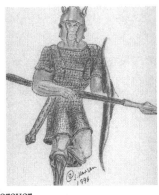

When Ben's awareness returned sensory awareness, rather than thought...... all around him was dark and cold. He couldn't locate himself in space and time. He felt no heart beat, couldn't feel his body or detect his breathing. Was he alive or dead.....or something else.......The thought of Dick Sand....the wolf skin mask, the agony of the deadly dust he spread....the nightmare rose again in him. What if he was a ghost now. Shackled to the cave.....to the Navajo Wolf. Suicides and witches had to live together forever,,,,,, Maybe he was in limbo.....waiting for the dine naaldloshi to come back and kill him again....and again... and again... forever.

Let me out. His thoughts howled through him like a dark wind. How do I get out of this? What can I do?

"You chose to die, Shonnie. You can do that. Anyone can do that." His Grandfather's voice was clear, cool and distant. Hardly caring. "You can't choose to un-die. No one has that kind of power......."

Bitter despair, fear, clutched his throat and threatened to cut of his breath again. There's a way. There must be some other way...... Then the discouragement returned in a wave. What could he do if he left the canyon? What weapon did he have to use against a man like Dick Sand?

At the thought of Dick Sand behind the wolf skin mask ice flowed into his belly and the nightmare arose again in him. Sand's grinning face, the burning, the choking, the awful fear of eternal suffering and loss, the anguish he felt at the moment he gave himself up to death.

A bitter, lonesome feeling filled him. A dream, he thought, became a waking nightmare generated in a brain that was drying out and hallucinating. But he had been robbed of the death he wanted.

It only felt like dying, he thought sadly. But I went through all that and I'm still alive, still suffering.

But soon, it has to be soon now.

The thought drifted through him like early morning mist. Softly, gently blanketing him in nothingness. He tried to turn over, shift his body a little, but he couldn't .

Then a thought thundered like an icy avalanche through his mind. What if he was a zombie? What if the Navajo witch has made me into a zombie. I could never die. Or ever live again.

But he found that he could still feel anguish. It did no good to tell himself that Navajos didn't make zombies. Just Hollywood did that.

Ben heard a noise and with great effort, turned his head toward the entrance, expecting to see the Navajo Wolf returning for his soul. Suicides and Witches had to live together in the afterlife. He felt overwhelming disappointment that the atheists were wrong. He yearned to simply cease to exist.

Ben fought to focus his eyes, it was lighter in the cave.   Fighting to concentrate, Ben saw a man standing just inside the entrance to the shelter. Huge, towering over him, broadchested and thick through the waist.   In the dim pre dawn it was hard to see details. Sword, round shield slung on his back by a leather thong. On his upper body he wore a leather shirt with round metal plates on it. His legs were protected by metal sheathes the old knights called greaves. For shoes he wore sandals, heavy with thick soles. Made for walking as well as fighting. Like, but not exactly like, pictures Ben had seen in history book of the ancient Vikings.

Ram-rod straight in the back, sturdy and self-assured. Everything Ben was not. Without saying anything he exuded authority, self-possession, self-confidence, something.   Ben's weary brain couldn't be sure what it was. But he felt a pang of envy, wishing that he would speak. Ben was acutely aware that he felt no fear of this man.

When it came the voice was deep, soft and friendly, "My name is Axelron but you can call me Axel. How's the vision quest going, Ben?" he said. "You seen anything interesting?'

Ben was stunned. He had no answer for that question. Young men were expected by some tribes to go out and fast and pray until they got a vision as part of their initiation into manhood, to become a warrior. Ben could admit now that he had simply come here to die. There was no honor in that. He felt the bitterness, the dishonor burning him with shame. But there was nothing in his future that he could see that was worth living for. He found himself looking at his feet.

He found he had nothing to say to this man.

Suddenly the wall before him glowed then he saw images.....people moving......Warren Valley College......he focused fiercely.   Sand.....and Terry. Walking together, headed to class. Ben propped himself up, ignoring the bite of rocks under his elbows, fighting down the nausea, ignoring the spinning room.

"Terry's lost, Ben. Doesn't know what to do... how to go on. She needs you. If you don't go back Sand will destroy her.....Just for his amusement. Are you going to let it happen?"

Ben felt the anger and resentment flush through him.

"How can I stop it? What can I do I haven't already tried?" Ben's throat hurt when he tried to speak and his voice sounded like a frog with the croup.

"So you came here on a vision quest? Looking for answers, for power to save those your love?"

Ben eyes slid away again, he gazed at his feet. He had nothing to say.

At best he had come here to wallow in his outrage at what his life had become. He had never expected to have a vision. But then he hadn't expected the nightmare visit from Dick Sand and the horrible way Sand had killed him. All that was still thrumming along his nerves like a January ice storm. If he wasn't dead now, death, when it came, would never be more real for him than what he had suffered. But there was no honor in that experience. He would be ashamed to tell it around the fire in Grandpa's hogan.

The man (apparition? ghost?) Tilted his head to one side and smiled. The smile was friendly, perhaps even sympathetic. Not the sneering, degrading grin of Dick Sand, but a smile full of warmth and good humor.

"Your name's Ben Singer isn't it?"

Ben could at least answer that question. But not trusting his voice he merely

Warrior's Way

nodded his head. It took a surprising amount of strength.

"You're Navajo, is that right?"

Again Ben nodded. He was close enough that technical details about all his ancestors weren't really important. He was pretty much Navajo by culture, if not by blood. The real question is, thought Ben, Am I dead or not?

Ben watched the man as he bowed his head and was silent for a moment, as though he was listening for something. Ben got the feeling that his visitor might be wondering if he had the wrong person. He straightened up his head and leaned forward a little toward Ben.

"Do you want to be dead, Ben? Did you come here to die? Is that your fate? To end your mortal life here among our ancient caves and canyons?"

The words jolted Ben like seven shots from a magnum pistol. He stirred, squirmed despite his weakness and felt a surging up-welling tide of raw emotion in his mind.

He had tried being dead and it was like living a nightmare. Was it even worse than living would be? Ben had no answer.

I need solutions resources power. Something to use on Dick Sand as effective as what he used on me. Some way to fight back without killing Terry I need a miracle and I don't have one. I'm powerless to change this fate.

Miracles come when you have faith in something. Ben placed his faith in the white man's law. The white man's way. No miracles there. For an Indian. It was just hopeless.

The life left to him wasn't worth living. Did he want to die? Maybe, maybe not. He only knew he didn't want to live the life Dick Sand had left him. So what was left?

"What do you say, Ben?"

Ben glanced at the man, felt his gaze slide away till he was looking at a worn spot on his Levis, feeling foolish, powerless, childish.

Maybe if he just sat quietly for a while this vision or dream would fade away.

"We know what Dick Sand did to you Ben", the voice said. The words jolted Ben. But it was the way they were spoken, with an overtone of concern, acceptance, and sympathy that softened a little the husk of bitterness that surrounded his heart. At that moment the implications of the words filtered into his exhausted mind. We? 'They" knew, without being told by anyone, what Ben had suffered?

"Who are you?" Ben heard himself croak. "How do you know what I'm thinking?"

Ben's voice sounded small, squeaky and ragged with emotion now as well as with thirst

"As I said, you can call me Axel."

This did nothing to reassure Ben, and his next statement only confused Ben more.

"Only One knows your thoughts and your heart Ben."

The voice was warm and assuring. Unreasonably Ben began to feel like crying again.

"But sometimes, for a good cause, others can be told a little about you."

Was "Axel" real? Could Ben reach out to him, rely on him? Or was he like the people who stepped out of Lennie's head in Steinbeck's story Of Mice And Men. Was Ben talking for Axel in his own voice, just not hearing it that way? Is this just some fantasy my dying mind conjured up to torment me? Was he Jimmy Stewart in

Harvey, talking to a six foot rabbit no one else could see? Or what's his name, in Heaven Can Wait?

"Warren Beatty," Axel said. His smile lit up his face. "I'm real, Ben. You can count on that"

Back to reading minds, too, Ben thought. If this is a real vision it's not an Indian vision.

Ben knew that in certain tribes, when a boy came of age he was expected to go off alone to fast and to seek a vision. The boys expected to see a spirit animal or person who would give them not only their adult name, and their warrior's name, but also the special power that they alone would possess to help them in battle. He knew that warriors fought by spiritual powers as much as by physical prowess.

Suddenly Ben saw his surroundings in a new light. The petroglyphs, the cave or shelter marked by a "blanket", the nearby water. This was a retreat, a sacred place to who knows how many generations of Native Americans who had come here and added to the petroglyphs while waiting to receive their vision of manhood. Of warrior hood.

To find the Warrior's Way.

"Axel" must know that. Ben was amazed at the thought of it, why hadn't he seen it sooner? Because he'd come here full of pain, disgusted with life, not seeking answers. Just discouraged and tired. Perhaps really just looking for a quiet place to die.

Do I? Do I want to die and really leave everything I love behind?

"You must feel like the Lone Rooster, as they say, Ben", Axel said.

Rooster? The Lone Rooster?

"That's Ranger. Texas Ranger, a special type of cop in Texas."

Somebody's fantasy, actually.

"Axel" talked like modern English was a foreign language for him. His armor and weapons hadn't been used in 500 years. Anywhere except Hollywood. "I know how you must feel, Ben". Axel's tone was so full of acceptance and understanding that Ben felt it even through the misery and despair and physical discomfort that gripped him.

"You're outraged that someone like Dick Sand should get away with what he's doing to you and to Lester and Terry. You also feel there should be justice, that someone should pay for your suffering and your loss. If Sand can't be made to pay, if he can't be stopped, then life is unlivable as far as you're concerned. You're outraged that this should be your fate. And it isn't, Ben. This fate doesn't have to end in being your destiny. Roads branch out from here.

"You think no one knows this, that the people you know best can't help you. You see no way back. and no light at the end of the pipe." Axel paused a moment and screwed up his face in concentration. Then his eyes lit up again and he said proudly: "tunnel".

Then, almost to himself Ben heard him say: "I saw a light at the end of the tunnel, but it was a train." He looked and sounded like a small boy reciting his lessons. But his face became serious, his look intense, as he continued.

"Your problem, Ben, is that you're sending the bill for your misery and pain to the wrong address. So, the bill doesn't get paid. The pain doesn't go away."

"Different people experience this in different ways.

"Mostly you're trying to pay the bill yourself. Blame yourself. When the chips were down you were too weak. You can't think of a way out of it because you're too

Warrior's Way

dumb.

"So you suffer, and even want to die because you see no way around what Sand has done to you. You've convinced yourself that you have to face it all alone."

Ben looked inside himself, behind the deadness, the emptiness and he saw the fathomless, red-hot lava of rage that burned there. Even this near death, the resentment was strong, unaffected by what thirst was doing to his body. Ben had never felt such anger before. Filled with awe at its power, he mentally, took a step back from it, the way one nervously steps back from the edge of a high cliff. Anger like that must be part of the evil that lived after one died, that became the dreaded Ch'iindii. And it was still aimed directly at him. This is all your fault, Ben.

"If this is really how life works, Dick Sand hurting me, my friends, ruining my life, and me helpless to stop it, then no, I don't want it "

"We see this all the time in Viet Nam veterans, veterans of any war", Axel said. 'They're in a wheel chair for life. They've given part of their body and some of the quality of their life for as long as they live. Naturally they resent it

'They resent it more when the people around them forget their sacrifice and daily suffering and go on with their lives. They feel, rightly, that they've made a huge sacrifice for their society, for America.

'They aren't getting the acceptance, understanding, and admiration that their sacrifice deserves from the people around them."

That's right Ben thought. My Grandpa wouldn't understand. Terry wouldn't. Lester is on the wrong side already. My mother might and destroy herself trying to help. But I won't ask that of her.

"Sand has no human feelings at all. Why is it that the ones who have no principles, no values, no conscience at all, always win?"

"Because they don't have to play by any rules except the ones they make themselves," Axel said. "They are the ones truly alone, with every hand about to turn against them.

'They think they can destroy lives and feel they will never pay for the evil they do." Axel smiled cheerfully.

What's so funny about that, Ben thought

"They don't always win, Ben. You know that most often someone stops them cold."

Ben felt his body beginning to stir again with the steady beating of his heart pumping the adrenaline-tinged anger through his bloodstream,

Axel moved around from the entrance and leaned against a sloping rock face and folded his arms. Ben noticed, to his surprise, that Axel left footprints as he moved. Do ghosts do that? As he got closer the shelter grew lighter still and Ben felt his body strengthen a little. The awful feelings dissipated and his mind seemed clearer. It was not a great change, but enough for Ben to feel it and wonder about it   Like ET, Axel seemed to exude some natural healing power.

He seemed to listen a moment before he spoke again. He didn't respond to Ben's thoughts this time. He seemed to have his own message.

"These people, like the veterans, are sending the bill for their sacrifice and suffering to the wrong address, Ben. That's why it doesn't get paid. Not because acceptance, understanding, and admiration equal to their sacrifice and more aren't available to them. But because they're billing the wrong people for it. The people around them are too often preoccupied with their own struggles to make their way in life to be able to give them what they need.

Axel looked at Ben again, his gaze intense, making Ben uncomfortable. Like he could will Ben to understand by the force of his concentration. Like a salesman who really wanted to close a deal.

"I don't suppose you've got that address with you by any chance?" Ben said. It was getting harder and harder to speak. He hadn't had a drink of water in at l east 80 hours, had passed out once. Now he felt great waves of weakness washing over him again, preparing to carry him away into the waiting darkness for the last time. The effect of Axel's presence could not put off for long the fact that Ben was dying.

"I do," Axel said. And a brilliant smile activated the wrinkles around his eyes. "I brought it along in hopes that you might use it."

"How do I use it to get Dick Sand?"

Ben felt the hunger. He couldn't look directly at Axel. But the desire in him made his hands tremble. He saw a look of caution enter Axel's face.

"Sorry, Ben. I can help you teach yourself some principles. That's all anyone has the power to do for you.

"We don't deal in formulas. Like 2+2 = 4. Something where you plug yourself and Dick Sand in on one side of the equals sign and automatically on the other side something predictable happens every time."

Axel moved around, closer to the front of the shelter. "The single most important thing in the Universe, Ben. is the right of every person to choose their own best way. And then take responsibility for their choices.

"I can tell you things that will help you teach yourself to see your choices more clearly. No one, absolutely no one, will make your choices for you. There's no formula. Only principles, that is things that are absolutely true for people like us, and choosing how to act on them. We can choose to found our lives on true principles or we can choose to ignore them. In which case , like Dick Sand, we use fantasy to measure our success. Justice always catches up to us. Learning to choose wisely is what this life is about But having chosen, you can't control the consequences of your choice."

"Dick Sand has chosen to be rich," Ben said. "He seems to be doing okay."

"Dick Sand's where his is because of the choices he has made, it comes with the territory, Ben. To be good it must be possible for you to be bad. For now, we have the Dick Sand's with us. But we don't have to be dominated by them.

"Look at the Whitehouse, Ben. It's one of many symbols of those who want to be good and do good."

Ben fought to understand what Axel was saying, the ideas were new, yet strangely familiar. But Ben's head was pounding now. His tongue was still swollen and blocked his throat. Thirst began to make him feel driven, almost desperate. The water glinting in the creek down among the coolness of the cottonwood trees mocked him.

Then he saw Sand's face again, gloating, as he looked from Ben to Terry and tapped the video tape in the palm of his hand. In an instant, despair, masked that of Ben's physical cravings. Sand had Terry while all Ben had was a rock shelter and dehydration delusions.

"I made choices. I made lots of choices. That's what got me where I am today, choices. Thanks anyway, but I just don't want to make any more. I've experienced all the consequences I can handle."

"Where are you today, Ben?" .

"Buried. Buried alive. Sand's taken everything that matters to me. And I can't get it back. That's where I am today."

Ben slid his hand down the seam of his levis, picked idly at a thread, stared at the dirt floor, and waited quietly for Axel to just go away.

"Do you want me to go away, Ben?"

Ben looked over at the huge man and felt his face twist with the irony of it and the sadness of it.

"Do you mean, do I choose to have you leave?"

"Yes." Axel's voice was soft. "And not to come back to bother you any more. Do you want to be dead, Ben? Or do you just want the hurting to stop?"

"That's what they say to suicides."

"If you decide to sit quietly here long enough, isn't that exactly what you'll be?"

Again the violent feelings welled up in him. Live, they said. I want to live! But I don't want to live without what I've lost. If you could show me a way to get it back, I'd do anything. If you can't, then let me die in peace.

Then a more reasonable thought fell gently into his mind. But I don't have to die right now. Ben thought. I can hear what he has to say first.

"No, I don't want you to leave. I choose to have you stay. But it won't do you any good at all to try and convince me that I should make choices again. What's going to happen will happen, with or without my help.

"But you are willing to listen?"

When Ben nodded slightly Axel's smile was bright again lightening the gloom in the shelter.

"There's a very wise man who lives near you in Utah", Axel said.

He was determined to talk to Ben before he changed his mind.

"His name is Hugh Nibley."

Ben could not remember having heard of him. He must not be teaching in the pre-law program.

"He tells the story of a person who has climbed mountains all his life. Finally, one day, he finds himself clinging to a mountainside with no handholds ahead of him and no way to go back down."

Axel moved around again to rest on the down sloping rock. Probably so he could monitor Ben's reactions better. Ben had climbed the broken-rocked Wasatch Mountains a little. He knew the joke about portable handholds. You grabbed a rock for a handhold, it broke free, and you carried it all the way down with you as you fell. Portable handhold. Convenient, easy to carry, but not much good.

"As he clings there, one slip away from eternity, he finally has to admit to himself that he's gone to far. He had kept growing, expanding his skills, practicing, with his skill always getting him down safely, even from places that had seemed worse than this.

"Finally he's overreached himself. Now there's nothing he can do to save himself.

"At this point the climber looks up to see a hand extended down to him, to pull him up to safety.

"A moral question here is: shouldn't he be allowed to fall? After all, he brought all this on himself. What do you think, Ben?"

Axel leaned forward a little presumably to get Ben's response. Ben shook his head slightly. Hanging by your fingertips from cliffs was not his thing. As he waited for Axel to resume his foggy brain began to tell him that he was much like the climber, hanging on by his fingernails, slipping faster and faster to the edge of a black abyss. Did Axel want him to think of himself as the climber? A little sliver of curiosity began to prick Ben's tired mind. He waited for him to continue.

"Do you study classic literature much, Ben?"

This must be a rhetorical question, one that required no answer, something to think about because Axel didn't wait for Ben to answer.

"The classic hero myth is about someone who refuses to sit at home and be ordinary. The hero does things, takes risks, and in the process learns until he becomes, for example, a skilled climber. Many classical heroes aspire to do the things the gods can do.

"Unfortunately, as Mr. Nibley says, they find out one day that they are only human after all."

"Most classical stories like that end in tragedy," Ben heard his creaky voice almost before he knew he was speaking. "To teach us what it costs to dare too much."

"They send the bill to the wrong address, that's all, Ben," Axel said.

"The key point here is that if the climber hadn't tried,, hadn't used his wits and his mind and his skills he would not have become the climber he is. Risk taking and growth go hand in hand. He didn't sit home by the fireside. He aspired to greater things."

Axel's voice sounded hushed and cautious, as though he had come to the edge of a section of thin ice.

" Will it ruin his character if he receives help? He has learned his lesson. Given his past, will he make good use of another chance?"

Ben was forced by the logic in him to say:

"Yes, he probably would. Like a fighter pilot who gets his plane shot up, but gets home to fly and fight another day. He would be more valuable because of what he had learned."

"Exactly," Axel said. "Such a person deserves our interest and sympathy. And our support."

Ben found his interest waning rapidly as another wave of weakness swept over him. I'm not like the climber, Ben thought. I made stupid choices. I played it safe so I wouldn't become like my father. I let myself go to pot physically. Then, when Sand got rough, I couldn't stand up to him. So I ran like a whipped dog. Ben rolled over on his back and gazed at the ceiling of the shelter. The rock up there was not fire-blackened as so many rock shelters were. He could see cracks in the rock and a yellowish lizard whose Navajo name he couldn't recall scurried across the ceiling.

When he heard Axel's voice again it startled him. It sounded a long ways off and Ben had forgotten for a while that he was there with him. As his will drained away into an abyss of sorrow and regret inside him, his body started shutting down again. Getting ready to close up shop. To bring an end to the tragic story of Ben Singer, the guy who wanted to do what the gods can do. Clinging weakly to the cliff of life. his fingertips getting numb, the muscles his arms burning, his mind telling him to just let go and get if over with.

"Ben," Alex was saying, "Ben, you've got to take another look at the choices you made. An honest look."

I'm not going to listen any more, what's the use?

He turned his head toward the back wall of the shelter. But the wall was gone. Ben was gazing again at the campsite where Dick Sand humiliated him and beat him and took away his humanity. Sand was again across the fire from him and Lester lay at Sand's feet. Prince stood beside Sand, grinning at Ben in the firelight.

91   *Warrior's Way*

"Look at him Ben. Describe him."

Ben heard his own voice telling Grandpa Tsosie: "He's the strongest man in Warren County and a deputy sheriff,"

"You attacked that man, that lawman, to defend Lester."

Ben saw himself, dusty, sore, full of humiliation, looking from Sand to Lester and then lifting his hand to his mouth and doing a ridiculous shuffling dance around the fire. He could taste the dirt in his mouth again.

"When you couldn't do anything else, you made a fool of yourself. And when you did you were thinking of someone else. Of Lester."

Ben saw himself, horrified, at the suburban. He saw Lester pleading. He saw himself signing his name on Sand's clip board.

"You did what you did because you couldn't deliberately hurt Lester or his family or yours."

The images were gone, Ben was back in the shelter. Alex was smiling at him.

"You care, Ben. You play by the rules. You act on your convictions.

"You decided to be an attorney, not for wealth or power, but to be sure your people had a friend in the taw. You left your own home and came here because you didn't want to hurt your family. All of your other major decisions have been of that sort. You want to be good and to make a positive difference. TJ's death was a catalyst in your life."

Ben still couldn't accept his logic. But he knew that what Alex said was true. Ben had wanted to help, and not to hurt. The greatest pain he felt he felt because he had hurt TJ and Terry so much and let Lester down. The people closest to him. That wound was the deepest of all, Ben realized. It was the one that was bleeding away his desire to live. He could find no way to take back the harm he'd done.

"You came to be hanging by your fingernails Ben, because you made choices. Your choices show your values and reveal what you are. Sand took advantage of your basic goodness as the wicked and perverted always do."

Ben was sure there was a flaw somewhere in Axel's thinking.

"Your choices, at the major turning points in your life, have always involved helping those around you. You've been grooming yourself to be a warrior with real battles to fight. To fight for justice within the law.   "You aren't perfect, Ben but you merit a little help. Because the good guys get to win this time.

"Why don't you reach out and take the hand that's reaching down to help you?"

Ben looked up to see Alex's hand above him, holding his tin cup, water running in crystal rivulets down the side. It looked so good to him. Water to make him live. But Ben had not seen a solution to his problem. He turned his head away.

"I can't fight Sand. I can't go on, knowing he's taken everything from me. Now you want be to buy into some dream that because I wanted to be nice that I can bring Dick Sand to justice."

"Well for starters Ben, how would things have been different that night, if you were as strong as your father? We can certainly do something about that."

Whoa. New alternatives. A way to even things up.

"You can be that strong, Ben. Even stronger. We'll show you how it can be done if you'll let us."

"Don't you see, Ben. If you'll send the bill to the right address you aren't alone. The hand is there. It's real. Take it and walk a while with me.

"Let me show you more clearly what your choices are by showing you what you can be. You can decide any day to die.

"But right now you have to decide whether or not to live. I can't interfere if you choose to die. It's your life, your choice to make. What do you say, Ben? Does helping Terry and Lester mean anything to you anymore? Or are you beyond caring."

Ben looked at Alex, at the smile, and again at the footprints he left. I want to live, something whispered inside him. I'd sell my soul if I can get Sand for what he's done. He felt the heat of his hate beating against the spreading coldness of death. Ben reached up and guided the hand and the cup toward his lips. He felt the water from his mouth to the bottom of his stomach. Cool. Refreshing. Living water carrying life and relief with it into his body. He couldn't remember anything ever tasting as good. He drained the cup three times and then lay back, exhausted by the effort.

From inside him came a singing feeling of peace. The hollow blackness was gone. Wondering, Ben fell asleep. It was the first real peace of mind he'd known since the day he agreed to meet Dick Sand at Tibble Lake.

Chapter 12
Ancient Warriors Walked Here

Each time Ben awoke, there in the darkness was Axel, offering water if Ben wanted it. He would take the cool water and lay back, falling asleep as Axel gazed out at the stars that seemed to fill every square inch of the heavens. Ben wondered once if Axel's home was out there somewhere.

Axel had turned to him and smiled and shook his head. Ben still felt anger and shame warring in him. Nothing had changed. But at least, this night, with Axel nearby, Dick Sand's ghostly presence moved back and gave Ben time to rest. "Good Morning, Ben," he said. His smile was as warm as the early morning sunlight and his concern modulated his voice. Ben wondered what he found to be cheerful about.

"Morning," Ben said. Not ready to say □good□ about anything at this point.

He hadn't made up his mind yet to take the helping hand Axel offered. But he remembered clearly the question he had asked.

How would things have been different, Ben wondered, if I'd been as strong as my father the night Sand beat me? That thought was as delicious to him as the cool water had been the night before. He replayed Axel's voice in his mind.

We can certainly do something about that .

If they could, how would that change things? If he could be like his father, and have another chance at Sand......

He felt the rage stirring in him, stronger now that his body was recovering.

He saw in his mind's eye his father lifting the Chevy sedan. He imagined himself lifting Sand easily and slamming him down, exactly as Sand slammed him. That terrible night at Tibble Fork. He imagined himself kicking Sand just as he had kicked Lester, and he could almost feel the impact.

He let the vision fade, and looked up to see a shadow of concern cloud Axel's face. It matched the sick feeling of fear of Dick Sand, and self-doubt that was floating up from deep in his bones. Sand had ripped something to tatters inside him and it was still hanging in shreds down deep in his soul. A coppery taste filled his mouth, the flavor of raw physical fear. Imagination was one thing. Dick Sand in the flesh was something quite different.

Reading my thoughts are you Axel?, Ben thought. How do you like them now?

He stretched and got to his feet, feeling the earth shift and rotate a little around him. He leaned on a wall of the shelter and gazed down at his bike forty yards below. Axel's voice broke the stillness of the shelter, bringing Ben back fully from his reverie.

"If you've decided to accept the helping hand we're offering then we need to start right away." Axel glanced out, looking up and down the canyon like he was expecting company.

"The sooner the better, Axel, but I'll tell you up front what's real for me about all this." Even Ben could hear the skepticism in his voice.

"I saw my father lift that car. I know it can be done, by him."

"You'll have to convince me it can be done by me. If you can do that, then I'm interested. That's getting me somewhere I want to go, to settle with Dick Sand."

It seemed to be Axel's turn to be nervous and unsure. He glanced across the canyon at the image of Whitehouse on the great red-rock wall. It glimmered only dimly, almost hidden in the morning shadow of the cliff. Ben wondered if Axel's determination to help was dimming too.

Whatever the source of his hesitation, Axel seemed to make up his mind. He turned to look at Ben and the smile was there again.

"For a day we can sit and talk. That will give you time to eat and regain some strength.

"You'll need it. I'm going to instruct you as warriors have instructed each other for thousands of years. This knowledge is usually only passed on within families or close-knit brotherhoods because it isn't something you want your enemies to learn. In a life and death fight you want anything that can give you an edge. This is it. It comes with certain obligations on your part, but we'll talk more of that later."

Axel didn't look at his watch. He didn't have one. But Ben got the feeling time was important.

"If you choose to use what I'm going to tell you about how to use the systems built into your body to develop a warrior's strength, to become a natural strong man, you'll need plenty of energy. I suggest you eat now and we'll get started."

Ben looked out into the canyon. It was empty, not a living soul. Just the smoking remains of several campfires and many signs and footprints in the sand. He looked questioningly at Axleron.

"They had to move on, Ben. We come here to refresh ourselves and renew ourselves. This place is holy to us.... As long as the struggle against evil continues we can come here. But we can't stay."

He looked again up the canyon, at the sky, and seemed to be listening.

Ben was too hungry to think more about it.

The food was down at the bike. The water was further down, in the stream. Ben realized now that he had never planned to make that trip back down, ever again. He looked at the steep hill and the twisted trail. He sighed. It was no steeper and no more crooked than the trail of his own life. As he started down he wondered if he could make it over either one.

*   *   *

Ben stoked up his body on Spam, dry whole wheat bread, some pork and beans and lots of condensed milk mixed with water and Nestle's Quick. Satisfied, he leaned back against his bike, still very weak, but feeling relieved. He wouldn't be dying today, after all. He would hear what Axel had to say that could help him beat Dick Sand. Ben felt again a stirring of hot rage that smoldered inside him. Like red hot lava, ready to burst out and burn up Dick Sand's world. He was prepared to change his mind about using force. His despair came from seeing no way out. Not from wanting to just give up. If the Law wouldn't serve as his weapon well maybe he could get his hands on something else.

Axel moved closer and sat on the ground, Indian fashion, except that his back was as straight as a cedar fence post. He bent forward a little from the hips and leaned his elbows on his knees. Ben had a feeling he was doing this to seem informal, almost cozy. Not because he needed to to support himself as most people Ben knew had to do when sitting that way. He looked at Ben and smiled his merry smile.

"I'm going to show you more clearly what your choices are, Ben. I'll tell you about principles, not formulas. General things that are true, not specific ways to use them. You alone will decide what you choose to do. You must take full responsibility for what happens as a result of these choices. So listen well, take your time, and choose wisely.

"Life is not a playground, as Dick Sand showed you. It's an earnest, life or death proving ground. So think carefully before you do anything."

Ben nodded his head. He had no trouble agreeing with Axel. Life was serious, to him, now. Natural politeness kept him from telling Axel again that he had no intention of making more choices. He would listen, nothing more.

HOW THINGS WORK-EXERCISE AND THE GREAT LAW OF ATROPHY

"The biggest problem people have, at first, is not knowing how things work. Once we know how the body was designed, with built in systems to maintain fitness and strength by forcing the body to exercise itself gently, steadily, 24 hours a day, then we have to have enough guts to do what it takes to make those systems work for us."

Ben puzzled over what physical systems Axel meant, but Axel wasn't waiting for questions. He moved in a direction that really mystified Ben.

"What happens to body muscle when it isn't exercised?", Axel said.

"Uh, what?", not asking what happened to it, but requesting a repeat of the question.

"What happens to athletes who get injured and can't move some or all of their body? Do their bodies stay fit, vital, strong and muscular?"

Ben had seen people in wheel chairs and hospital beds. Even a few days in bed sick caused Ben to feel weaker when he tried to get up and get started again. He saw an image in his mind of the muscles of limbs shrunken or withered away from lack of use. A leg or an arm in a cast for a long time could grow dangerously weak. An inactive muscle did not stay strong and fit. Ben knew he'd lost seven to ten pounds over the last four days, and, weak as he felt, all of it was muscle mass.

"No", Ben said. "Something happens to them. The muscle disappears and the arm or leg gets weak, and even useless."

Why do you want me to know this, Ben thought. Where is this leading? How does it help me with Dick Sand?

"Does Dick Sand lift weights with the football players and wrestlers?"

Ben felt the shock hit him again. Axel knew what he was thinking.

"No. He claims he grew up on a ranch and worked hard when he was young and that he's just naturally strong."

"Just naturally as strong or stronger than the weight lifters?"

Ben didn't answer. Sand had a reputation for being stronger and tougher than anyone in Warren County. And he never said it himself. The people who did must know what they were talking about.

"Do you know other people like that? Just strong, enduring, and "well built" as they say, but just a "natural build"?. They don't do anything special to stay that way?"

Ben looked at Axel. He could qualify, Ben thought.

"Yeah, I suppose, though I never paid much attention to that kind of thing."

"We noticed."

Axel's smile took the sting out of his words, but Ben still felt his emotions as they took the long dive back into the black despair he'd felt the night Sand ridiculed him in front of Lester. His stomach felt like he was in free fall after jumping off a cliff. Shame, and rage welled up in him, anger at both Sand and at himself. He felt weak and powerless again, and he hated it.

"Well, why do you think that is? How do you explain the apparent contradiction there?"

Axel gave him no time to brood. Ben found it very hard to both be angry and to think clearly at the same time.

"I'm afraid I don't see a contradiction. What do you mean?"

"You know that unexercised muscles atrophy, shrink, get weak, and so on when they are not exercised regularly. Yet you have people who are very strong who say they don't do any special exercises. If they don't why don't their muscles shrink or turn to fat or both? With most people they do. So why not with them? Most people exercise just to keep from getting out of shape. If these people exercise it's only to perfect their physical or athletic performance."

CAN YOU INHERIT MUSCLES THAT DON'T NEED EXERCISE TO BE STRONG?

"I just assume that they inherited it from their folks."

Ben knew little about exercise and fitness. He had no use for it. He never intended to push anybody around. He'd always avoided physical things since the day he saw his father. He didn't want to be anything like him. One way to make sure of that was to avoid athletics in any form.

"You mean there's a different kind of people with a different kind of muscle, muscle that does stay strong even if they are injured or even just plain lazy?"

Axel looked at him like he was being asked to believe that there really was a Santa Claus. Ben knew of no instance where anyone, no matter how athletic and well built, had become injured or paralyzed without losing muscle tone and strength and muscle size.

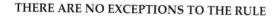

What's going on here, he thought. Even if he's right, what's he leading up to? Where's this conversation going?

"This is the first step to understanding, Ben. You've got to confront your fuzzy-headed thinking on this. It's part of seeing your choices more clearly. Part of coming to know that the body has systems designed into it that can operate to make a man `naturally strong'.

"I've never known anyone who was injured or paralyzed who didn't suffer muscle atrophy," Ben said. Even he could hear the boredom in his voice.

THERE ARE NO EXCEPTIONS TO THE RULE

"Okay, now we're getting somewhere. To be fit, strong, and enduring a skeletal muscle has to be exercised regularly. There are no exceptions to that rule. It's a law of nature.

"Another one is that we don't get more muscle when we exercise. The muscle fiber we have expands and grows larger and stronger."

"Okay," Ben said. He gazed off down the canyon at the ravens crying and circling over the water. Have it your way, his voice tone said. So what?

"Okay. Now the next thing," Axel said, as though everything was settled about muscles, "what holds the body upright?"

97   Warrior's Way

That was an easy one and Ben couldn't help but smile a little as he said:

"Bones, of course. Everybody knows that bones hold up the body."

"They do?"

Axel sounded genuinely amused. He turned and pointed down the canyon.

"Look," he said, the smile in his voice as plain as the merry look on his face.

Ben felt a chill run up his backbone and slam into the base of his skull hard enough to raise the hairs on his neck and to tingle his scalp clear to his forehead.

What Ben saw, walking up the canyon, was a grinning skeleton.

Ben thought of the `Anaa'i Sani who had lived in this canyon. He thought about Ch'iindii and the danger the dead were to the living. He rubbed his hands on his pant legs and began to slide away from the bike, getting ready to run.

"What's that," he said.

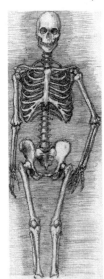

He sounded exactly like he did when Grandpa was telling ghost stories and young Ben heard something moving in the dark outside the hogan. Ben glanced at Axel. His grin, coupled with all his strange behavior, did nothing at all to reassure Ben.

"Those are bones, Ben. Holding themselves up, like you said. Everybody knows that's how it is, you said."

Ben discovered that he was backing up a slow step at a time. He realized it when the handle on the bike suddenly jabbed him in the kidney. He grunted and turned his head, actually expecting to see another skeleton behind him. He didn't have time to feel relieved that it was only the bike. By now the grinning, flesh less monstrosity was striding into the campsite. Ben looked at Axel. Axel only smiled and nodded his head and said:

"That's just some more of your fuzzy-headed thinking at work, Ben."

Ben was startled by a dry clacking sound and looked over in time to see the skeleton fall into a dusty heap. Ben stayed alert, expecting the thing to get up at any moment, afraid of the danger it represented even just laying there. He imagined he could see a ghostly mist of Ch'iindii rising from the bone pile, leaking out

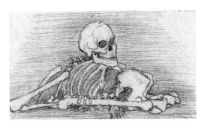

of the eye holes and from the grinning mouth. Ben found he wasn't bored anymore. His mind was remarkably clear and concentrated. The hair on his neck still tickled him a little.

"Now, Ben, again, what is it that holds up the body?"

"Uh, if not bones, I guess I don't know how its done."

At this point Ben was prepared to believe Axel if he told him it was done with smoke and mirrors.

MUSCLES DO THE JOB

"As you can see, bones hold up nothing by themselves. It's our muscles, specifically designed, carefully engineered, acting in concert together, and using the bones as points of attachment for leverage, that actually hold us upright."

Ben looked at the heap of bones. Half of him was watching warily for any hint of movement. The other half was thinking about what Axel had said. That's logical enough, when you think about it, he thought. But it's amazing that bone and muscle and nerve, in a self-contained unit like the body, with only two feet on the ground for leverage, can press down, lift up, twist, contract, and hold a human body upright in a standing position. It was a miracle of sorts.

"Pretty impressive, huh?" Axel said. He sounded like he was showing off his new car.

"Now that you understand those two ideas we can move on and get to the good stuff."

Ben could see no connection whatever between muscles getting weak if they weren't used and the fact that muscle, not bone, was used to hold up the body. But I'm not going to say so, he thought. Axel might make that thing get up and walk again. He glanced over at the pile of bones, but could detect no sign of movement. He looked very carefully.

"Relax, Ben," Axel said. "You got the idea. We don't need the bones anymore."

Ben glanced from the bones to Axel. When he looked back they were gone. But the marks they'd made in the dirt were still there. Ben felt the hair rise on his neck again as he turned back to Axel. This guy is strange,. He's quite a teacher. He certainly knows how to get my attention.

ISOMETRIC AND ISOTONIC

"Now, let's get down to the nitty-gritty on this."

Axel looked at the sun, like time was still important.

"There are two general kinds of muscle exercise that makes muscles fit, and strong. One is isotonic and the other is isometric. Isometrics were big a few years ago. Everybody was pushing against walls and doorways or contracting muscles in ways that made them pull against each other. When you push hard or pull hard against an immovable object, you're getting isometric exercise. Charles Atlas is still selling a program that uses what he calls "dynamic tension". The idea, the knowledge, has been around a long time.

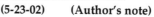

Or, and this is a key piece of knowledge, when a muscle contracts and holds the body against the pull of gravity, but doesn't actually move anything, that is isometric exercise too.

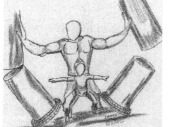

(5-23-02)   (Author's note)

Actually, many exercise physiologists, including Covert Bailey,(CovertBailey.com) speak of two kinds of skeletal muscle, not just one. One's called "fast twitch" muscle and is used for short sprint, quick movements as in playing a sport. The other type is called "slow twitch" muscle. It has peculiar characteristics and a larger blood supply and can contract and hold for a long time."

Trying to hang your body on its ligaments and using fast twitch muscles where they were not meant to be used makes you tired quickly. Raw strength and endurance emerge almost as a by product when you learn to allow the slow twitch muscles to power up and do what they were designed to do, thus freeing the fast twitch muscles to do their job.

Most fat is burned by slow twitch muscles.

Ben saw himself trying to push and pull Dick Sand to get him away from Lester. I got lots of isometric exercise that night, Ben thought. Pushing against an immovable object. He felt the blood creeping into his face as the shame came awake in him again. The feeling of helplessness came back, strong and raw.

"Yeah, I know about that."

Ben felt himself pushing the words awkwardly past his clenched teeth.

Axel looked at Ben with a quietness in him. Like the hushed reverence at a funeral. Like Axel knew Ben's pain, and respected it.

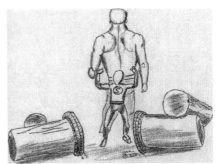

"Isotonic exercise means moving the muscles against a load, working, in other words, as we commonly know it. Weight lifters work with progressively heavier weights to build muscle mass and strength. But anytime we use muscles to move a load, even if that load is just the weight of part of our own body, we are doing isotonic exercise. As long as we are active and moving everyday our body muscles gets some exercise. If we stop moving, or don't move right, atrophy takes over.

'And Ben, you need to realize that atrophy is selective. In other words, it attacks the muscles you aren't exercising. No matter how much exercise selective muscles get, others can be weak and flabby."

Ben raised a hand and Axel paused.

"Okay. That makes some sense. But I'm sorry. I don't see where all this fits. How does knowing this stuff get me closer to settling with Dick Sand? I don't see any way knowing this does me any good..... If there are connections here between unexercised muscles getting smaller and weaker, the fact that bones don't hold up the body, muscles do, and the fact that there are two kinds of exercise that make muscles fit and strong I just don't see them."

Ben shook his head to show his bewilderment. But he did nothing to show Axel that he wasn't interested. He peered around furtively to see if anything was approaching.

They were alone in the canyon. Insects hummed, a warm breeze blew by gently bearing the scents of sand and water and greasewood and sage. It was a quiet spring day, and Ben wanted it to stay that way.

WHY IS IT A SECRET?

Axel smiled again and said:

"Practically no one does see a connection, Ben, in spite of all the interest in sports and physical fitness. And the ones who do are mostly dead now. The others aren't talking because it isn't in their interest to tell anyone."

Axel moved over near Ben again and bent over without curving his spine at all and smoothed a place in the sand. As Ben looked it became a T.V. screen or a crystal ball. Ben saw men in ancient leather armor with shields, short swords and long spears marching along a sunlit, dusty road.

"In the old days, Ben, before guns made men equal, a fight was something to behold. We'll talk about it more later. But one thing here, among these early Romans, and among all men who marched off to fight hand to hand. They often fought together as clans, uncles, nephews, brothers, sons, big extended families. Then battle was an individual test of endurance and of raw physical power and of athletic ability. Gymnasiums and regular physical exercises were not available. In battle the weakest died first and the mighty men of war ruled the world."

Ben looked at the huge man across from him. Mighty man of war was a description that suited him exactly......Ben wondered how much of this Axelron knew about first hand......

Ben immediately thought of his own clan. Every Navajo of his clan was a relative of sorts who could call on him for help under certain conditions, including warfare. In the past, even in Grandpa's time, they had gone on raids together and had fought together against the Spaniards. For a fleeting moment Ben pictured his father. What a magnificent warrior he would have been if he had only lived in those times.

ANCIENT WARRIOR SOCIETIES

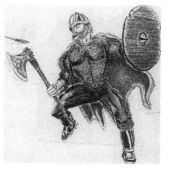

"No matter what the war was about, the main goal of the clans was for every person to survive. They trained together, and the experienced men coached the younger men, their sons, nephews or cousins. They told them everything they could that would give them an edge, help them survive. Knowing about body systems that could build great strength and endurance, even when you didn't have time or opportunity to keep the body fit with regular training exercise were closely held secrets. Yet they are used even today. But few who know about their existence are willing to talk about them. They are mostly men who survive by their strength. Why should they help a potential rival?"

Ben saw the ranks line up and march toward similar ranks and lines across a broad valley. He heard a muted roaring, unlike anything he'd ever heard, coming from thousands of throats as the battle was joined. The image faded and Ben was looking at the sand again.

"Men who know the "secrets" of how to force the body to exercise itself every moment, 24 hours a day, to build great natural physical strength and athletic power, don't share them with outsiders.

"These things became a part of the secret lore of warrior societies. But because they are also natural and normal some people accidentally fall into using these habits to build vitality, fitness, and sometimes amazing strength into their bodies. Often they have no real idea what they are doing or why it works. Your father was one of those."

Ben looked at Axel. So you knew my father, he thought. A dozen questions came into his mind. But he didn't ask any of them. Axel was gazing at the sun again. The day was passing swiftly and this seemed to make Axel uneasy.

Ben had his own worries. He saw Terry again, driven into Sand's arms, her heart broken, her hopes wrecked by the very man who held her.

What was Dick Sand doing right now. Was he working on Terry? Still lying to her about him, telling her he was dead? Talking her around to his way of thinking. Taking advantage of her pain? Ben felt his finger nails biting into his palms. He consciously relaxed his hands and wiped them down his pant legs. Time was short. No question about that. Ben felt the tattered place inside him that Dick Sand had made when he broke Ben down and made him dance. Ben felt the fear again, just as strong. No matter how bad he wanted to help Terry, the thought of going back after Sand suddenly made no sense at all.

Chapter 13
Where In The World Is Benjamin Franklin Singer?

"Well, Herschel", Dick Sand said. "What do you know? Where you at? Why haven't I been hearing from you?" His voice held the whiplash edge it could take when Sand was getting nervous.

"Well sir, right this moment we're in Kanab headed south to Arizona. Virg wants another wife like Tom Greene and we figure there's a place there where he can get two or three."

"Don't try bein' funny. It's been a week with no sign of Singer. Like he fell off the earth. Nobody's seen him anywhere. Not even down on the reservation."

"We haven't seen him either, Dick. But we hardly been looking. We been real busy checking on your mule pens and keeping everything going. That part is going good. Lotsa people moving through and no glitches so far. They'll be working their way into Warren County in a few more days."

"Yeah, yeah you guys are doin' okay. Singers got me hearing footsteps in the night."

"Who you gonna call? Ghostbusters, that's who."

"I told you already, stop fooling around. I'll tell you when it's time to clown around. Now ain't it."

"Sorry, Dick. You know how boring Virg is to be around after awhile."

"I'm going down to Chinle. I'm taking a chopper down and back tomorrow. Private flight, on my day off."

"You got an idea he's down there somewhere, Dick?"

"Naw, I'm sure he's not. We got tribal police looking for him too. But I'll bet his grandfather knows where he is. Maybe I can get a clue from him."

"He know you're the one sent him the tape?"

'How you know I did?'

"Cause that's how you work, Dick. Besides, you said you had it covered, that he wouldn't be welcomed and invited to stay. That seemed like the surest way to do it. Send his family the tape."

"Yeah, I did. But the old man, he don't know it was me."

'Well, have a nice flight. We'll be starting home tomorrow, case you need us for anything. When you go over Muley Point you might take a look at our handiwork and see, if just by chance, there's a big Goldwing off down in there somewhere. Sure would make things easier, wouldn't it?"

"Yeah. It would at that. I'll do that. Stay in touch, Herschel."

"Yup, can do, Dick." But Herschel was speaking to a dial tone.

Herschel looked over at Virgil who, as usual, was driving.

"Want me to drive awhile, Virg?" Herschel tried to hide his grin for the sake of the joke, an old, tired joke that lay between them for years.

"Nope. I'll keep on truckin', thank you. I have no desire to see what life's like on the inside or on other side just yet."

"Aw, gimme a break. One little fender bender and you won't let me drive no more?"

"Herschel, that fender bender involved bumping a very hostile highway patrolman into the borrow pit ."

"That's what gets me about you, Virgil, truth be told. You're picky. Small minded and picky."

"You're too big hearted and generous. Someday you'll get us killed, trying to yield the right of way to a cop."

Hershcel sighed expansively and changed the subject.

"Sand's going down to Chinle to see Singer's grandaddy. Seems that man just can't let things rest."

"Always picking at the sores instead of letting them scab over."

"Putting his oar in the water."

"Stirrin' the soup."

"No, what he does mostly, is he stirs up a hornets nest. That's what he usually ends up doing. Just can't leave well enough alone."

"Can't let things happen, has to try and make them happen."

"He don't think nobody's smart except him."

"Most especially not Indians."

"There is that ..You got any Injun blood Virg?"

"I guess everybody has some, but me, well the blue eyes and blond hair sorta disguise it, don't you think."

"Pretty much, I'd say. How 'bout you Hersch? Sand gonna take you for Native American?"

Herschel grinned a big, toothy grin that lit up his dark face. ☐I reckon the black hair and brown eyes might be mistook by some. Mostly my folk was unwilling immigrants to this country. Made the crossing flat on our backs and worked ourselves to death in the south, learning agriculture, stuff like that."

"Made you big, ugly and mean, all that farmin'."

"I'll go with the big and ugly alright. But mean? Dick Sand's got me there any day. That man invented a whole new meaning for mean."

"You're sure right there, Hersch. Best we don't go around looking too much like Indians the next little while. We don't want him mad at us."

"Like he's mad at Ben Singer."

"'Cause Singer was inconsiderate enough to stay alive and disappear."

"Instead of biting the dust the way he was supposed to."

"Like them Hollywood Indians do in the movies."

"Guess nobody told them Navajos they was supposed to lose."

"I'm just glad Sand's going down there in person. Not sending us. What I hear Ben's daddy is a rip snorter when he isn't sucking a bottle and his grandaddy actually raided the Mexicans and Utes when he was young."

"They never took kindly to people coming into their country. Not ever. Now Sand thinks he can run his Mexican mules right under their noses."

"Yeah, you know, Herschel, when we get paid again we better find us a hidey hole to run to and put a huge chunk of cash away."

"Words to live by, Virg. Words to live by. I also think we better get to know Sand's boss a little too. We can start by sounding out one of them segundos Monterro sends along to check up on things from time to time."

"Lay off a little side bet, just in case Sand decides to self destruct over Singer?"

"But carefully, Virg. Oh so carefully. Sand best not find out."

"As you like to say, Hersch. Words to live by."

****

When Ben drifted out of his melancholy reverie he saw Axel looking at him, a wistful smile on his face.   Whatever he was thinking, he chose to go on teaching Ben about muscles.

THREE KINDS OF MUSCLE WORK

"Muscles make three kinds of movements and there are three types of muscle action. (1) They are simple, but they are important to know if you're going to become your own physical fitness trainer.

"Muscles can move concentrically." Axel extended his arm out then brought his hand to his chest. "When muscle shortens to make a bone move, its moving concentrically."

Axel lowered his hand slowly to the ground.

"When you allow gravity to help, but you use muscle to slow the action, that's eccentric movement. The muscles are gradually lengthening to allow controlled downward movement."

Author's Note: In the panel A points to the muscle at the back of the leg, which is contracting (concentrically) to move the leg. At the same time C points to the front muscle which must relax and lengthen (eccentrically) to allow this movement. In other motions each would take the opposite role. (See Warrior's Walk later for details)

Yes, for you purists, Dave Berry says the scientific nomenclature for the front leg muscle is "front leg muscle".

Axel straightened up and looked at Ben, his eyes almost glittering.

THE GREAT SECRET

"The next kind of muscle work is where the great "secret" is, if there's any secret at all."

Ben felt the irony of his situation. Here he was, sitting around in an ancient Indian burial ground, in the warm sunlight of an April day, talking to a guy who did weird things with skeletons and who thought muscle work was important. Well, it was unreal. Now, apparently, he was about to learn the great secret of the Universe. Ben tried to prepare his mind and not let his bitterness and fear show.

"The third kind of work muscles can do is static or isometric work. This is related to eccentric movement."

Axel shifted a little and sat up straight. Ben became aware again of his military bearing, upright, and powerful looking.

"But rather than lengthening gradually against the downward pull of gravity, the muscles contract and hold in one position, at a certain length and resist the pull of gravity. If they tire and weaken, there is a gradual, or even a sudden eccentric lengthening, lowering, letting go. We call it "de-programming" or "de-energizing or de-patterning". If you decide to grow naturally strong like your father you'll get to know isometric/static holding against eccentric movement and its effects intimately."

Author's Note: This is hard to create a picture of. See "sitting" for a better idea of how it works because when you sit the Warrior's Way you will find many muscles holding your body up isometrically. And yes, it is the same in many ways as the old isometric exercises we all learned to hate. But with an important twist. This is done nature's way, and that makes all the difference.

Axel's smile was a little lopsided. Ben concluded that this was not to be an excessively enjoyable pathway to knowledge.

"You'll find out soon enough why few people bother with the body's isometric muscle systems. It's not like winning a hundred yard dash. It's steady, often boring physical effort that takes more strength and endurance than you can imagine. But most of all, Ben, it takes guts. Going through the build up period can be tough.

"And once you get there the law of atrophy just hangs around like a scavenger waiting for the first sign of weakness or neglect to move in and weaken the muscles if you stop using them isometrically to hold up your body."

"Strong men lose strength as they grow older or as their habits changes. Others fall into the right habits and build strength and vitality almost overnight, and lose it again because they don't know its source.

In between strong and weak you have infinite gradations between right and wrong that account for all the muscular body-development types that you see around you. Because these systems are under our conscious control, and we all tend to control them differently.

"Only rarely, in a man like your father, does it all come together correctly. As you know, the results can be impressive."

I've seen my dad, Ben thought. And I've fought with Dick Sand. Anything that will let me take him on one more time with my dad's strength, I'm going to do. I don't care if it's pleasant or not. Ben felt his face getting hot. He wanted to clench his fists and punch something. Someone. He wasn't about to look Axel in the eyes - to let him see the hate and the fear he knew glittered there.

Ben got up and drank some water and stretched. He felt stronger already, but still lightheaded. He was happy to set back down by the bike and listen to Axel.

REMEMBER THE THREE KINDS OF MUSCLE ACTION?

"Part of understanding the difference between raw physical strength and athletic power lies in understanding that muscles, at different times can do any of these kinds of work. They can also perform three kinds of action. People who are "muscle bound" are often very strong. But they are not athletically powerful. (1) In many ways Dick Sand is one of these."

Ben took note. Anything that had to do with Sand, he wanted to hear.

"Muscles can be prime movers, that is, they are moving the body or parts of it.

"They can also be antagonists."

Axel moved his arm out and back again.

"Moving out, the muscles on the inside of my arm, the biceps, could stop the action if they contracted. They have to relax to allow the other muscles to pull my arm out. Coming back, the biceps are prime movers,

"But rather than lengthening gradually against the downward pull of gravity, the muscles contract and hold in one position, at a certain length and resist the pull of gravity. If they tire and weaken, there is a gradual, or even a sudden eccentric lengthening, lowering, letting go. We call it "de-programming" or "de-energizing or de-patterning". If you decide to grow naturally strong like your father you'll get to know isometric/static holding against eccentric movement and its effects intimately."

the others have to relax and not impede the movement. One part of sports training involves making sure that antagonist muscles are not interfering with the athletic movements of the sport. That the athlete is not literally "fighting himself". Muscle bound people have this problem, and the third kind of action, isometric holding, the operation of muscles in the fixator mode can add to it."

Axel leaned over and looked at Ben again with the glittering intensity that seemed to say: This is important, Ben. Pay attention.

Ben looked around to see if anything spooky was coming and wiped his hands on his shirt. Whatever you say, Axel, he thought. If it's important to you, it's important. Even if I hardly understand it

"Again, Ben, if there is a secret to natural strength, grace, and bodily beauty, its here, in the third muscle action. That is, fixating on isometric holding makes a rigid platform for the prime moving muscles to operate from.

"Muscles can act as fixators. That is, they contract and hold, statically, isometrically, to just hold a joint steady and tight against the pull of gravity while other muscles act as prime movers and perform some movement of the body or its parts.

"Remember the skeleton, Ben. Here is where it comes in, as rigid points of attachment for muscles and with the capacity for articulated joints."

Axel leaned back, like Lincoln contemplating what he'd said after giving the Gettysburg Address.

Ben sensed that he'd just heard something that Axel thought was really significant. Important in ways that only mystified Ben. He went back over, in his mind, what Axel had said. Ben was good at remembering, good at any kind of brain work. This was something he could do. But Axel wasn't waiting for him. With another glance at the sun, which was now well down in the west, Axel went on speaking.

"The bottom line on this, Ben," Axel said, "is that the human body is beautifully engineered. Bone and muscle are designed to work together. Some muscles use bone and ligament attachments to work isometrically.

"They contract and hold the bones and joints tightly, if not rigidly, in their proper position, resisting the pull of gravity, so that isotonic muscles can contract or relax and work as prime movers to make the body move in certain ways. This has to be done even when isotonic movements put extra stress or "G" forces on the joints, as when an acrobat does back flips.

"Picture the complex movements of acrobats, dancers, and a thousand other specialties that show what the body can do using these great natural systems."

`NATURAL' ATHLETES? NOT REALLY

"We can't change our basic physical inheritance. We inherit certain body types.

"But aside from these genetic gifts (things you get and don't get from your ancestors, especially your parents) you can consciously or unconsciously, energize isometrically certain muscle groups to "temper" body movements, to make them strong, athletic movements. This means that they use part of their muscle system to hold flexible body parts, such as joints and the spine, more or less rigidly while the isotonic muscles move the body. When you are seeing real grace and real power, smooth, powerful, graceful body movement, it is always being created by the supportive role isometric systems play.

"That means, that if you learn to use them, you move gracefully, powerfully, athletically. The use of the systems is what makes a powerful, graceful athlete. Not the other way around. This way of managing your body makes you strong and athletic. You don't manage your body this way because your are strong and athletic. More fuzzy-headed thinking, Ben.

"The isometric system holds the body and at the same time tempers and smoothes the movements of the isotonic or action muscle groups engaged in making the proper athletic movements. Swinging a bat, diving from a high platform, competing in a karate bout, and so on.

Natural athletes are people who hold their bodies isometrically in ways that build strength, co-ordination, smoothness of movement. They may also have inherited genetic tendencies toward body type, muscle and bone mass, nerve reflexes, etc. That gives them an edge, but you can have all those genetic gifts and have nothing if you don't acquire the capacity to hold your body isometrically to form the platform for the prime movers to operate from. You can also have few of those gifts and still be strong and fit."

Axel paused momentarily. He seemed to be listening. But not to his inner voice. He glanced up the canyon and then looked back at Ben.

Ben started to make some connections between what had seemed at first an unconnected set of facts about bones, muscles, and atrophy. But he couldn't pull it all yet together and Axel wasn't giving him time to think about it.

"The problem is that, unlike animals, a large part of this isometric/isotonic system is under our conscious control. That alone is enough to account for the wide variety of human bodies you see around you. It also means you can make marvelous changes in your physical body by using these systems in the way nature intended them to be used.

YOU HAVE TO CHOOSE

"People have to make a choice. They have to decide whether to hang the weight of their bodies on their bones using the joints and ligaments, and practically no muscle effort, just letting the isometric systems go un-energized. The only real exercise some people get is isotonic movement-walking, etc. Others are exercising their bodies isometrically and isotonically 24 hours a day.

"Or they have to decide to hold their bodies up using the isometric systems, using the muscle that was designed for the job.

"Everyone was supposed to be as strong and fit for their body size as a cat is for his. Freedom of choice enters in here too, though, and sadly, most of us choose not to make the effort. "Using the system means that they use muscles that contract and hold, isometrically, as fixators to hold joints rigidly in position against the pull of gravity so that isotonic muscles sets can act as prime movers with the proper foundation or support from the rest of the body.

"When that happens every movement is smoothed by muscle contraction. It means that the body is compact and that organs and bones get the support they need all the time, not just when we "exercise". This gives our movements the smooth, graceful look we admire so much in naturally strong, graceful men and women. So much more muscle power is being used that it burns huge amounts of energy and virtually eliminates weight problems in many people. It also tones and strengthens large parts of the body's muscle system that usually goes unused. This results in an increase in endurance and energy.

"They have to choose to move their bodies using unsuited muscle and again lots of joints and ligaments unsupported by the work of the fixators. Or to move their bodies with the muscles designed for the job and with the bones properly fixated to allow a platform for smooth and powerful prime mover motions. That decision makes all the difference in the world to what kind of physical body they'll live in."

Axel was giving Ben his glitter-eyed look again. Ben began to think about his father and Dick Sand. The two real natural strong men he'd known. He'd never thought about what made them strong. But he could now see in his mind's eye, the kind of thing Axel was describing. Could it really be possible that doing these things could create strength like that? He touched again the bitter despair still lodged inside him. The despair that had driven him to Whitehouse canyon. If it didn't work, if it wasn't true, then he was still out of options. There was no way to regain what Sand had ripped away from him.

Ben saw Axel shift nervously. Maybe he was mind reading again.

"If they hang their body on their ligaments, the muscles designed to do the work get no exercise. What happens to muscles that don't get exercised, Ben?"

Despite his mixed emotions, this was actually starting to make sense to Ben and he was pleased to show that he had a right answer.

"Atrophy! The muscles weaken, get smaller and weaker," he said. "Then you'd slump and you couldn't hold yourself up. As he heard the wonder in his voice he felt like slapping his forehead in an "Oh my gosh!" gesture. It's like a vicious cycle!

"Right," Axel said. His smile was a great reward to Ben. He badly needed to do something right. Even if he wasn't sure where all this was leading, he could at least show that he was learning something.

"The beauty of all this is, that if you start using these systems they build strength, in an upward cycle, the muscles growing strong isometrically and isotonically, till you have a Dick Sand, and sometimes, very rarely, a Frank Singer.

Ben's thought turned inward at that. Can I be like my father? Is this the way? Never in his limited experience with athletics had Ben heard anything remotely like the physical management process Axel was talking about. But it made some sense. And if it worked?

Ben felt a jolt of adrenaline hit him. It would be so nice to visit Dick Sand again, on his turf, and introduce Dick to his father's strength. Ben felt heat from the rage inside him reaching into his face. He discovered he was clenching and unclenching his fists. But the fear of Dick Sand, though diminished, didn't go away. Ben found that hopes and wishes couldn't cancel raw physical fear and self-doubt.

Axel went on.

"In the animal world, especially the world of the predators, these isometric systems are not left to the control of the beast. Their isometric, fixator systems work automatically.

"Then every movement they make is cushioned by muscle contractions. Not like people can be. Not a lazy slapping of uncontrolled limbs and loose-hung joints. Not a teetering, barely erect carriage that is clumsy and scarcely keeps from falling over altogether. Only human beings can do that. Look at this."

Ben started to look down at the sand again, but caught himself as he saw Axel looking up toward the shelter. Ben's stomach churned as he found himself looking into the yellow-rimmed eyes of a huge mountain lion that lay on the rocks just outside the shelter.

The big cat stood and moved along the rock shelf that ran by the shelter. Part of Ben went cold when he saw the cat turn and start down the slope in long graceful, powerful leaps that covered a dozen feet at a time. He marveled at the grace, smoothness and at the same time the terrible power that the big cougar displayed as it moved.

Seemingly without effort it leaped forward and upward at least ten feet to clear the entire campsite, sailing over Ben's head as he sprawled backwards in the dust, clearing the bike, landing lightly on the bank of the stream and then leaping across it in a single, massive display of strength and grace. Ben tasted dirt as he turned to watch the cat lope along the far bank and out of sight among the Tamarack brush down the canyon. In a moment it was gone.

" But animal muscle is the same as human muscle."

Axel had this irritating way of going on in a normal tone no matter what was happening. As though nothing unusual had happen.

The thought hit Ben. Maybe this is a normal day for him, he thought. How would I know? One thing he did know, the cat tracks were there, real, as substantial as Axel was. Now Ben had two apparitions to watch out for. He felt Axel touch his arm and he turned back from gazing after the cougar to see Axel smiling his merry, Santa's Elf smile at him again.

He's enjoying this, Ben thought. I'm glad someone is. He looked around again, but quickly. He didn't want to give Axel the impression that he wasn't paying attention.

"If animal muscle doesn't get exercise it will shrivel and weaken just as it does in humans. Crippled cats, for example, often become man-eaters because they can't capture their normal prey anymore.

"But under normal conditions Nature takes over for these animals and sees that their isometric systems give them the exercise their bodies need. Big cats confined in the zoo for years can still take off your head with one swipe of their paw."

Ben had no trouble believing that. And he had no desire to prove it. He took another quick look down the canyon. At least that cat didn't seem to be crippled. Even so, he didn't feel much better.

"You have control over the kinds of food you eat. Most people feel that choosing to eat one kind of food over another can make a difference in your health.

"In the same way how you choose to hold and move your body can have a huge effect on the strength and endurance of the body you live in."

Ben was becoming uncomfortable. He felt an uneasy stirring in his mind. A part of him was starting to evaluate his physique. To think about how he carried his body. He wasn't happy with what he was finding out about himself. He glanced over at Axel. Axel was quiet again, still and seemingly respectful of Ben's thoughts, giving him time to digest what he was learning, to make some connections among the ideas Axel had taught him.

Ben also began now to see just how erectly Axel held his body, how powerful his body looked despite his small size. Maybe that's why he was sent, so I wouldn't be totally discouraged right off the bat.

"This isn't all that complicated, Ben. Don't start getting intellectual on me. Remember Lenny in Stienbeck's famous story "Of Mice and Men"? He was prodigiously strong. But he was certainly not an intellectual giant. You don't have to be a space machine man," Axel paused and his mobile face screwed up into intense concentration. Then his smile return in a rush.

"You don't have to be a rocket scientist to do this, Ben." He seemed pleased with his control of slang. Ben wondered again just where Axel came from. He surely wasn't from Ben's time.

Axel's voice took on almost a pleading note as he said:

"Don't outsmart yourself on this, Ben. Muscle doesn't grow strong when you think about it. Understanding is important so you can choose and so you can act intelligently.

"But in the end you must choose to do it and then find enough gumption to carry it out and do what needs to be done. That's what counts. It takes effort and action to overcome the wrong habits and join those who are "naturally" strong, fit, and vital."

Ben looked at Axel and nodded. He was painfully aware that he had made a habit out of carrying his body around awkwardly suspended from joints and ligaments, exerting as little physical energy as possible.

Axel looked at him like the couch potato he was. Like the coach looks at a bench warmer in the closing moments of the biggest game of his life.

Can I send you in his look said to Ben. Will you play? Or will you fold and not even try?

Ben didn't like the feeling. But he had no answers either. Axel went on speaking.

THE BOTTOM LINE-KEY MUSCLE GROUPS
ERECT FIRST! STRETCH AS TALL AS YOU CAN - THEN EVERY THING ELSE

"By learning how to "energize" or "program" (contract or use, if you will) key isometric muscle groups you can choose to fully utilize the isometric\isotonic\ and mixed functions of muscles that are designed to stabilize joints and to move your body. When you do, the muscles designed for these jobs will get the exercise they need to do their job.

"Right off the bat you'll think it's easy. After you've tried to do it 16 to 24 hours a day for a few days you'll see why naturally strong people don't need any special exercises to stay fit and maintain good muscle tone.

"Nor to keep from gaining weight in the form of stored fat. You can be sitting quietly watching T.V. with the proper isometric muscle systems energized and be sweating like you were doing a full body work out in the gym."

THERE IS NO SHORT CUT

"There's no short cut, Ben. The law of atrophy is supreme here. Gravity is the power that makes you either weak or strong.

"The muscles must be exercised, constantly, and correctly. If you decide to do it this natural way, it will still be hard work. But it will be done in the way your body was designed for it to be done. By putting the work on the correct muscle systems that were designed to do the job, at the pace that is correct for your body.

"The muscles getting the exercise will be the ones designed for it. That's how you reach the full genetic potential of strength and vitality.

"If you want to match up to Dick Sand you'd better settle your mind on this right now. There's no easy way. We're talking about science, not magic and fantasy."

Ben shut his eyes. He didn't need Axel to conjure up Dick Sand for him. Sand was there inside him. Smirking. Calling him the Pillsbury Dough Boy. Hugging Terry while Ben ran like a scared rabbit.

It seemed that two paths lay open to him. One tinged with anger, the other with fear. One was the downward path of degradation, weakness and death, taking in death one drink at a time till he died. All the time blaming Sand and all the time knowing it was his own unmanliness that was really to blame, allowing himself to die, not with Sand's poison but of fear and self-loathing.

That left Sand the winner. It left Terry and Lester and Ben and TJ Davis, and who knew how many more people, the losers.

Ben saw his father, his coat splitting as he lifted the awesome weight of a car in such a smooth and effortless motion. Ben saw the mountain lion. He heard himself saying to Sand on that awful night: My dad could pull your arms off and beat you with them.

But my father's dead, Ben thought. He can't help me now. If someone is going to yank off Sand's arms it's just going to have to be me. Axel's trying to get me to see that. Common sense told him that it just might work. The strange things Axel did added to his glimmering faith. And the pay off, if it did work, the pay off was that he could go after Sand. For just a moment, no more, he opened the red hot pit of hate that burned in him and immersed himself in it. It felt good. He knew he didn't dare bask in its warmth yet. Daren't let himself hope too much too soon. But he wanted it all to be true so badly he felt himself trembling a little as he opened his eyes and looked at Axel.

"Why don't you tell me how to get started," he said.

He was surprised at the edge of emotion that colored his words. Determined and terrible.

Ben realized that he was back from wherever he'd let Dick Sand drive him. He had a cause, people needed his help. He wouldn't walk away and just abandon them if there was a way he could help. The blood of warriors was coursing through him in time with the pounding pulses of his heart, like the steady beating of a war drum.

I'm just not that kind of person, Ben thought. Not a quitter and I hate to lose....

Thinking back to what Axel had said about climbing cliffs, trying to help people, and getting in serious trouble because of it, Ben found some comfort. Should I try? In the end that was all he could do.

Yes he would. He would try hard. He'd die trying if it came to that.

Chapter 14
Ben Does His Homework

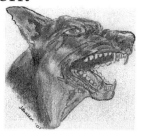

"That's right," Dick Sand said. "He's still out there somewhere." He leaned across the hood of his Lawman suburban, looking at Herschel and Virgil, who had just come in over Currant Creek to the top of the grade above Sleepy Hollow. Remote, seldom visited, all roads could be seen from here for five miles in all directions. Half a dozen forest roads led away, making it easy to avoid meeting anyone. Sand couldn't be seen associating with the likes of these scruffy, bearded, camofluage covered men.

Below them to the south, beautiful Strawberry Reservoir glinted in the late afternoon sun. Grey-black thunderheads climbed to the stratosphere, their tops eye-achingly white in the late spring sunshine.

Sand toyed with the key chain that normally dangled from the ignition. It had a .338 Winchester Magnum bullet drilled out, hanging from a chain. He imagined Ben Singer centered in the scope of his rifle and himself taking up the slack in the trigger, pulling gently till the recoil surprised him and Ben Singer disappeared behind a cloud of gun smoke.

Gone forever.

If he was found, still being stupid, un-alerted, just wandering around in a stupor, as his grandfather had implied, maybe he would take the time to go down and take him out personally. He felt a grin stretch his face. Do him, as the TV bad guys would say, and then go out with Terry. Not saying anything, just knowing

Neither Herschel nor Virgil offered to get out of their Land Rover. They left the engine running until Sand signaled them to shut it off.

"Yeah. I went down to Chinle and interviewed his grandaddy.☐ Sand's eyes went slightly out of focus, like he was seeing something besides empty forest and dusty road.

"Funny old man. Hard as flint. I walked in, he took one look at the badge and said: "You're the Billy Goat, huh?"

"Just like that, in English. Then he moves a piece of bed sheet or something on the table and starts acting like he's cleaning this honest to goodness old time western single action Colt. It could easy be a hundred years old, has a tie-down holster with silver dollar conchos on it, all over the belt too. Worth a thousand if it was worth a dollar.

"But he wasn't cleaning it. It was loaded. I could see the bullets through the front of the cylinder. After that he wouldn't talk English. Made the Navajo policeman do all the talking."

Sand faded out again. Seeing the old man. Seeing death in his eyes. Which was something Sand always recognized instantly. Realizing suddenly he was on this old man's turf and that the old man didn't like him. The accidental shooting of a visiting lawman might not receive as much attention out here as it would elsewhere. And he had sent the old man the tape. The old man couldn't know it was him, of course. But it seemed to have made him generally mad at white men.

He felt his belly crawl a little again as it had when the old Navajo passed the gun muzzle back and forth across his middle while they talked. While the officer talked and old man Tsosie had answered in little more than grunts and an occasional nod of his head.

Yes, Ben had been there. Looking like he'd been in a fight. (When he'd said that was the first time the gun muzzle passed across Sand's belt buckle.) No, he had nowhere to go, just didn't want to stay here. He was embarrassed to stay here and see his family. (The muzzle passed by again.) He talked about his father and the prison down in New Mexico. He might go there, even though he knows he's dead. Or he might go to Navajo Mountain to see his father's people. (Sand had checked that out with the helicopter on the way back to Warren Valley. No sign of a Goldwing out there anywhere near any of the major camps. He'd asked the Navajo Tribal Police to check further, but nothing turned up.)

There was a good chance he was just riding around somewhere feeling sorry for himself, the old man said. He liked to ride. Maybe that's what he was doing now. What do you want him for, the old man had asked. Sand said they only wanted to talk to him about a case, that he might know something about the death of a little boy.

The gun muzzle passed again, slowly this time and the weathered old thumb of the gun hand had rested on the hammer. Sand found he had taken a step back and sideways, had put the Navajo policeman between himself and the old man.

His face burned now as he thought of it.

You come down in a helicopter just to talk to my grandson. The old man shook his head. If he comes back I'll be sure and tell him that you were here to talk to him. With that he had cocked the pistol, a sharp, grating, metallic sound in the quietness of the big hogan. The Navajo policeman suddenly stepped away from Sand, leaving him staring into the flinty eyes of the old Navajo. They jostled each other a little, both trying to go through the door at the same time. The interview was over. Sand had learned all he was going to from Grandpa Tsosie. His skin crawled between his shoulders as he walked toward the helicopter. Would a Navajo shoot you in the back? In the old days they'd shoot you any old way and then eat your heart. Nobody had free passage across their lands. They still controlled them today, and these old men were less than a generation away from those who so ably defended their own against all comers.

Sand tried to maintain a little dignity and hurry up at the same time. So he only stumbled once on the way back. Ears burning, face red with shame, he'd heaved a huge, involuntary sigh of relief as the chopper cleared off old man Tsosie's land. When he caught up with Ben Singer........ Somebody was going to pay.....

He learned in Chinle that Ben had gassed up. bought food, and driven northward, toward Round Rock most likely. But the roads branched and he could have gone anywhere from there.

"Nobody has a clue about Singer's whereabouts at this time. Tribal police checked Navajo Mountain, no one else has seen him."

"You looked at Muley Point, then?"

"Yeah. For sure. That would have been the simplest. Had to stay back far enough so the pilot didn't spot two bodies by a wrecked truck. Congratulations, by the way .. There wasn't no bike there."

"Strange. Like the earth just swallowed him up, or something."

"He could pop up anywhere, anytime. He wasn't supposed to live. Not after the beating I gave him. What he knows about me. We got to get him."

"I don't see how we can find him by ourselves. This four corners country is just too big. Besides, we got a business to run. What you want us to do?"

"Run the business. I got plans for Singer. He's my special project. I'll set enough fires that no matter where he's holed up he'll get smoked out and have to run for it."

Virgil poked Herschel and pointed. Far out across the flat of Strawberry Valley a rooster tail of dust marked the progress of a vehicle toward their position.

"Somebody's coming, Dick. Our end's doing okay. We could sure use a payday, though."

"Okay, okay. You done good with things. I'll give you yours and half what Blinky had coming. That will keep you afloat for a while. Won't be long at all now before that big river of money gets aimed our way and you guys are my main men around here. We're going to be Warren Valley Developers ourselves. Whatever we put on the street there we get to keep outside of any deal with Monterro to ship stuff through here."

"Yeah, Dick. Sounds real good and that'll do us just fine .. for now. Thanks."

"Stay close to your phone. When Singer bolts from his hole I might need a little backup."

"We can do that. We'll be back in Fairfield in two days to re-supply and check over the equipment. That way we can come with what's best, depending on what you find out."

Sand swung the chain with the rifle cartridge around with a sharp twist of his hand. It smacked hard into his palm and his big hand closed over it. He glared at Herschel as he turned away.

"Maybe I'll just do it myself. I owe him something for all the trouble he's been "

Sand whistled up Prince, climbed into the suburban and drove away without a backward glance.

"He's doin' it again, Virg. Sure as sunrise Sand's getting tunnel vision and spending too much energy and attention on one little detail."

"I got a bad feeling about this. When that money comes in we best go to Devcon Ten and get us a hiding place to run to."

"We'll start with that segundo Monterro has looking out for northern Arizona. See if we can open an embassy there ..Just so long as Sand doesn't find out."

"We're walking on the dark side from here on out, Virg. Sand is nobody to have mad at you. If he finds out what we're doing he'll sure be mad."

"The only way we're likely to find out is when he starts shooting."

"Words to ...'

"Yeah, I know, I know.'

Virgil put the Rover in gear and the left by the back road that led eventually to Heber Valley and home.

****

"I just don't get it", Ben said. "Whereas the justice in this world? Dick Sand is a sociopath wearing a badge and a gun. How'd he ever get past the screening interviews and get hired?"

"Simple answer, Ben, is that he's not what he seems to be. He isn't stupid, just incredibly warped. He's playing a role, and doing it very successfully. What you call a sociopath is a genius at deceiving people."

"People like that have to be stopped. I always thought the law was the answer. I don't believe that any more."

Ben looked away, not meeting Axel's gaze, trying not to register the concern he saw in his eyes.

115

'Sand has murdered to get gain. He has crossed a river that cannot be recrossed. He has taken a darkening path that is its own punishment. But it leads to a far greater punishment in the end."

"He doesn't look to me like he's suffering at all. He's rich, powerful, and has a lot of influence. So much that he can get away with murder. And he can beat and humiliate people, torment them endlessly ..threaten the people they love. "The fact is people like him can't be touched by the law. They are the law."

"Stop dreaming, Ben. Get your head out of the clouds. This isn't a fairy tale. Life isn't a playground where you make your own rules. Choices have consequences. We have power to choose given us. We are not given the power to chose the consequences of our choices. Wisdom lies in taking counsel from those who know the attendant consequences. Bad, Ben bad, thinking like this."

"Yeah? Well it's hard to think any other way when I see what's going on."

"Men are left to choose, at first. Having chosen, as you chose to do good and try to prepare yourself to help other, consequences follow. You aren't dead. You have new choices to make that you earned the right to have. Part of those choices can prepare you to check Dick Sand and stop his evil."

"Bring him to justice? Put the law on him? Or just end his miserable life?"

Ben felt his voice shaking with the power of the hate he felt for Dick Sand.

"Just as there is a way to do evil there is a way to do good. You are being offered a chance to learn that way."

"To get Sand."

"To learn how to check evil in the world."

"Yeah, whatever."

Axel gazed off up the canyon. Withdrawn and distant, like the dark hump of Navajo Mountain. He sighed heavily and turned back to Ben.

"You can acquire two things from this, Ben.. One, the physical power your father had. We talked about those theories yesterday. You'll have to suspend your judgment until I can teach you how to apply them yourself. That's the test of all truth. How it works for each of us."

Ben looked squarely at Axel, masking, he hoped, his disbelief.

"The other?"

"The Way of the Warrior. The true Warrior, not the bloody butchers of story and legend. The way of men who fought for good causes and defended the defenseless. Not men constantly at war, but those who knew how to make and keep the peace."

"The good guys."

"Just so."

"The knights in shining armor."

Axel frowned, sensing ridicule in Ben's voice. He rose effortlessly from his sitting position and strode to the stream, fell forward into a push-up position and lowered himself to drink deeply. Ben was impressed by the amount of muscle such a relatively small man had in his back and shoulders.

If I were as strong as my father . If I don't have to sign up for some army of Boy Scouts to get it .maybe I should let him tell his story. What he's said so far about muscles and stuff makes some sense. But where does it go from there? How does it affect me?

Axel came back and sat down again, crossing his legs, leaning forward with his forearms on his knees, his back ram-rod straight. He gazed directly at Ben and for the first time, in the mild sunlight filtering through the trees, that Axel's eyes were golden brown, the gold appearing as flakes in the rich brown iris. Ben had never seen eyes like that before

"After you are tutored you will be tested. Physically and mentally, to the limit of your knowledge and power. To the level of character you must have to be accepted as a true warrior."

Axel's voice was sober, but firm and vibrant.

"To find out how you'll choose when you have power, when you can make things go your way.

"But remember this, Ben," Axel's look was so direct that his eyes fairly glittered in the morning sunlight. "If there's nothing in you, no true dedication to the right, if you're only playing a role, you'll end up only a strongman like Dick Sand, and your father. If you serve only your selfish interests you'll never find your way to the powers and the influence and the honor of a true warrior for the Whitehouse Society. When the time comes, you won't be fit to join them. You'll be checked, just as Sand will be."

Axel shifted again so that Ben could see that the twinkle and the smile were back.

"You've chosen well this far, Ben. If you hadn't I wouldn't be here now. I just want you to understand that you will now get new choices. Make them carefully. Don't be casual or off-handed about anything. Watch out for the pit falls. I know you can do it."

Ben almost got up then and walked back up to the shelter. There he'd given up the struggle to choose and it was tempting just to go back and wait quietly for the end. That would be the easy way.

Then he saw TJ again, in the hospital bed, wired up for his short journey out of life and he saw Terry's face, white, pulled out of shape by the emotions loose within her as he pulled away that awful day he left Warren Valley. Ben felt his old sense of injustice and outrage well up in him again. There's more than one way to die, he thought. I'm going to die trying.

"I don't know if I can or not." He still couldn't bring himself to call this man "Axel". "But I want to try. For TJ and the others."

And for myself, he thought as the blood leaked back into his cheeks and made them burn with the shame he felt. If there's a way to destroy Dick Sand I want to know what it is. And how I get it.

"Just show me what to do and I'll do it."

Axel smiled a wistful smile like he had just heard a small boy swear to kill the bogey man.

"Fair enough, Ben. Lets get on with it.

BEN SINGER STARTS LEARNING HOW

"We talked theory before, Ben. Now we'll start working. These are some of the things you need to know to start building the power your body is capable of creating for you."

"First, there are, for all practical purposes, two major muscle systems that hold and move our bodies. Though you must remember that some muscles can perform in either system.

"One system is isometric, primarily pulling against bone and the opposition of other muscles to hold some part of the body in a certain fixed position. This provides a platform or a foundation for isotonic muscle groups that act as prime movers. They move the body and assist the body to move other things. They also do important repetitive functions such as breathing."

Axel pointed to the smoothed sand patch again. Ben looked and saw a world heavy weight champion weight lifter. Ben had seen him on TV. at the Olympics or somewhere. He was huge. With a massive belly that struck Ben as being ridiculous and out of place in a man who was so powerful.

"That's right," Axel said. "But think it through now. The central set of bones in a body is the spine. It has to support any weight that he lifts. The huge belly muscles are the isometric secret of his power."

Isometric, Ben thought. That means that they hold the bones of the body in place while the isotonic or work muscles move things. In this case, he's moving the equivalent weight of a small car.

"They support the spine, take the forward curve out of it and make it straight enough to support the tremendous downward pressure of the weight he's pressing over his head. The size and strength of those muscles are a measure of his ability to fixate his spine and to lift the loads that make him an unbeatable champion. Without them to support the spine and hold it in line he would crush the spinal discs and the nerves they protect. No matter how strong his arms, shoulders and back, without them to work isometrically to hold his spine and other major joints in place he would not be able to lift the weight he does."

Ben watched the solid steel bar sag under the weight of the great metal plates he was lifting. He thought of his father lifting and pushing over the old car at Navajo Mountain. He saw again his father's coat split and saw the corded knots of muscle standing out in his father's back and shoulders. He knew now that those were the isotonic muscles at work. Then, the sudden insight hit him and he saw his father walking past the truck again. How flat his belly was, but how thick his body was also.

The isometric muscle was there too, holding and supporting the body, liberating the strength in the isotonic system by holding the body correctly while they did their work. He had a new understanding and respect for the display of raw physical power he'd seen that day.

Ben snapped back from his reverie to see that the sand was sand again and to hear Axel speaking to him.

FIRST THINGS FIRST

"Isometric first, to hold the body correctly. Isotonic can only be properly learned and used after that. In fact, some muscles cannot really contract and perform their role properly till they have been stretched into position by the bones and the isometric system. That's why "natural" athletes get their reputation. They operate from a much better muscular foundation, with far better isometric support, than average people do."

Ben could see in his mind's eye how pathetic his own attempts at athletic activity had been. Weak, uncoordinated, embarrassing. Like your fight with Dick Sand. The shame was still there in him, just below the surface.

BODY "ZONES"—SHORTCUTS TO ISOMETRIC HOLDING

"A good way to think about this is to think of body "Zones". Areas of the body that have inter-related function. The body (torso, etc.) is a good example.

"The human torso has three parts: The pelvis area, the chest and upper body area, and between them the mid-section. The pelvis and the upper body have lots of bone to serve as points of attachment for the muscles. But the midsection does not. And that's where most people go astray."

Axel reached behind the picnic table and brought up the upper part of the skeleton. Ben's nerves started to crawl again, but he noticed that the bones were lifeless and he let himself relax a little. Axel arranged the bones so that Ben was looking sideways at the upper body.

"Most of what I'm going to tell you is common knowledge in one discipline or another. It's just that people don't make the connections they should to tie it together into a system. And ordinary people are pretty much like your. They just don't think about it. That's because they don't know what it could do for them.

"The spine is the foundation of the body. It has to be supported properly or nothing else works right. As you can see, the lower spine here has a large forward curve. Too large. Weight bearing down from above puts great pressure on it. To take out the bad part of the curve and just as importantly, to support the spine properly so that the isometric muscles of the rest of the torso can do their work properly, you have to do two things."

Axel took hold of the pelvis and lifted up the front of it. As he did Ben saw the lower vertebra of the spine move backward and the curve became smaller. He noticed that the upper part of the spine took on an upright, gently curving arc and that the head of the skeleton came upright above the spine instead of hanging forward.

He also suddenly became aware that his belly was sagging limply outward and that his upper body was bent forward, his chest sunken in and he was resting almost the full weight of his body on his elbows, which rested on his knees. He tried to set up straight.

"If you want to get it right I'll show you how."

Axel's smile was still accepting and friendly. Ben looked again at the straightness of Axel's body and felt the rumpled, lumpy thing he called his own. I'm a mess, he thought.

"You need to be very careful from this point on. We'll talk about the basics, but you need to consult a doctor before you start re-arranging yourself, especially your back. It can be dangerous to try to undo the habits of a lifetime in a short time. Remember, I'm not Yoda, and you aren't Luke Skywalker. I can give you choices. But you must choose and assume the responsibility for your choices."

Axel pulled Ben's tarp off the bike and smoothed it out on the ground.

"Most of what I'm going to tell you is common knowledge in one discipline or another. It's just that people don't make the connections they should to tie it together into a system. And ordinary people are pretty much like you. They just don't think about it. That's because they don't know what it could do for them."

Axel lay down on the tarp. He raised his knees and pressed his backbone against the ground. As he lowered his knees his backbone stayed flat against the tarp. His belly not only didn't stick up, it seemed a little hollow. He arose in one smooth movement and said:

"If you want to try this you can. People are told to do it against the wall sometimes too. Now days, with camcorders, people have a great opportunity to see what they are actually doing."

Ben saw a camcorder/VCR assembly and a small screen T.V. setting on the ground near the bike. The red light was on on the camera. He shook his head a little as he lay down on the tarp. For him it was awkward, he had to roll from side to side a little and when he lay back it seemed to cut off his breath. He felt ridiculous and uncomfortable. His knees were already raised because he felt an uncomfortable strain in his lower back and his belly.

"Notice the position of the hips, the pelvis, Ben. Most people let the front of the pelvis sag forward. To make your spine touch the tarp you have to pull up the pelvis with the muscles in the front of the lower abdomen. You flatten the upper middle part of your spine by pressing backward with abdominal muscles higher up. You might get it right by pretending that you are trying to gently push your belly button up against your spine."

Ben felt this, a definite muscular effort was taking place down there somewhere.

"Whole sets of abdominal and lateral muscles are designed to act as fixators just to hold the spine."

Ben was trying to listen, but his breathing was coming in painful gasps and muscles in his chest were starting to burn and hurt. He realized that he was now using those muscles to breathe with and they weren't used to it.

"Try pushing down with your diaphragm, Ben, to relieve some of the pressure on your breathing."

"Huh?" Ben didn't know he had a diaphragm, let alone how to push with it.

"The muscle right at the bottom of the ribs."

"When you grunt you push down with it. Push it down gently but steadily and hold it there."

Ben did, grunting lightly to get it right. Pushing down relieved some tension in his chest, but he still had to breathe with the muscles on the sides and back of the rib cage and they didn't like it. And pushing down seemed to force some of his belly muscles to lock up hard and tight and the ones pulling up the pelvis and the ones pushing back on the upper middle spine were strongly contracted. He used the muscles in his middle abdomen to push his spine down against the ground. In a few moments he felt absolutely miserable from all the muscles that were aching. But he also felt a peculiar sense of rightness, of proper alignment and support for his body. He felt like more of a unit instead of a collection of parts flapping around.

Axel helped him stand up. He immediately felt all the tension leave his mid-section as the muscle groups relaxed. He felt more awkward than ever.

"I notice that "abs" and "ab"crunches are all the rage today.

"There's more to stabilizing the spine properly than this. It helps to think of the body in zones. You couldn't do anything else if you tried to keep your mind on the activity of each muscle. Muscle groups are interrelated and you can learn to consciously energize or pattern key muscles that will 'force' the rest to do their jobs. That frees your mind to take care of your daily activities.

People instinctively know this is a key area of the body. They just don't know it takes more than sitting up exercises to bring it under control."

Axel looked at Ben again, in the direct, calculating way he had sometimes.

Axel patted his behind.

"These muscles are called "glutes" in the weight training game, or buttocks. They are a key factor in the body zone that extends from the knees to the bottom of the rib cage. This is the critical zone because so much of how we handle it is under our control. And what we do with it determines whether other muscle groups have a fixated platform to operate from, whether we are forced to breathe with the muscles designed for breathing, and whether or not we do things with the muscles designed to do them or if we simply hang our body on our joints and ligaments."

"You contract these muscles to roll the front of your pelvis up, smooth out the front of your lower abdomen, and to fixate all the joints in the hip and pelvis region. These, and the muscles they cause to energize, cushion the movements of the walking and sitting muscles and keep the pelvis centered correctly under the lower spine."

"When you sit, you sit on the buttocks like pillows. If you have to, raise yourself up off the seat on your hands with your feet straight out in front of you, energize those muscles, and then sit down with them under you. You'll then have the spine sitting properly on the sacrum and you can use the abdominal muscles to push the lower middle spine backwards, just as you do when laying down. That takes the forward curve out of it. It calls into play the muscle groups below the rib cage. If you push yourself up by pushing down hard against the seat, push the spine back with the abdominal, and push the diaphragm down and far as you can and hold it you'll have it just right."

Axel demonstrated, sitting on the tarp and gathering his buttock muscles under him. He sat taller than Ben expected. Ben had often noted that people who were shorter than he was when standing actually were on a level with him, or even taller when sitting.

He sat down and did an awkward imitation of Axel's movements. He found that by pushing down against the ground he could push himself upright. Pushing down his diaphragm locked up the muscles in his abdomen and he then used them to force his lower spine backward. He again found himself almost panting as the muscles around his chest started working to do the breathing for him. He felt muscles that he'd only felt before when he was out of breath from exercise or rapid walking.

In a few minutes his whole torso was one burning, hurting column of pain. Not sharp, but pervasive. And he noticed that he had to concentrate almost exclusively on the middle abdomen muscles. If he didn't, they relaxed.

And when they did, the results were interesting. His chest immediately stopped working to pump air in and out of his lungs. Instead, the relaxed abdominal muscles moved in and out to breathe for him. The diaphragm became involved also, and when it did, the whole middle part of his body sagged forward and outward, even though his buttocks were still supporting his pelvis, except that he could feel it tilting forward on him.

> "There are no shortcuts, Ben. Atrophy is a basic principle of life. Muscle has to be exercised or it grows weak. Naturally strong people are getting exercise. They pay their dues just like the weight lifter. It's just that they use the systems the way nature intended for them to be used. The muscles that get exercise are the ones designed to do the work.

He had to lean back on his hands as waves of nausea and weakness swept over him. He hadn't regained even his normal strength after his long fast, let alone enough strength to keep up this physical effort. He looked over to see Axel smiling at him in an

Warrior's Way

"I warned you" way.

Axel gave Ben the canteen and he took a long swallow. He was surprised to see that he was sweating, and the cool water felt great going down.

"Those muscles will grow strong incredibly fast if you eat well and get plenty of rest. I'm surprised that you can do as much as you can already."

Yeah, Ben thought. I was great. The Dough Boy rises. He smiled to himself. Maybe he could take some yeast, rise like bread dough. He looked up to see Axel rewinding the tape on the VCR. In a moment he saw himself, sitting up, pushing up tall. He was amazed! Flabby as he was, he saw that a lot of what hung on his body was muscle tissue that was simply being allowed to dangle when it wasn't used. When stretched and held upright by the isometric system he assumed almost an athletic shape. He noticed the breathing barely showed, just a rising and falling of the shoulders and upper chest.

But he remembered the power he had felt in the upper shoulders, upper chest, neck and back. It was fleeting, but the memory had lasted.

"Now you can begin to see what I've been saying," Axel said.

"You need to start watching people, analyze what they do. You'll see the whole spectrum of humanity from people who simply hang their bodies on their bones to men and women who use both systems of muscle management almost to perfection.

"Jack Palance, the movie star, naturally does a lot of this. You see him at his best in an old move "The Silver Chalice" with Paul Newman. Palance almost gasps as he breathes and you can see costal breathing at its best. When he played in "City Slickers" he was in his seventies and could still do one arm push-ups. His isometric systems are locked on day and night and the strength goes on year after year without any special exercise on his part.

"Few people are in to isometric exercises. Standing around holding yourself in certain ways is not exciting. Nobody denies that they produce power. You hold the muscle against the pull of gravity. It fixes joints and bones and forms a platform for prime movers like the breathing system built into your chest and rib cage.

"Without the isometric systems the isotonic systems just don't work right. You end up exercising them to keep from getting flabby and out of shape instead of working out to increase your athletic performance."

"When you have to work out to "get in shape" and to perform at your sport you're at a great disadvantage to the people who have ..are you ready for this? A great, "build" Your term for a "naturally" athletic build or body that lends itself to training for sport."

Axel was looking at Ben again like his was a pirate telling Ben where he'd hid his greatest treasure.

"Most people don't know how to do this. And if they did, the vast majority are too lazy to do it. In fairness - its hard and uncomfortable and tiring. If you don't have some idea of what it can do for you, it just doesn't seem worth the effort. It takes time to build up the strength to do it 24 hours a day. Most people won't go through the hassle unless, like in the old days, it's a matter of living or dying.

Axel looked wistfully up the canyon. Perhaps he was thinking of the people who lived and fought and died here a thousand years ago.

"Lots of athletes get "out of shape" as they get older. The "pot" belly is almost a standard with men. All it shows is that they've lost the patterning in their abdomen and pelvis. Usually it comes from sitting poorly and from inactivity and loss of muscle tone.

"But there are older people who still have the natural trimness and fitness, and energy that belies their years. "

FIT NOT FAT - IGNORE THE FAT - DO THE MUSCLE -

1. TAKES MUSCLE TO BURN FAT
2. CONCENTRATE ON NOT GRATIFYING YOUR APPETITES.
3. THE EXERCISE WILL CUT DOWN ON THE APPETITE

"You can feel the difference between the calories you've been burning and the number you're going to burn to keep just these systems energized. You now have some idea why people who do even only parts of this don't have a weight problem. Its the person who does none of it who puts on weight while eating less than other people do.

"Think it over. I'm sure it will answer lots of questions for you that you never thought to ask before."

Axel looked at the western sky. The sun was down and the canyon was quiet in the twilight.

"I suggest you eat some more, Ben. You understand why now. I'll be around tonight to keep an eye on things again. You get all the rest you can.

"But, Ben?" Axel's face looked sober again and Ben felt a sinking inside him.

"As much as you can, lay so that you can gently energize your buttocks and abdomen and start pushing out on your lower back all that you can. You'll know when you have it right. Even when you can't do it all right, do all that you can, every bit will add to the building up, to the strength. It's not a matter of all or nothing. Half a loaf is better than none, every single thing you do helps."

Axel paused. Ben thought. No time to waste, that's what he means. Something's up with Sand . When I have it right? Yeah. When I'm forced to breathe with my chest. He nodded and got up to fill his canteen and find something to eat.

Choices. Chances. Something I can do. Instead of drink. Instead of dying It probably couldn't work. But it was something, a way to go on.

Ben turned back to Axel.

"Thanks, Axel. I appreciate what you're doing. Not just teaching me, but for being here when I really needed someone."

Axel said nothing, but his smile deepened and he nodded, a big, dynamic man, charged with something more than physical energy. What Ben said seemed to affect him, to add to his energy and his cheerfulness. Ben's words mattered. Ben's gratitude was received like a gift. As he moved away Ben decided that Axel came from a society where every person was an important individual.

His Grandpa Tsosie would approve of that. It was a good Navajo thought.

Chapter 15
Death Is In The Details

Note To The Reader:
Before beginning this chapter you should read Appendix A which is placed at the back of the book. I have found that most readers need more explanation than can be woven into the story. This detail will be found in the Appendix.
Now, on with our story!

"Terry!"

Terry recognized Rhettas voice and put her head down, trying to lose herself in the crowd headed for the Student Union Building. It was lunch time and young appetites were driving hordes of students to the food lines. But, of course it didn't work. With Rhetta it never worked ..

"TEEREEEE! Terry! Now you stop girl. This is important."

Terry's face burned as she saw the glints of speculation and interest in the eyes of those who knew her. Who knew what Ben had done to her. They fairly salivated as they waited for the next episode of the ongoing scandal of Terry and Ben.

Terry let out a big sigh and stopped and turned to see Rhetta almost levitating in her rush to catch up.

"Terry, honey you got to start listening for me. I can't be chasing you all over creation."

She put a fluttering hand up to her chest. With the other hand she made a dramatic, sweeping gesture pulling her rusty-red hair back over one ear. Getting her story straight in her mind, obviously pleased she had an appreciative audience hanging on every word.

Terry turned and started walking rapidly away from the crowd, intending to lead Rhetta someplace quieter. But Rhetta would not be denied her moment of glory. Terry felt her hand take her firmly by the elbow, almost spilling her books as Rhetta stopped her and turned her half around. Terry balled up her other fist and the look on her face knocked Rhetta back a step.

"Terry, why won't you let people help you. We all know your pain. You just won't let us in .."

"What is it, Rhetta."

Terry felt the bite in her voice, getting past her determination not to give Rhetta anymore excuse to lecture her in front of her classmates.

Rhetta smoothed her hair again, making sure she was ready, on stage, to deliver her lines.

"Ben's alive, Terry-"

Shock radiated through Terry like a level 8 earthquake. Suddenly her knees went weak and she tottered sideways. Rhetta reached out and put an arm around her waist for support. She bent over, looking earnestly into Terry's face.

"They said he was dead. It was on the news. Dick said so too."

"Dick Sand called to tell you, but you weren't home. I thought he knew your schedule, that you'd be in class. But maybe he couldn't wait. He didn't want you to hear the rest of it on the news."

"The rest of it? What are you talking about, Rhetta. The rest of what?"

Terry had forgotten her classmates, had forgotten everything in the sudden rush of conflicting emotion that stormed over her when she heard Ben was still alive.

"They got a manhunt out on him now. He's wanted for murder. Maybe more than one murder. Two men found at the bottom of a cliff in Monument Valley and .and maybe TJ. Oh, Terry. I'm so sorry. I just always told you there was something about him that wasn't right. Didn't I tell you that? Oh honey ."

Terry jerked away, struggling to juggle her books and papers and fled across campus. Headed for her room. She didn't see Rhetta, feet splayed, hands on hips gazing after her, sadly shaking her head. Finishing an almost perfect, triumphant tour de force performance.

Easily one of her best ever.

****

"Good morning, Ben. How did you sleep?"

Axel's voice startled Ben from his delicious vision of Dick Sand's destruction. Quickly he emptied his mind, then fought to bury his rage. He glanced up and then quickly away. Axel could read his thoughts, or somehow knew what he was thinking

"Fine .I guess. Yeah, it was a good night. Thanks for keeping watch. I guess you didn't sleep much "

Why Axel seemed to need no food or rest was just another of the many mysteries about him. When he rolled over to get up Ben felt stiff and several muscle groups around his chest and shoulders were sore.

He had arranged himself each time he woke up, tucking his buttocks up under him to tip his pelvis up in front, and pushing back with his stomach muscles to push his spine outward, taking the forward curve out of his middle back and locking his diaphragm down so he could only breathe in his upper and lower chest. Each time he woke up he found that he had to do it all over again. As soon as he stopped concentrating and dozed off, the muscles in his torso, around his belly button, relaxed. When that happened he stopped breathing with his chest. The isometric system dropped out and he was his old, flabby self again.

But finally, toward morning, muscle cramps in his rib cage and upper back muscles woke him up and he found that he'd actually been holding himself properly even while asleep. Good enough, at least, that he had to breathe with his chest instead of his belly. That explained the sore muscles. He'd been exercising even when he was asleep

He felt pleasantly tired. Like he had done a day of yard work or had followed the family sheep all day. And he was hungry, almost ravenous.

Axel smiled from across the shelter.

"How's the body today?"

"I can feel some muscles talking to me, but it sure isn't the way I feel when I overdo it at work and end up with sore muscles that hurt for three days."

He stopped a moment and consciously tucked in his buttocks, which brought up the front of his pelvis, and pushed down with his diaphragm and back with his abdominal muscles toward his backbone until he felt everything lock up and he was breathing in his chest. There was some muscular strain, but it felt like mild exercise feels, stretching, limbering, good. And he felt an absence of pressure on joints, ligaments, and nerves that was very pleasant.

WHY YOU GO TO "POT"

"If you do it right, put the load on the right muscles they will grow strong surprisingly fast. You body's circulation, digestion, and metabolism are all designed to support you when you do it right. No artificial exercise can even come close to exercising every key muscle group in just the right amounts the way energizing your isometric systems can. That way moving and working with the body, a firm platform of joints and bones being held in place by muscles, function isometrically, statically."

"The other benefit is that it forces other muscles to exercise and strengthen themselves isotonically. When you have to breathe with the chest it develops strength in the chest, shoulder girdle, neck, and back.

"The first step downward for aging athletes is usually that they let the belly sag, the pelvis tips forward, and the breathing drops out of the chest. In a matter of a couple of weeks the muscles atrophy and weaken to the point that many lazy people just slack off and let nature or gravity take its course. An injury, even a temporary one, or a sick spell that keeps you in bed for a while can trigger this let down. If you don't understand these principles you can't recover your former fitness. You often go down hill from there."

Axel glanced at the early morning sun. Then he looked down the canyon, the way Ben had come in. Ben wondered if he was hearing something from his directors.

Then Ben heard the far-off sound of a helicopter. Axel reacted by scooping up the tarp, throwing it over the bike and camp gear, and running for the shelter.

Ben had been conditioned too well by his Navajo upbringing to stand around gazing open mouthed at the sky or asking stupid questions. He followed Axel as quickly as he could, feeling clumsy, his shoulder, not fully healed, still burning a little as he pulled himself upward.

Maybe Axel was concerned about time, or maybe he'd been expecting something like this all along, Ben thought. He clambered into the shelter and moved into the shadows near the boulders at the back. The air burned in and out of his lungs as he labored to get his breath. His heart was beating so hard he could feel it in his chest. Axel was not even taking deep breaths. He peered out of the shelter, a worried look had replaced his normally cheery countenance.

Then the chopper crossed the canyon a hundred yards away and several hundred feet up in the air. It paused briefly above the canyon. Ben imagined someone looking for tracks along the bottom of the canyon. The witch wind took care of that, Ben thought. They won't see anything unless they spot the bike.

The chopper soon moved on.

"Just a sweep search," Ben said. "Who would they be looking for, anyway?"

Axel didn't answer, he only motioned toward the back wall of the shelter. Ben saw it glow and turn into a video screen.

He felt the skin crawl on his neck. Every time I start to think of Axel as human, Ben thought, he does something like this.

Ben saw himself stopped at Deer Flat. The new Ford truck roared past, followed moments later by the sheriff's patrol van.

Then the scene shifted. Ben saw the truck at the turnout at the top of the Muley Point cut off. Two men were scanning the road a thousand feet below with bulky looking binoculars. The police van pulled in behind them, the bumpers almost touching. Ben saw the deputy behind the wheel reach down and shift into four wheel drive.

"You see him?"

The voice crackled with radio static. One of the men in the truck picked up a microphone.

"Not a sign of him."

The voice held the strain of a man who had lost something of great personal value.

"He must have gotten through. We'll have to run down to Chinle. See if we can catch him there."

It dawned on Ben that they were talking about him.

The backup lights went on as the driver put the truck in reverse. Both men turned and looked back at the men in the police van.

"What did Sand tell you about that?" the deputy said.

The van pulled forward with enough force to slide the truck to the very edge of the drop off.

"He told you he'd have to give you up, didn't he."

The van surged forward as the screaming men in the truck dove for the doors. Ben felt the shock rip through him as he watched.

The truck shot over the lip and began its seven hundred foot plunge to the sandstone and junipers below. The men made it out of the Ford only just in time to fall alongside it.

The sheriff's van shot down the grade, racing to overtake Ben, even as he was riding up behind them. Ben saw them again, charging across the flat, lights flashing, turning left toward Bluff and the cutoff he had planned to take.

As the scene faded Ben felt sweat leaking down his back, wetting his forehead and hands.

Hanksville was no mistake. The deputy there had reported seeing Ben. When they learned Ben was alive, not dead in the campground, they had rushed to find him. The men who failed were executed. Ben shook a little as his scholar's mind started seeing how neatly the pieces of the puzzle fit together.

He was supposed to die all along. Sand had run him off, fully intending to kill him. Everything he had done to Ben was to get him to leave. Sand had never meant for him to live out his life somewhere else.

He sat down abruptly. They knew he was still alive, that he was not at Chinle. The chopper was looking for him. If they found him, they had the poisoned hand. They could kill him. Ben was sure Sand had never intended to let him live. Only to get him away far enough to kill him and make it look like an accident.

He was deeply insulted. He refused to excuse Sand's actions just because yesterday Ben had been killing himself. He knew the emotion was strange. But it was powerful and deep. Who did this Dick Sand think he was, anyway?

He looked at Axel, who looked back, very sober for once, the smile wrinkles almost gone.

"Why me?" Ben said.

"You're in the way, Ben. Not so much for what you know as for what you are. What you'd do. The intelligence with which you'd do it."

Ben shook his head. Unbelievable.

"What do we do now?" he said.

"I don't know," Axel said.

"You don't know?"

Ben heard the rising note in his voice. Surprise? Panic?

"I guess first you need to know that there is no `we', Ben."

Ben was flabbergasted. He felt his face slacking around his mouth and realized that his mouth was hanging open. He shut it abruptly.

"You said trust me, walk with me, let me help you. And all the time you knew they were trying to kill me."

Ben tried to put disgust and outrage in his voice. It came out somewhat like a mouse squeaking defiance at a tomcat.

"You don't understand yet Ben. There are limits to what I can do, to what I can know. Within those limits I will help you every bit that I can."

Ben heard himself snort.

"Why don't I feel better?"

"There's much you don't understand yet. That's where I can help."

He paused, as if listening again.

I hope you hear something useful, Ben thought. He was hungry and aware that he'd forgotten all about isometrics and isotonics. His body sagged like a gunny sack full of bones and guts. It didn't seem to matter much, if he was going to be dead sometime later in the day. Part of him listened intently, straining to hear the sound of rotary wings beating the air.

Axel turned to him.

"Can you be trapped in this canyon? Is there only one way out?"

Why are you asking me? You know so much. Didn't you notice on your way in? Or did you just pop out of thin air?

"There's only one way out if I take the bike. If I climbed out on foot anywhere I'd be miles from water or help, out in the open on the desert. An easy target from a chopper."

Ben liked the feel of saying `chopper'. It made him feel a little like Rambo. Except that he knew he was a rabbit being hunted by professionals. By professional murderers with wings.

Ben thought it over, adding up what he was learning about Sand's operation. Obviously Sand monitored the law enforcement radio net, maybe over several states if he was up high and had a powerful radio and listened at night.

Ben didn't have to puzzle for even a moment on that one. Sand patrolled the high country, claiming that he loved the outdoors. He lived in a palatial mountain cabin somewhere up behind Mount Timpanogos. He had back road access from there to the rim of the Colorado Plateau at 11,000 feet to the east, or Mt. Nebo out in the valley, which was just as high and looked off to the west and south.

It seemed he also had an organization in Utah, and perhaps in other states. Some of his people apparently were in law enforcement and some were not. The one's in law enforcement seemed to be planted in sheriff's departments. Ben puzzled over what Sand was engaged in.

What advantage does Sand gain by having people who travel out in the counties, away from settled areas? I don't know what he's doing. Without knowing how can anything else make sense? Ben could find no immediate answers.

He also couldn't figure out where he could go to escape from Sand's people or to keep from being spotted by them as he moved over the few roads that stretched through wide open country where in places you could see for a hundred miles.

"How can I stay alive?"

His voice startled him.

"I don't know, Ben" Axel said. "What I do know is that we have time today. Here. But you should be giving some thought today to what you'll do tomorrow, and the day after that. They're eliminating places where you might be very quickly.

Apparently they have the manpower to do that very efficiently."

Ben felt a sinking feeling in his stomach. Something had shifted in their relationship. Yesterday Ben had been almost helplessly dependent on Axel. Now he found that he couldn't lean on him at all. For just a moment he regretted his decision to live. Then he deliberately straightened up and re patterned his body.

But I don't want to die now, either, Ben thought. A feeling of muted anger filtered through his body. Axel is a trainer, or perhaps a coach. But he can't play the game, he can't tell me what to do by looking in his version of the Crystal Ball. Axel is just a tool. Maybe a weapon I can use against Sand. He's not my savior. Just my friend.

"I guess I was lucky. Getting this far I mean. The storm, being afraid to be seen near Warrren County, pulling out at Deer Flat, even not staying with Grandpa."

"Whatever it was, Ben, you can use it now."

Axel smiled as he glanced up at the sun.

What else do you know that you haven't told me about all this, Ben thought. Why are you holding back? Who sent you, and if their power is reflected in your power why can't you help me against Sand?

Axel looked at Ben, a little wistfulness crept into his eyes, even though the smile stayed firm and friendly.

"Why don't you eat, Ben. I have a lot to tell you, some of it is just as important and just as little known as what I told you yesterday. You can't make good choices till you see more clearly what your choices are."

Ben nodded. He stepped to the entrance and started down. The great white house seemed to float above the cottonwoods, highlighted strongly by the sun that had at last risen high enough to clear the eastern rim of the canyon. The great building seemed distant and majestic, and unreachable to Ben as he trudged down to the bike, still half listening for the sound of the metal wings that carried killers with poison hands.

* * *

Ben couldn't find a lot to eat. He usually only carried some canned goods and a few things to make a meal or two out of if he broke down somewhere. But he had pork and beans and plenty of chocolate and powdered milk. He soaked dry bread in the milk and made a reasonable meal. But tomorrow he would have to leave here to get more food or start to starve again.

When he finished he leaned against the bike again, leaving it half covered by the tarp in case the helicopter came back. He noticed that clouds were building in the west again. It was spring and good weather never lasted more than a few days. He saw the high cirrus clouds coming that always moved in ahead of a cold spring storm. Tomorrow or the next day it would storm and then turn cold again. He wasn't very well prepared for that.

He also knew that the weather might give him cover so he could move. If he could decide where to go.

He felt his arms and hands tingle. He had realigned his midsection and pelvis as he came down the slope. He liked the feeling of the solid, integrated power he felt in his movements when the isometric system locked in his spine and hips and back.

Now, looking down he saw the veins in his arms and hands standing out prominently. That was something he'd noticed in strong men and in some athletic or graceful women. He'd seen it in himself only while exercising. As his mind checked the sensations coming from various parts of his body, one by one, he could feel muscle working all over. Legs, chest, upper back, and especially in the abdomen. He found he couldn't slouch backwards against the bike and still keep his back and pelvis in balance. He had to sit up fairly straight, like Axel did, and rest lightly against it.

Muscles in his upper back, shoulders, and neck were starting to burn and hurt. Exercise is exercise, he thought. As Axel says, there are no shortcuts. Just smarter ways of doing it.

AXELRON TELLS ABOUT THE WHITE HOUSE SOCIETY

Axel walked over and sat down, Indian fashion, in front of Ben. He was warm and friendly still. But Ben saw him now as a visiting foreigner who might soon return home, leaving Ben alone to struggle with the war against Sand.

"Not alone, Ben. Trust me on that. But right now we need to get your physical development underway.

"The Whitehouse stands for an idea, Ben." Axel spread the sand smooth in front of him. "Sometimes it's easier to see an idea by looking at it's opposite. People associate together. We don't like to live alone. It's hard to survive by yourself."

You got it, Ben thought. I'm alone. I wonder if I can make it.

He felt himself nodding in agreement.

"When people live together in groups a couple of things can happen. There has to be rules, and with rules there has to be enforcement. Some way to handle those who won't work by the rules.

"The only real peace and freedom come when individuals control themselves, voluntarily live the Golden Rule and then move beyond it, to love others first, and to serve them even if they haven't yet developed their potential for goodness. That requires an enlightened conscience and great self control.

"Too often you have men like Dick Sand. Driving, envious, ruled by passions and appetites, determined to rule at any cost. They create a Hell on earth for themselves and everyone who falls under their influence. I guess I don't have to tell you that." Axel looked at Ben.

Ben felt his eyes snap back into focus and realized he'd been reliving the events in the campground that night. He was feeling again his amazement at how callous, inhuman and unfeeling Sand was.

"I felt I was in the presence of evil that night," Ben said. "I didn't know there were people like that. I've met bad men. But no one like him."

"Like the Marines say, Ben. Nobody wants to fight, but somebody has to know how. Or as someone else once said: For evil to triumph it is only necessary for good men to do nothing.

"In every age good people have had to fight. Not always physically. Often they had to struggle to find and support good men and women in government. Look at Columbia today, nearly overrun by the drug cartels, judges and others guarded day and night, risking their lives to create a society that will nurture and protect its citizens and let them develop into decent human beings. (A more recent example is Iraq)

To simply be left alone, to live in peace. To build a society based in justice, honor, compassion, and personal liberty. Afghanistan is a perfect example of what happens when a group of tyrants get control and can impose their will by force. They have to be checked and resisted. Whether they are a nation or just one single, evil man."

Axel pointed up at the white house pictograph.

"The people who came here knew something of that. They lived peacefully with one another. But they were trained warriors, prepared to defend themselves. And they were running away from societies and governments like the Aztecs had in Mexico when Cortez arrived.

"The Aztec leaders were sacrificing people at a rate of ten thousand or more a year. Cutting out their hearts to make sure the sun rose each day. They were running away from societies like that."

Ben nodded.

"Most societies everywhere had governments that fed power to the few and misery to the many," he said. "Hitler is a good modern example of that."

"But many lives have been lived in peace, in compassion and love, also," Axel said. "It's just that history records the wars and repressions and ignores the good. The society expressed by these people here in this pictograph has existed many times and in many places."

Axel's smile lit up like fourth of July fireworks. His voice had a breathless quality about it.

"Now we're preparing to bring it back, permanently. A thousand years of peace. It will take the efforts of many great people. It will be done. You can be part of it. You can be a true warrior, Ben. One who works to establish justice, peaceful union, and equity among mankind."

"If Sand doesn't get me, you mean?" Ben felt the corners of his mouth pull down and a pucker gather between his eyes.

What good is high sounding words if I'm dead tomorrow? What is Axel? Some kind of cosmic recruiter looking for a few good men? I'm not a good man. I don't even like to fight. I just want my father's power. No more no less. And Dick Sand in front of me one more time ..

"If that happens, Ben, it happens. But we really need mortal men to help fulfill the promises and to help bring this about."

Ben shook his head, bewildered.

"We need you to try, Ben. If you want to. No one can force you, nor would we if we could."

Axel's smile seemed a little lop sided. Ben felt great uncertainty in the air. There were no guarantees.

No, that was wrong. There was one iron clad certainty.

Dick Sand was going to kill him. There was no remote and peaceful canyon where Ben could go to live out his life in peace. Sand was his enemy. Sand was hunting him even now.

And I don't even know why, I don't have a clue.

He felt a warm rage flood through him, warming his limbs and flushing his cheeks. Maybe I can't stop him from doing that to me. He felt his mind shutting down, narrowing its focus and closing off some of the more civilized parts of him. Something of the old Apache coming to the front of his mind. But I don't have to die like a sheep. I don't have to lay down belly up and show him my throat.

Ben felt his body harden as muscles that had been steadily exercising themselves while he and Axel talked, suddenly contracted strongly, pulling his body into line, raising his head erect, setting his neck against the back of his collar. Making his arms and hands tingle. Making him feel the beginnings of power and strength. He imagined his father, his erectness and grace. He imagined himself becoming like that. It felt good as he clenched and unclenched his fists.

He saw Axel move back a bit as he stood up. He locked his knees and felt his body growing longer as he stretched himself to his full height with his gut and pelvic muscles taking the forward curve out of his spine, making it feel like he was stretching his lower back wider, from side to side.

His breath came in almost panting gasps as the breathing started high in his chest, just under the collar bone, and lifted his chest high before the sides of the rib cage expanded to finish the breath. He felt the pull in chest, shoulders, and back. He felt power.

He looked at Axel.

"I don't have to play rabbit for Dick Sand's dogs."

He was amazed at the tone quality he heard in his voice as it reverberated in his chest and was supported by the strength of his breathing. And his anger.

"Maybe I'm a dead man. But I can make Sand pay a price to get me under the ground. He'll know I wasn't a push over. And if he makes a slip ."

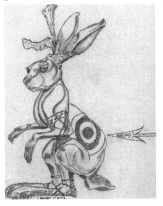

Ben felt his fingernails digging into his palms until the pain shot up to his elbows. His vision was narrow, focused, and red-lined with hate.

When he turned his gaze to Axel he saw a worried look had replaced the grin.

You're sitting on the sidelines on this, aren't you, Ben thought. You can't play, and you can't tell me how to play. If I take care of Sand do I get the credit? How does this work, anyway?

"Be careful, Ben," Axel said. "New choices always open up new roads to your destiny. Not every path should be taken. Some things should never be. Choose carefully because you can't choose the consequences of your choice."

"Sounds mysterious, Axel," Ben said, well aware that this was almost the first time he'd used Axel's name. "I don't see that I have all that much choice. Dick Sand's going to kill me if he can.

"That simplifies everything. I get him first. Or I make his life miserable before he gets me. Not many options there."

"Simpletons boil their options down to simple choices, Ben. Then its easy to just forget yourself in action, pretending that you are only responding to the threats around you.

"That means your reacting, not acting. Others are dictating your actions and the pace at which you move. You're not free. And you won't be effective, Dick Sand will still be guiding you."

Axel stood and moved back, partially behind the bike. He stood with his feet planted firmly and his right side rotated to face Ben, his right arm hanging straight down from his shoulder. Ben got the impression that Axel was prepared for things to go either way, for Ben to come at him, or for them to go on with their conversation. Somehow it didn't seem to matter to him which way it went. He was ready.

Ben's muscles began to burn like they were near a fire. He felt the energy drain created by energizing his isometric systems. He wasn't strong enough yet to keep it up for long. Certainly not for twenty four hours a day. He had a feeling now for the strength that it would take. And he wanted it so bad it was an ache in his heart.

But he decided to let it pass that Axel had called him a simpleton. He let the anger drain down inside him to the reservoir of red hot lava that burbled deep in him. He let it simmer there and warm him with its glowing fire. But he put the lid on and firmly held it down with mental effort. Axel says he can☐t help me. I☐ll keep my own counsel, then. Just see what happens. I don☐t have to sign on with Axel and his silver knights I'll choose when the lid comes off. When I want it to, not when someone else tries to do it for me.

"I think I understand," he said. "I'm just a little off center. I could accept dying quietly, as my own choice. I can't get used to the idea of rolling over and playing dead for Dick Sand."

Axel nodded. The smile crept back, hesitantly.

"It's tempting to take the vengeance trail, Ben. That☐s one way open to you. You will be enticed in that direction, as part of your journey. I hope you'll think carefully as the new avenues open up to you. Freedom opens up possibilities for great accomplishment and miserable failures. Remember your father, Ben. Not just the power he had to lead and to fight."

Axel's voice was soft, almost like he was speaking at a funeral, talking about the dead. His eyes were a little glazed, unfocused for a moment as he gazed at some inward picture from the past, Ben supposed. Then they were boring into him, glittering again with fire and passion.

"The proper use of power is to defend the rights of the powerless, Ben. That's the straight and narrow path for the strong of heart. Any other way leads to becoming like Dick Sand and his kind."

THE GREAT SECRET OF BUILDING RAW PHYSICAL POWER

Axel smiled and shrugged a little and looked on down the canyon.

"Let's take a walk, Ben. When the isometric systems are on line, fully energized, walking is the exercise that forces the whole body into isotonic movement. Walking properly, under these conditions, is the activity that builds athletic strength and raw physical power into the body."

Ben felt himself grin ruefully. His muscles ached and burned and were slipping out of pattern on him until he felt like a juggler keeping ten plates spinning on tall, flexible sticks, running back and forth frantically as various ones began to wobble. Every time he took his attention from one area to try and correct the muscles sagging in another area the ones he wasn't watching would "wobble" and fall out of pattern on him. "I'm practically exhausted already. I don't know how much more I can do."

"You'll be amazed, Ben. Most fatigue is caused by muscles running out of oxygen and fuel. When you use big muscles, large muscle movements, your movements speed up blood circulation and help distribute new supplies of food and oxygen. When you use your back and shoulders to chop wood or saw with a buck saw you can keep up the movement much longer than if you put the stress on just your arm muscles.

"You need to learn the tricks, how to use the right muscles to move. You'll be surprised at how much strength you already have. You feel weak because you try to use the wrong muscle systems in your movements. And you don't support your movements with an energized isometric system so you can't unleash physical power.

"You're tired now mostly because you've been inactive. You need large muscle movement to spread the fuel and oxygen through your body and to clean up your system."

Axel moved around Ben and took a few steps down the canyon. He turned around and looked back at Ben.

"Lots of people exhaust themselves at work and then go home and work and play half the night. A change is as good as a rest, as they say. When you get tired doing one thing then do something else.

THE KEY THAT MAKES EVERYTHING ELSE WORK

"But you have to keep the isometric systems tightly energized. The pelvis has to be tilted up, the diaphragm locked down, the chest held high, shoulders pulled down, aiming for that slope shouldered look that marks the truly powerful natural strong man, the head held erect, on top of the spinal column, not weakly tilted forward, the breath high in the chest, the belly muscles and the lateral muscles pushing back against your backbone to take the curve out of your spine and to lock the bones and joints in position so the isotonic muscles have a rigid platform of muscle and bone to support their movements. Then the isotonic systems is forced to do its job. This makes you breathe, for example, with the chest muscles. You can't breathe with your belly if you are keeping the excessive curve out of your spine. Energizing the isometric system doesn't just exercise that system, it kicks whole isotonic muscle groups into gear too.

"You're better off to move around and try to keep it all going than you are to simply sit. Regular movement will clean out the circulation system and re-oxygenate the muscles. You can come to have the good, warm, relaxed feeling that you get after moderate exercise with you all the time.

BEN LEARNS TO WALK

"If you forget how it feels you can always lay down and get your spine down on the ground, lock your buttocks, then sit up or stand up and walk, holding as much of the pattern as you can for as long as you can.

"As soon as you can, start studying people. Find those who do some of this, observe how they sit, stand, and walk. You'll understand quickly and easily. That's the simple part. Paying the price to do it is another matter. At first it's hard. As it becomes more of a habit and the muscles grow stronger the feeling of power and grace become addicting. Then you're on you way."

Axel came back and stood looking up at Ben.

"You need to pick out people with body types like yourself to study the most."
BEWARE OF THE GENETIC CELEBRITY
"The old saying about horses is true of humans too: **TOPS MAY COME BUT BOTTOMS, NEVER.**

"Artificial exercise can build muscle in men and in horses. A horse may have magnificent muscle development if it's exercised right. But the place to look is at the bone structure of the legs, ankles, and feet. Good bone structure is a matter of genetic inheritance. Poorly aligned bones in a horse's leg causes an inborn weakness that no amount of exercise can overcome.

"Among people, genetic inheritance of bone, muscle, and body type limits what a person can become. Not every man will be a Tom Selleck in Quigley Down Under.

"You, like many men, are a descendant of men who had to survive in close hand to hand combat just to go on living. In many societies, built by selfish, greedy, power hungry men like Dick Sand, people had no choice but to fight well or die. There was a process of natural selection that weeded out the weak, the timid, the inadequate in many societies all over the world.

Ben imagined his father in armed combat, with sword and shield. Ben shivered a little as he imagined himself aligned against his father in battle. He felt a coldness in his belly, as though he were shrinking away from cold, cutting steel.

Axel looked at him soberly, a little respectfully perhaps.

"You inherited your body-bones, sinews, lung capacity, muscle size, basic disposition- from him, from your father, and from your fathers back through time.

"You'll never be tall and narrow hipped like Dick Sand. You'll never square up to him in height or reach. You're what people call, when they speak of horses, "close coupled". You have relatively shorter, heavier bones in the arms, chest, and shoulder and legs and back. You can unleash vastly more power than Sand can ever hope to command because of the mechanical efficiency of the power of your isometric systems to hold the shorter bones and joints more rigidly and the shorter, stronger isotonic movements that are possible for you.

"Sand could never make his body rigid enough to support the muscular effort needed to lift up and tip over a car. You could, if it suited you.

"Study yourself and others, develop the body you have to its peak potential and don't spend time mourning what you don't have.

Axel's smile was warm again.

LEARN TO BE THE BEST YOU YOU CAN BE

"Watch out for the genetic celebrity syndrome, Ben. The media people search for some sort of `perfect' body type and exploit it until everyone who isn't that type feels guilty, inadequate, unsure, worthless. That's just so much hype. Is that the word?" Ben nodded and Axel continued.

"The systems are there and work to some degree for everyone. The idea is to use them to be the best person you were meant to be. Build to your strengths, Ben. Ignore the weaknesses."

I suppose he's happy to be doing what he's supposed to do. He's more comfortable when he doesn't have to try to tell me how to survive long enough for any of this to do me any good.

"You have to be active for short periods every hour. Also, you need to get plenty of rest, a nap or two during the day if necessary, during the build up period. And a good diet that offers nutrition and building blocks for your body. It's not just muscle that has to get stronger. Ligaments have to thicken, and so does bone to support the new isometric strain. You have to furnish the raw material and rest your body enough to let the natural systems do their job of feeding and growing. This is especially true of ligaments that connect the glutes to the tail bone. You can hurt a lot if you don't give this area time to get strong before you get too active physically.

"But you are never as tired as you feel. Isometrics are boring and tiresome. That's why so few people benefit from them. Often, when you think you're exhausted you'll find that you are only hungry. A good nourishing meal will set you off again.

"Men can come to the gym tired from a day of work and still systematically lift ten tons as they go through an exercise routine. Remember that. Someday it could save you. You're never as tired as you feel."

WALK ON

"As with every physical movement, you have to support the effort of walking with a strongly energized isometric system. Especially the glutes and the obliques in the waist that take the curve out of the spine. This gives the walking muscles a strong platform to operate from and forces you to walk correctly, using the muscles designed to do the job.

"You will see an endless variety in walkers. I leave it to you to study them. But there's only one way to do it right.

"You stand with the pelvis pulled up in front, the gut muscles pushing backwards toward the spine strongly, the diaphragm pushed down and held as low down as possible, the glute muscles strongly energized and rolled up and forward.

The Diaphragm Is The Great Secret.

"Locking down the diaphragm is the real secret of getting things right. When you do it strongly it forces all the other systems to pattern themselves. You concentrate on the diaphragm and the rest takes care of itself.

"That's the beauty of the human body. If you had to think about every muscle it would be impossible. But anybody can think about one.

"But remember, if you don't push the belly button back strongly you can end up with a deep forward curve in the spine. You might be relatively strong and well built, but you'll have a bay window if you get fat and a major weakness in your body all the time. Dick Sand has this potential defect though at this time it doesn't show up."

Tell me about it. I sure didn't notice any defects that night at Tibble Fork.

"Every vital, naturally strong person, man or woman, has that gentle outward swelling of the middle and lower back.

"You've got to lock it down so you can't breathe in your belly. You've got to feel that chest working day and night, every breath. It is the foundation of muscle development, ligament growth, and real power.

"I think you can imagine what would happen to someone in a fight if they had to weaken their middle body in order to breathe. That's deadly. Literally.

"You feel the isometric contraction in three places:
1. In the buttocks
2. In the diaphragm
3. In the muscles of the stomach area as they push backwards against the spine. This modern exercise focus on the abdominal muscles is an instinctive recognition of their importance, but sit-ups don☐t even begin to strengthen them properly for their real role.

"If one and three are strongly done #2 locks the breathing into the chest and you have to breathe costally, that is with the rib muscles. Doing it 24 hours a day is the kind of gentle, steady exercise that can build strength incrementally, to amazing levels.

"And just as important, it builds the breathing capacity so that when you have to make extreme physical efforts the lungs can provide the oxygen you need. Again, a matter of living and dying. Isometric exercises build lean, enduring muscles that are powerful without being bulky. The many repetitions involved build in an ability to keep going long after others are exhausted. In a fight for life that is the difference between winning and dying.

"When you stand you rotate the buttock strongly up under your pelvis and hold it. That, plus pushing back with the lateral and obligues does the trick on the spine, then the diaphragm comes down and you lock your legs and push down hard and pull yourself as erect as you can. You won't feel that you are getting taller as much as feeling that you are puling the shoulder girdle down, and away from the neck, into the slope shouldered look that goes with real strength. You can actually stretch taller by relaxing the gut and diaphragm. But it's a false feeling.

"What you are actually dong when you do it right is pulling the shoulders down and back as you press the curve out of the spine and breathe in the chest. It details the upper body, pushing and pulling things into the right alignment.

"Study Woody Strode in Ghengiz Khan, Jack Palance in any movie. Arnold Schartenegger and Hulk Hogan are weight lifters so they've added muscle mass by artificial exercise. But both bodies are built on a powerfully energized isometric system that holds their bodies upright and undergirds their other movements.

"When you stand upright this way, with everything patterned and strongly energized, breathing in the upper registers of the chest and the middle part of the body locked up tight, the spine held tight and straight, you are putting out amazing effort. People who do this constantly seldom have a weight problem unless they gratify their appetite for food like a drug addict does for drugs."

WHY YOUR BODY BECOMES A FAT-BURNING MACHINE

"When you are ready to move you use what physical culturists call the "heel and toe" stride. There are books on the subject if you want to study more about it. But if you are properly holding yourself, walking correctly is natural and easy and you don't need a college degree to get it right.

"Like I told you before, you have to be careful not to out smart yourself and get your head into this too much. It's just something you do until it becomes a habit. It takes guts and dedication, not brains and money.

"When your middle body zone is locked in properly you'll have a tendency to use your upper body, from the hip bones up as one unit. You'll have great power in your back because of this. And when you walk, you'll tend to walk from the shoulder blades down.

"Many people, especially men, walk from the knees down. But when you are walking correctly you will feel the muscles working in your back clear up the to shoulder blades. At the same time your breathing is forced up into the chest. You'll find chest, shoulder and neck muscles are also getting a work out. Done properly, walking is a great strength developing exercise.

"And in front the gut muscles will be contracting and relaxing with each step. That's what makes walking properly such a strength producing activity. It strengthens and develops the muscle that has to support the spine when you unleash the power in your body.

"The isometric systems being energized is already creating strength in those muscles and then the isotonic exercises add to the exercise load and this can create the kind of power you saw your father use.

"The human body is an amazing thing, Ben. Designed by a Master. We use it so poorly. Just as we use the life we're given so badly sometimes. So little of our

Warrior's Way

potential is ever achieved during our stay in mortality."

Axel looked wishful. Did he miss being alive? Was he, therefore, dead? Ben couldn't answer that. It made him nervous.

"Anyway, to walk right, you have to use a key set of muscles that work for walking just like the diaphragm, properly used. It's the key to holding yourself properly with the isometric systems.

"You must learn to use your hips to throw your leg and foot forward. As you do, the leg joint bends naturally. Like a hinged board, flapping forward until the muscles in the front of the leg contract to slow it down, smooth out the movement, and as the muscles in the front of the lower leg contract to pull the foot up so the heel touches first, not a slapping, flat footed, clownish walk. But a movement cushioned by muscle. Think of the tiger. In the meantime the other leg has rotated backward, locked the knee and the foot is rolling onto the toes and the back foot is pushing off distinctly with the ball of the foot. The hips turn, the shoulders don't. You do a smaller, modified version of the famous hip/shoulder rotation exercise with every step you take.

"It exercises muscles all around the waist.

"Then the body moves out over the forward leg and the hip with the back leg is "thrown" forward sharply to throw the other leg out ahead.

"You can imagine this being jerky and stupid. But in a powerful man or a graceful woman it is not jerky. Muscle contraction smooths out every motion. The movement is steady, sedate, calm, regal.

Ben saw his father striding across the parking lot and nodded.

"There is nothing "sexy" about this, either. It isn't the exaggerated, mincing walk of a model. You can see it in football players and it is manly, graceful, and utterly powerful. The power of the muscle contractions is the key to this.

"Toddlers often demonstrate the walk perfectly. And they hold the buttocks muscles together properly. Few adults even come close. And more women than men tend to walk correctly this way.

"Start watching other people now that you know what to watch for and you'll find lots of bad examples and occasionally very good ones.

"You have a natural sense that physical trainers call the kinesthetic sense. Your body can tell when it's doing it right. You'll feel it."

CHAPTER 16
Escape From Whitehouse Canyon?!?

Axel was gone and Ben was all alone again. The silence of Whitehouse Canyon was deeper, more oppressive, than before. As though the ghosts were loose again. Ben was lonely. In a way he'd never felt before. He was alone. In a dangerous world. Alone and unsure.

He could still see the look in Axel's eyes as they shook hands and said goodbye. Hopeful, doubtful, friendly, but now reserved, withdrawn. He walked up the canyon, around the corner, leaving tracks in the soft sand that ended twenty yards beyond where the wall curved north toward the river. Just out of curiosity Ben had checked. He didn't know what to make of what he'd learned.

One way or another, he'd had his vision in this canyon. Fact or fantasy? Real or not? The only thing he had to cling to was what he'd learned. That was fact because he could use it and it worked. He didn't see how his fevered brain could have come up with such an elaborate fantasy so on some level at least, Axel was "real". He was also gone.

Graduation. Ben had received his lessons. Now he was going back. To Sand's world, before Sand's world came after him. The rabbit was about to leave his hole and start running again. Somehow he had to find a way. Avoid the fate Sand planned for him. Change the game from "everybody chases Ben Singer".

Ben loaded the bike and then glanced again up the canyon where the helicopter had crossed. He strained to hear the sounds of a helicopter or truck out beyond the canyon rim. If they caught him out in the open, racing along the bottom of the canyon, building speed to climb back up out .

Then he turned and studied the western sky. It would be full dark in an hour. The purple thunderheads that loomed over him blotted out the sun and seemed so full of rain and lightening that they would burst at any moment. To get the heavy bike back up the trail he would have to leave now, before the clay soil got soaked and became a giant slippery slide. He wasn't sure he could drive the heavy road bike back up to the head of the canyon even on dry ground. He hadn't really planned to ever go back up that trail. Now he wanted to, he wondered if he could.

He looked around the canyon, his mind flooded with the events of the last two days. It was unbelievable, the turn his life had taken. Without Axel Ben could almost believe it had never happened. Except he had Axel's voice tape, and his body was patterned tightly, strongly, as it never had been before. He felt a power and control in his movements that was thrilling. It was hard to maintain, but the benefits were so great he hated to stop to rest. He knew that in a matter of days he would have the strength to keep himself patterned all the time if he was not required to put out much extra energy.

The big bike started smoothly and idled quietly while Ben removed all signs of his stay. No sense making anything easy for Sand. It was hard to turn the bike in the sand of the canyon floor. He had to rock it back and forth, turning a little, gaining some each time, careful not to let the bike tip. It was too heavy to manage easily in these conditions. He doubted he could get it upright again if he lost control.

A rumble of thunder echoed up the canyon and he felt a trickle of fear start down his nerves. He was losing time. He'd have only one shot at the grade. He had to be going just fast enough to steer in the sand and to climb the grade without having to accelerate the engine. If he spun out in the sand and began sliding backwards down the hill he would never be able to recover. The rain would catch him and hold him in the canyon without food for days, perhaps long enough for Sand to find him.

He fought the bike up to a speed where it rode upon the sand, accelerating a little across the hard pan to build up momentum for the hill. Way too soon he rounded the last turn in the canyon and saw the hill 75 yards away. It would be like climbing to the top of a 3 story building on a slope at least as steep as a playground slide. There were alternating stretches of hard pan and blow sand. The big front wheel would plow down into the sand and then jump up onto the harder parts of the slope. At any point the wheel could kick sideways or the rear wheel could spin out and throw him out of control. He had to go fast enough to bounce into and out of the soft spots without being kicked sideways ..it would be like trying to stay with a bucking bull in the rodeo .. His hands started sweating but he couldn't take the time to wipe them off on his pants. He was fully committed, no turning back now.

He had to be going fast enough at the bottom to be able to climb to the top without having to give the bike any additional throttle. If he was going too fast at the bottom the slope would knock the bike over before he even started to climb. A sudden flash of light followed almost immediately by a booming clap of thunder told him that he'd have at best, one shot at the hill.

He adjusted his speed, accelerating smoothly, the bike running powerfully, skimming the ground. Ben worried about the sand pile right at the bottom of the hill. If he were riding a trail bike he would have jerked up the front wheel and accelerated almost into a wheel stand to be sure the front wheel didn't bury itself in the sand. But not with this big Honda road bike.

He was getting closer rapidly now, his hands sweating, his heart beating strongly. He spotted what looked like a ridge of clay dirt running up through the sand. He adjusted to hit it straight on, accelerated another 5 miles per hour, and committed everything he had to the hope he was right.

The bike hit the clay strip and the ground was hard enough to start the front wheel up the slope. In a few seconds Ben was half way up the slope, but now in blow sand. The bike began to slow alarmingly. At this rate it would lose all forward momentum before it reach the top. Ben felt himself rising a little in the seat, almost willing the bike to keep going.

Within another ten feet Ben was fighting the impulse to gun the engine. His nerves were screaming, and a booming pulse of thunder slammed in to his ears, disorienting him for a few critical moments. Then the bike's wheels sank far enough into the sand to find the underlying clay of the slope. Ben felt the change instantly and added a few rpms to the engine. The bike held a steady speed, but by now it was so slow Ben could barely balance the it. At any moment now he would have to twist the wheel one way or another to regain his balance. In the process he was sure he would dump the bike.

Just then several large drops of rain spattered down on the windshield. Ben felt his body start to sag. Despair started to flood through him.

Then he felt a sudden burning surge of anger that galvanized him. He thought of Sand at the top of the hill, watching him, a big sneering grin on his face. At the same time he pulled his body back into its pattern, back flat, chest high, legs and glutes pulling strongly. He felt his balance return. He shot the big bike another jolt of gas, and he and the bike came up over the crest in a shower of sand, small rocks, and chunks of clay.

He fought the bike down into the track that led him now away from the storm, from the canyon, from where he'd last seen Axel. From where the people of the Whitehouse Society had built their refuge. Now he was moving towards people who wanted to kill him. There was no refuge anywhere for Ben Singer unless he settled things with Sand.

He accelerated strongly, until the bike skimmed the sandy spots in the road and rumbled powerfully along the hard pan. He knew now that if he was careful he could out run the storm. He thought about flipping on the lights so he could see better.

Then, without a conscious thought, he suddenly found himself pulling up, waiting for the shocking curtain of cold rain to overtake him. He was now simply running on his Indian mind, civilization's veneer melting away in the rain. No fancy words or involved intellectual concepts, just instinct served him now. He felt an urge to absorb nature into himself and in turn to be absorbed until he was so much a part of the land that he was invisible.

In a few moments he could see only a few feet in front of him. He slipped into his rain gear then he dropped the bike into low and drifted along the road that would lead him back past `Oljee' Toh, around the big monument, and back to the highway.

He was careful not to outrun the rain. And as the darkness settled in around him he didn't turn on his lights. He would travel, he thought, like male rain, storming across the land, full of power and destruction. Let Sand's dogs hunt him in this.

At the highway he cut south into Arizona. He made better time because he was headed across the path of the storm so he couldn't outrun it. He just ran in it. There was almost no traffic and he went too fast to be caught from behind. The few vehicles coming toward him had little to see but a flashing blur as he swept past. He turned left again on Highway 60 and powered up the bike to get him to Mexican Water in under an hour. Then he turned back into the reservation, turned on the lights, and covered the 35 miles to Roundrock in twenty minutes. Every foot of the way his eyes strained ahead for the hint of movement or the glint of headlight in the eyes that would warn him of horses on the road.

At Lukachukai he headed Northeast on a dirt road leading to Red Rock trading post. There was an all night gas and go there and he quickly stocked up on calories, eating as he drove, confident that the sleepy man behind the counter scarcely noticed him. He passed over the Carizzos Mountains through a high mountain pass on a narrow gravel road that led down to Shiprock, New Mexico. He arrived there about 2 A.M. and glided through town without seeing anyone. Since Shiprock was the Northeastern sub-capital of the Navajo Reservation it was totally Indian governed. He had bypassed all state and federal highways to get there and had leapfrogged a hundred and fifty miles from Whitehouse Canyon without giving any Anglo policemen a chance to spot him. The storm that had covered him in Monument Valley was drifting along to the north now, rumbling and slashing the dark sky above

Warrior's Way

Ute Mountain with massive jolts of white-hot power.

Ben moved through town, ignored the turn of to Cortez, Colorado, and drove the 45 miles or so to Farmington. This was a big Anglo town, a trading capital, the home of many Indian traders who drove the lonely miles to their trading posts on the reservation rather than live out there. It was where the Tsosie family did their business and their banking. It was where Ben needed to be.

Only two motels were still open at three in the morning. Ben ignored them both. On the eastern edge of town he turned down along the San Juan River and entered the KOA campground. He selected a spot down in the willows near the river that was isolated and well screened from the other campsites. He went back up, paid his fee for two days, took a shower and changed clothes without seeing anyone and went to bed.

As he slipped into a dreamless sleep the silky sound of the river purred in his ear. But it was not reassuring to him. He had nearly drowned in the rapids on the Colorado one summer and this river was also big and powerful, with undercurrents, quicksand, and nameless threats that would have nagged at Ben even as he slept if he had not been so weary from the effort of driving the bike and of keeping his body rigidly patterned.

Without Axel's comforting presence his work in holding his body correctly, feeling the power building in his muscles, the smooth integration of each movement, was the only connection he had to what had happened to him in Whitehouse Canyon. His only ray of hope, the tinniest light to hold up against the black despair that surrounded him moment by moment. It had driven him beyond what he normally thought of as his limits of endurance. He was amazed to learn that what Axel said was literally true. When you throw the work on the muscles designed for the job they grow stronger. You don't exhaust or burn out the smaller, lighter muscle groups that were never designed to hold up a slumping body. You feel athletically tired, not frazzled and nerve weary.

There was little else to raise his hopes. He had probably made the trip without alerting Sand. But he was a hunted man with only death to look forward to unless he found a way to stop the Utah deputy. And Terry . He felt a tightness in his chest. Terry was still forever beyond him. He had not the glimmer of a plan, no course of action he could think of made sense. He cleared his mind, forced the black feelings inside him to retreat with an effort of will, and let his tired body slip down into the soft world of sleep.

*　　　*　　　*

Ben woke with the late morning sun shining on his face. He felt rested, but hungry. He ate, packed his gear and left the campground, avoiding the occasional campers he saw. It was too early in the spring for the campground to have many patrons. Everyone he saw was preparing to leave. By nightfall they would all have gone their way and forgotten him. He by-passed the campground office and store and took the highway back to town. In the bustle of a business day in Farmington he blended in unremarkable and unnoticed. Communications between the western states lawmen, even the Highway Patrols, was notoriously relaxed. He behaved normally, and since he knew the town well, in fact, he felt quite secure. A plan of sorts was forming in his mind. He felt a quirky smile twist his face behind the dark glass of the helmet he wore.

Not a plan so much as a simple determination. If he was going to die, to be murdered by Sand and his henchmen, it was going to happen close to Sand. Not in some far, lonely spot where they ran him down and left him like so much garbage on the roadside. No, Sand would have to do it personally. That was Ben's only real plan. He'd have to do it himself while Ben was doing everything he could to find out why Sand so badly wanted him dead. He'd make Sand's life miserable in the process. Except Sand had Terry and Lester ..

He was going to do his best to warn Terry and Lester. (And at the same time vindicate himself if he could.) How he was going to explain that he knew about Sand because Axel turned a sandstone wall into a video screen was a problem he'd handle when the time came.

He drove to the Farmington Interstate Bank where he had his `home' bank account. He used the Warren Valley branch in Utah, but he had a long-standing account here, in the same bank his Grandfather Tsosie and his mother used. He talked to Ms. Ferguson, an assistant manager that he knew well. She showed no sign that she was seeing a ghost so Ben assumed she knew nothing about his problems in Utah. Not yet. But Grandpa had said he was picking up the money in the account. Both he and Ben could sign on it. Ben felt his hands sweating and tingles ran along his nerves each time Ms. Ferguson stopped to take a phone call.

I'm taking $8000 out now, he told her. He asked for a cashier's check. That left $2000 in the account so she wouldn't get suspicious. I need better transportation, he said, and I'm going to summer school this year.

The more he talked the more guilty he sounded to himself. He was waiting for her to ask the fatal question of why he couldn't operate out of his bank in Utah, with this same account. He said something lame about traveling for a while too and then shut up. In twenty minutes he left the bank with the check, made out to himself. In another hour he had a new bank account in his name only at the new Western States Bank that also had branches in Utah. But he took back $5000 in traveler's checks and drove back to the ATM at his old bank and pulled out the maximum allowed, $200.

After recharging his body with a large lunch he toured the bike shops out along the Bloomfield highway. He soon found a shop owner willing to sell his bike for him. Farmington was a college town, it was spring, and the bike was in first class condition, despite its recent hard use. Ben left the bike, promising to come back in a week or two and talk about getting something more suitable. The shop owner seemed happy, and he should, Ben thought. He had let him talk Ben down in price till he would be making nearly a thousand dollars more profit on the sale than he could usually expect. But Ben wanted a quick sale, and the shop owner had a good reason now to sell the bike fast.

Ben glanced back as he walked away and saw the owner looking after him, a calculating look twisting his face into a disquieting mask. He thinks I'm a drug runner, Ben thought. Then another thought shook him. What if he puts the bike out on the highway patrol net to see if it's stolen or has been used in a crime. That could get back to Sand. Just having title papers was no guarantee the bike was clean. Ben waved and walked on. His story that he was selling the bike for money to go to school would hold up or it wouldn't. He couldn't do much about it now. He shifted the lumpy load of gear he was packing and hiked back down the road toward Farmington.

In the next few hours he rented for cash, not using his credit card, a small white economy car with an unlimited mileage package from a local place called ☐rent-a-Wreck☐ that he could leave anywhere in the area to be picked up. Then he had purchased additional camping gear so he could stay out in the open comfortably

Warrior's Way

anywhere, despite the raw spring weather and enough food to keep him for two weeks.

He also acquired a fine set of small military binoculars and a bulky 20 to 100 power spotting scope. He planned to buy weapons too, but he would do that in Utah. No waiting period, he could use his Utah residency to take immediate possession. If Sand found out about it? Well then he would know that Ben meant business. That he wasn't just going to lay down and play dead.

An emotional mixture of rage and fear kept pulsing through him. Making his bones seem to melt, destroying his attempts to keep the key muscle groups energized. He'd feel his belly sag forward, his chest drop, his shoulders hunch as his fear of Sand welled up inside his mind. Then the deep-seated anger would bubble up out of the depths and death itself was not enough to keep him from trying to wipe out the insult Sand had given him. He would feel his body pull down hard, till his muscles began to burn and his vision got misty red. Then he would take a deep, shuddering breath and try to get on with what he was doing. At any moment he could run into somebody who knew him. He hurried with his preparations and went back to his campsite at the KOA.

He spent the rest of the day around the campfire, sorting gear and food, loading various sized packs for different situations and preparing a survival fanny pack that he would wear constantly. He put on tough Redwing hiking shoes and soft whip cord pants that would not make noise as he moved through the brush. He cooked a savory pot of stew with little meat and lots of vegetables, had a good green salad with French bread and drank some milk.

In the evening, by the light of a neon camp light, he began reading the books and magazines he's selected. Perhaps he knew little about survival. But he was a good reader and a fast learner and he had a lifetime of practical experience to draw on since he'd grown up in a desert where his family hauled all the water for fifteen miles and lived in a dry camp. Where his grandpa had actually tried to pass on to him the skills of Indian survival. What a fool he'd been not to listen better.

He found himself adding to or taking from the ideas he was reading, based on his own experience and what he could recall of his Grandfather's instruction, which probably came down for a thousand years through his people. He paid attention now.

It was a matter of life and death now.

He was searching for was a way to live. Sand wanted him dead. Sand had money and power and the will to use them. So Ben's life was greatly simplified. Just go on living. That was the challenge.

His mind absorbed everything he read. He read fast and widely and late that night he fell asleep, his body exercising itself as he kept the key muscle groups energized, as he thought about western Colorado and eastern Utah. He had to pick a route. A lot depended on the choices he made. There was no reservation land to hide in. he'd spent years exploring Utah back roads and forests. Now it would serve him well. When he crossed back into Utah he could be sure Sand's net was still in place, watching for him to surface like wolves circling their prey. The one thing he couldn't do was call the police. He'd have to get from place to place through the back country. But not in a little white car

    *   *   *

Ben left before dawn. So far as he knew, no one from the campground staff had seen him. He had changed clothes, gotten a new vehicle and now wore a large brimmed, deep crowned Australian type hunting hat that he contrived to have shade his face and hide his dark hair.

Taking no chances, he headed east toward Bloomfield and then turned north to Durango. There he turned left, back toward the west, passed the entrance to Mesa Verde National Park, the huge collection of Anaa'i Sani ruins that seemed to contribute spectacular pictures of cliff dwellings to almost every calendar he'd ever seen. As he drove through Cortez and on west on highway 666 toward Utah he thought about the Ancient Ones and the Whitehouse Canyon. As the crow flies, Mesa Verde was only 150 miles or so from the Canyon, but Whitehouse was far north of the major Anaa'i Sani settlements. Close, but not too close.

Fifteen miles west of Cortez Ben passed a Colorado Highway patrol car. It brought him up sharply, cleared his mind, reminded him that in less than an hour he'd be back in Utah if he kept going. He planned to cut north at Dove Creek, stay in Colorado and take the secondary roads to Montrose. He wasn't ready for Utah yet.

The scenery was spectacular as he skirted the western edge of the Colorado Rockies. From time to time he became aware of just how beautiful the land was. The snow capped peaks gleamed in the evening sun and he saw the snow line was retreating up the mountainsides. Much of the really high country would be closed for another month but the foothills were almost dry now.

Mostly, however, he worried. His fear spoiled the day and when he got to Montrose he was exhausted physically and emotionally.

He again selected a secluded spot in the local KOA, this time down along the Gunnison River. He hated water, especially moving water. But he knew that most people would not cross water to come up behind someone. Especially not a river in spring flood that was bitter cold. On the other hand, in one pack he had a small inflatable ring fly fishermen used and canned air to inflate it and the insulated wet suit they wore. He positioned it so that in a matter of moments he could quietly slip into the water and be gone, with a good chance of surviving. He knew the fear of the water would not overcome his hate for Sand, nor his determination to haunt him, to sell his life a dearly as he could.

It was a surprisingly balmy night and he walked for two hours or more, up and down along the bank, out to the country road and back, never leaving his campsite for too long at a time, carrying his survival fanny-pack on his belt. Several times he wished he had a dog like Sand's to walk with him. For the company, and so he could watch the dog's reactions to sounds and smells that were beyond his senses.

Mostly he walked to blow out his body just as Navajos believed that every so often you should take a car out and run it down the highway to blow off the junk that accumulates in the motor and in the oil. He wanted his heart to pound and his lungs to work to clean out his system. He felt changes taking place in him. Stored fat was being converted and burned, the by products that had been accumulating in him for years were being expelled. He often had a mild headache and it seemed that vigorous exercise helped.

He found it a challenge to keep his hips tilted up level and his back flat and his diaphragm locked down in place and at the same time to concentrate on walking correctly. He stopped often to stand and re-pattern his isometric systems. Then he would begin walking again, the ball of the back foot pushing off against the ground, the forward foot swinging briskly out until the muscles at the front of his leg tightened, the knee opened out, and his heel touched ground.

After 20 minutes or so, when the blood was coursing through him and the key muscles were well warmed up, he again experienced the thrill that he had felt when Axel took him walking in Whitehouse Canyon. As the hip rotated forward to throw the leg and foot out ahead, he felt one layer of his belly muscles harden and he felt the muscles in his back clear up to his should blades taking part in the action. He began to see clearly just how much correct walking could strengthen a body. Legs, stomach, back, all the breathing muscles. The neck, shoulders and chest as the head was held high and the spine stretched straight and the whole body became erect. He felt regal. He felt like what he saw in his father. He began to understand how warriors who had to walk to their war, and who knew these things, could create incredible power in their bodies while 'simply' walking along.

Ben thought of a young man his own age who worked as a smoke jumper in the forests of Idaho during the fire season each summer. He was small, yet every bit as straight and erect as Axel. He's made the casual remark that he could put on twenty pounds of pure muscle in two weeks of working the fire lines and of eating the huge meals served to the fire crews. He thought of what he's heard about Abraham Lincoln. He'd been a champion wrestler, taking on all comers when he was young. He was tall and very straight and seemed thin, but they had marveled at how powerful his body still was in his sixties, when he'd been shot and they undressed him to treat his wound. He had carried much of his physical power all through his life.

He could also see more clearly now, drawing on his own past and on the things he was seeing in people all around him, how most people walked with their isometric systems more or less shut down, with their body parts hung from their bones mostly by the attachment of the ligaments, that they avoided exertion and reaped the benefits in back aches, weakness, overweight and health problems. With no one to show them how, they just did the best they could.

He was passing the campground, his body warm and glowing, and he couldn't resist stepping up to the back of the rental car. It was small, an economy size car, and had front wheel drive. Really nothing to compare to the car he's seen his father move. But he grabbed the rubber lined bumper, adjusted his body, bent his legs and heaved. The feeling of power flowing through him seemed to focus on the key muscles of arms, back and legs, and with a little groaning sound the car body rose higher and higher. He felt the power of the shorter, close-coupled bone and muscle groups in his body. The car stopped moving upward when the springs extended fully and it was time for the wheels to come off the ground. But not until then. Ben felt a little awed by it all. No less by the fact that he felt no sense of straining or tearing or compression in any part of his body. Just a sense that the power had run out. This time.

I wish Axel would write a book, Ben thought. Everyone could benefit from knowing this, even the naturally strong. For if they change their habits, they will lose their strength. They won't find it again because they don't know how to do the right things consciously, deliberately, explicitly.

Thinking of Axel, Ben was reminded again of just how alone he was. What powerful enemies he had. He had taken the helping hand Axel held out to him only to learn that Axel was not his savior. Only his friend. He could use a friend right now.

Then he saw Terry's face floating gently in his minds eye, bathed in the moonlight. She had been his friend. Sand had taken her away, had broken both their hearts and left them to walk through life alone.

Suddenly, Ben was very tired. Weary of the world. Alone and afraid and unsure. Unsure anymore if the effort was worth the cost. If he ran far enough and hid well enough Sand might give up on him. But if he did that, he'd be looking over his shoulder the rest of his lonely life. Terry would be left with Sand.

No, he promised himself, I'll see Terry one more time. No matter what it costs. And when I leave her at least she'll be able to live her life knowing that I did love her, that I didn't deceive her. Even if I die she can build a life for herself on that. Wearily he walked back to camp and settled in for the night. It was a clear, star-filled sky that drew the blanket of darkness over him. He was scarcely aware of its beauty. The ugliness of the world around him, of the private world Sand had made for him, seemed drown out the beautiful stillness of the night. Alone he sought his bed and sank into sleep. Hoping, wishing, some outside intervention would give him the break he needed.

That night he met a new Mentor.

Warrior's Way

Chapter 17
Ben Singer Meets REX

Ben found himself in a long hallway, like a castle, stone walls sucked the heat from his body and he shivered. He heard a series of sounds, unnatural in their sum, and felt the air stir around him like some vast door had opened and then closed again. Next his skin crawled as some sense in him screamed that he was no longer alone ..

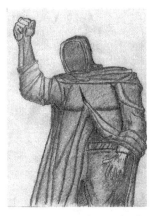

The moon was casting long shadows when Ben woke with a start. For just a moment he thought Dick Sand was standing across the fire pit from him, just beyond the picnic table. The fire was still glowing, but it seemed not to reach out far enough to illuminate any of the details of the bulky shadow man across from him. Ben felt his hair crawl and gooseflesh ran down his legs. This man was much bigger than Dick Sand. He was at least as big as Axel. His body was draped in a cloak, with a hood that made him look like something out of a Halloween horror movie. Like the ghost of Christmas Future in the movie Scrooge.

Spooky.

In one smooth motion Ben brought himself up in the sleeping bag and drew his feet under him. He was wide awake and the adrenaline was beating steadily through his body. He could feel the empty, almost hungry feeling it made in his middle and he felt his hands shaking a little. He no longer thought of these reactions as fear. He knew from his reading it was only his body being prepared for fight or flight. The survival magazines had taught him that.

The dark figure was between him and the road. No way to get around and away from him. He could slide into the cold river, but the thought of the icy water sweeping him away made him pause.

Fight? he thought. If I can't beat Dick Sand what possible chance do I have against this guy?

He pulled his body into line, wondering if this man weighed as much as the back of his car. He was wishing he had bought a gun. He wondered if he really could get to the river faster than this dark apparition could come across the fire pit. He had no answers, just the nervous pounding of his heart.

"What do you want?" Ben said.

He was pleased to hear his voice vibrate deeply, almost a rumble in his chest. The neighborhood dog growling at the invader of his turf.

The man moved slowly around the table and towered over Ben, even from across the fire pit. His shape seemed to blot out the stars and make the shadows darker. He was easily the biggest man Ben had ever seen.

"To talk a little," the voice was cavernous, hollow, strange in Ben's ears. "If you like."

Ben untangled himself from his sleeping bag and sat on his camp chair, a little closer to the riverbank. With the fire pit still between him and the other man. His visitor promptly sat down.

"Who are you?" Ben said. What are you, he thought.

"My name is REX."

"Why do you come to see me?" How do you know I exist? Ben asked himself.

"To ask you something."

Ben had heard enough now to know that this man was shifted somehow out of Ben's space and time. His voice was plain and deep to suit his size. But somehow the voice just didn't sound like it was created by a set of vocal cords vibrating against the same air Ben was breathing. Axel's voice was like Ben's. REX's voice was strangely altered. Darth Vader was the only name that came immediately to mind. Breathing and talking at the same time

Ben felt gooseflesh again on his legs and upper back. The adrenaline kept right on pumping through him. He could feel a strong pulse in his temples. He knew now that part of that was simply the operation of fear on his body along with the effort of patterning the muscle systems. He was fully awake now, ready to go. REX was still there. He was not a dream. A nightmare, maybe.

Ben folded his arms across his chest, right arm over the left and not tucked under, but laying on top, his hand lightly gripping the back of his left arm. He was ready to defend himself instantly. Another thing he was learning from the books. He tried not to think about the fact that he had only been in one real fight, with Dick Sand. Not exactly a personal best worth bragging about.

"What did you want to ask me?"

Ben's voice was starting to sound spooky and thin to him. He was feeling like he did when he was small and Grandpa told midnight stories about the Dine Naaldlooshi who turned themselves into were-animals that could run as fast as a car and snatch children right out of the truck window on a dark, moonless night. Or run the 90 miles from Shiprock to Gallup, New Mexico and back in one night. Or come into a rock shelter in Whitehouse Canyon and kill Ben Singer with agonizing spirit fire.

"We're wondering about you, is all".

"We?"

"Some of your fathers, and some others. Why you let Dick Sand do things to you. And to those you say you love."

Ben was stung by the biting edge of scorn REX put on the words you say you love. His voice dripped with anguish and contempt.

Concern for Ben's manhood.

"We would not let any man treat us the way you are letting this man treat you."

☐Even as the words slammed into his mind, the contempt cut him to his soul. All the feelings and fears he'd had that night at Tibble Fork erupted and flushed through him again. He felt his belly sag outward as the muscles released and went slack. Ben uncrossed his arms and leaned forward and put his elbows on his knees. He felt naked even though he'd worn his clothes to bed, just in case. He felt the fear in him strengthening as it was fed again by the creeping feeling of shame and unmanliness he felt that night in Tibble Fork Campground.

"I was weak then. It would be different now."

"As you say. You're are growing very strong. Soon you will be formidable. So, then, why do you suffer this man to do these things?"

"Dick Sand isn't alone. I am. He has influence and money and that means power to do what he wants."

"Just so."

The voice carried approval. This puzzled Ben.

"Are you saying I should stand up to that power network alone? That's like spitting in the wind. It's senseless. Stupid even. He has all the cards. He dealt me out of the game."

Ben's voice sounded bad to him. Thin, almost a whine and he'd lost the patterning in his middle zone. The muscles sagged and his breathing dropped out of the costal region of his chest. This, he knew, was the real symptom of fear and in a fight it was deadly. The isometric systems would not be there to provide the firm, steady platform the isotonic muscles needed to unleash their power. Ben knew if he tried to lift the car right now he would barely budge it and might hurt himself trying.

"Now you are beginning to see."

Ben saw the massive head nod in approval. Where was this guy coming from? He didn't seem to be able to grasp that Ben meant that he was helpless to do anything to Sand. It was too dark to see REX's features. They were like dark granite seen through deep water. Unable to read the metamessage of the expressions on the face Ben was at a loss to understand his words.

"A man cannot stand alone against other men who have combined their power. Dick Sand rubs your face in the dirt for all your friends to see and his allies help him by producing the pictures that move that he used to drive you away. By hunting you with their machines and their firelocks.

"He shows you the power of his combination. He makes you howl and dance like a Hollywood Indian and drives you away like a cur. And you go. And you decide to die. Thus you only make him stronger, more confident in his power."

The voice was shaking, the huge body seemed unable to sit still, but moved about under the strength of the emotions REX was feeling. Ben felt anger rising again in him and the thoughts of vengeance flooded him with strength. He felt his body repattern itself and he sat up straight to allow his breathing to move high up into his chest, to become almost a pant. To breathe like Jack Palance breathed. But he could find nothing to say.

"And so we ask." REX now shifted forward and seemed to be studying Ben's reactions. "Why do you accept this? A man must have a man's pride. Not even life is more important. But a man need not be a fool. He need not fight alone. Shall we think you a fool, Ben Singer?"

The words hung in the air like circling vultures, ready to consume the last scraps of Ben's manhood and pride.

Ben thought fast. Can't do it alone. Must combine with other men.

"I don't know anyone who has any power who hates Dick Sand like I do" he said.

REX snorted in dismay or disgust. Ben plodded on trying to make REX see how powerless he was. His voice sounded small in his ears. He looked down into the glowing fire pit, not at REX.

"What good is it to fight with overwhelming odds against you?" But that's just what I'm going to Utah to do.

"What king ever said that? Kings rule, but they are upheld in their power by a circle of men who profit from their rule. Open your eyes, Ben. Do you think those who uphold Dick Sand love him? They profit from what he does. Not just in gold, but in power. The power to bend others to their will, to have their way, no matter what they want to do.

"Buy your allies as Sand does. Give them the spoils and the power to destroy every hand raised against them. They will uphold you in all your desires. They will never ask to be your friend or to believe in your cause. But they will make you very powerful."

Ben felt some new thoughts coming into his mind as he listened the man who called himself REX, which was Latin for `king.' He felt a coalescing of thoughts, impressions, and intuition and knew that a part of his mind had been actively pursuing the burning question: What is Sand up to, why is he doing this?

Sand was rich. Assume for a moment it wasn't his grandmother's oil money, like he said it was. Then add to that the fact that he obviously had some kind of organization, or to use REX's word, combination, behind him. A organization with killers. A combination ready to do anything, no matter how sleazy, no matter how much it hurt innocent people. Dick Sand was right in the middle of it, REX implied he was the leader of it, though Sand might have superiors somewhere that he had to account to.

What kind of illicit business in America today generates large amounts of money and attracts degenerates who will do anything for a price? Ben saw the pallid face of TJ floating in the air between him and the glowing embers of the fire pit. TJ accused of supplying drugs to school children, now dying of an overdose of drugs himself. Ben heard Sand's voice on the phone saying TJ had been murdered. Inviting Ben to join him in a hunt for the killers. Actually setting him up so Sand could drive him out of the county. Not send him away to live his life somewhere else, as Sand had said that night. Just to get him far enough away. To help him have a fatal accident, but not in Dick Sand's back yard.

Sand's a drug runner.

With that thought many things fell into place. The size and the pervasiveness of Sand's organization became clearer. He was heading up a major effort to establish something in Utah. A backwater place full of quiet towns and villages, filled with people who were peaceful and law abiding and often pathetically naive. Utah was known as the scam capital of the United States because so many trusting people had been cheated.

He's infiltrated at least part of the law enforcement community, Ben thought. And he's probably deluded the others. Sand was a man's man. He came across almost like a hero to many people. He was the perfect plant.

Ben's mind worked at light speed as he sifted, filed, developed implications, followed trains of thought in several directions at once. Then he smiled inwardly, an ironic, bitter smile. I'm doing just what Sand was afraid I'd do, he thought. No wonder he tried so hard to kill me.

He was afraid of me! The thought left him thunderstruck. A little trickle of pleasure, pride, leaked into his heart. He sat up a little straighter.

Sand's not alone so he makes a bigger target than I do, Ben thought. There are flaws in his plans somewhere. I'll be trying now to find them while Dick Sand is busy trying to kill me to keep me from finding them. He felt the ironic, twisted grin light up inside him again. It will be a king hunt, like at the end of a chess game when most pieces are gone from the board, each player is chasing the others king, and the first to make a wrong move loses. At that, it was a better chance than Ben had had when he went to bed last night.

Ben decided to see what else he could learn from REX. Sand has an organization behind him. That's how he got the tapes made. Somebody owes him. Who do I know would join me if the price was right? Maybe there are those with a grudge against Sand. Maybe there people who, just like him, want power and wealth but are afraid to act alone. But who am I to run such an organization?

"But how could I lead such men," Ben said.

"First you must be strong, as you will soon be, now that you somehow have learned the secrets of the old warriors. Also, you have a certain intelligence, though you have not used it wisely.

"Now you must be willing to dominate men and make them conform to your will. First one, and then the two of you will get another, and soon you will have your small band of leaders. The rest of it, the unifying organization, we can teach you. The principles have existed for a long time. Many men have used them. You can do it too, Ben Singer. If you have the will to do it."

Where were you when I was weak, silly old Ben Singer? Ben asked silently. I could have used you at Tibble Fork. Why are you showing up now?

Ben gazed at the glowing coals and saw a flickering TV screen in the back of Dick Sand's van. Okay, maybe I'll die, but I was going to do that anyway. Why not go out trying to even the score with Dick Sand, or to do him some hurt no matter how small.

"Why don't you do something to that man?"

Ben looked up, startled, and then realized that REX was not reading his thoughts but rather speaking to the issue between them.

"Why do you let him win? Will Terry respect you more because you are a weakling man of peace? When what is called for is war? What good is your intelligence and your great strength if you don't use it to get what you want? When what you want is only what is right?"

REX was shifting on his seat now, back and forth and seemed to be looking for something to hit with his massive fists.

"We can help you Ben. You can be one of us. One of the great ones. You have it in you from your fathers. But you must choose carefully what you will do. And you've got to strengthen yourself. Make your heart and mind strong, not just your body. Make up your mind to make war on Dick Sand and his people. Win the peace with honor and with pride. And make yourself rich and powerful so that you can continue to fight and win."

Ben had a picture in his mind of an Indian war chief stirring up his men for a raid. He felt the same stirring deep in his bones and in his mind that he always felt when he heard the big drums start to beat in a Pow Wow. His people did not dance a war dance as the plains Indians did. But he always envied the men who arched their bodies and danced in the powerful, proud, warriors stride.

"Physical strength is only a beginning. Some men haven't needed it at all if they had good minds and strong spirits.

"Will is what counts. Implacable will. Dominating will. A heart and a mind set on succeeding at any cost. A willingness to direct and use and even to sacrifice others if you must to attain your ends. It will be worth it and those you sacrifice will be seen as heroes in your cause.

"You can give people peace. You can bring the order of your will to an evil and disorderly world. You can force people to build a better world. You can forcibly create a place where the young learn from the beginning of their lives to serve your cause and to defend your plan. To serve your peace and defend you against your enemies with their very life's blood."

REX paused, like a man who sees a familiar and pleasant scene.

He knows what he's talking about, Ben thought. He's been there. He wishes he was still there.

I wonder what happened.

"You can have more power than Dick Sand has to reward your enemies properly. Your name can be respected, Ben Singer. If you want it to be so. If you want it badly enough to act, to use your gifts and our help."

The silence lengthened between them. Ben could still feel the emotions gusting across the fire pit from REX. Ben began to wish he could see REX's face, gaze into his eyes and see what sort of soul was looking out at him.

"Why do you let Dick Sand do this to you?" REX asked again. "It should not be so. Will you accept our help?"

The last seemed almost a pleading rather than a straight forward offer of help. Ben felt that REX and Ben's "fathers" had a big stake in Ben's answer.

"Who's we?" Ben asked. Since they think I'm an Indian George Washington I might as well play my part.

"We are legion, Ben Singer. A numberless host. Some of us know your fathers. We have much experience in human affairs. In dealing in power. We have helped to build many mighty men of influence and power."

Ben was intrigued. Maybe REX would give him a written resume along with references from some of these great men.

On sudden impulse Ben leaned forward and threw a handful of bark on the glowing embers in the fire pit.

"Who were some of these people you speak of, REX? Ben said.

Before the bark caught fire and began to throw more light on him REX stood up and stepped behind the picnic table, burying himself again in darkness. Ben's breath stuck in his throat as he saw the imposing size of the man across from him. Ben had no trouble believing that REX had done what he said he'd done. Ben felt small and foolish. Challenging such a man. He wondered if he'd recognize him if he could see his face.

REX was through being polite. The lash of contempt came back to his voice. The implication that if he was a man Ben would do what REX suggested. The suggestion of a doubt about Ben's will and pride, even his manhood..... but not his ability.

"Think, Ben. Think about getting smart. About getting even. Think what Sand has done to your manhood. To your pride. To your friends. If you decide to take your revenge and if you want our help then move back to the Diamond Fork area, out of Dick Sand's reach. We'll visit you again there, when we know you have decided to make Sand bend to your will. We will help you then."

REX turned and walked into the night. Ben stared into the trees around the campsite. The firelight hid more than it revealed. Like REX's words, Ben thought. A little light, but too many things still shifting with the shadows, out of sight in the dark.

Spooky and worrisome.

Ben stood and walked to the road. The shadows were deep in places, but he could see well enough. He was not really surprised that there was no sign of REX.

Ben sat down again by the fire. No use trying to go back to sleep. As he went over in his mind what the huge "man" had said, what he had implied, Ben's daydreams of vengeance took on a new force and a new direction. as he began to think in specific terms, to consider concrete plans of action.

Not just to go back and warn Terry and die ..

He began to toy with the delicious idea that he might get the power to strike back hard at Sand for the filthy things he was doing to children like TJ and good people like Lester and Terry.   And to Ben Singer.

His fantasies of revenge became more real. He wasn't alone. He had an offer of help from some pretty impressive people.   Unlike Axel, who couldn't help when the going got rough, REX seemed ready to jump in against Sand at any moment.

People who thought that Ben could lead them!

Ben began to consider the idea that somehow he fit the criteria REX had named for being the kind of leader men like REX wanted to follow. That was a powerful and compelling thought. A new note began to sound inside him, a note that was trying of offer a counterpoint to the gut-wrenching fear that tried to dominate him when he thought of challenging Dick Sand.

He crawled back into his sleeping bag. His restless brain had much to assimilate now.   New resources to help him against Sand. Twisting paths of logic and implication he had to follow.

The sense of aloneness was there too. He couldn't stop himself from wondering about Terry.

Where was she? What was she doing?

What was Dick Sand doing to her?

It took Ben a long time to fall asleep.

Chapter 18
Ben Meets Bud

Ben was jolted awake by an icy shot of adrenaline that screeched along his nerves like fingernails raking a blackboard. The foggy vestiges of emotion and image, of hate and fear and doubts evaporated in an instant. His mind was as clear as the starlit night sky.

Why?

He heard the sounds of the night. crickets, a breeze in the tree tops, the occasional sound of a fish feeding in the river. The silky sound of the water sliding by in the dark

The normal sounds of the night had not startled him awake. Something had.

What?

He felt a trickle of fear. Had Sand found him? Were they creeping in on him in the pre-dawn darkness? He was sleeping like a brainless sack of straw, right in camp, alongside the fire.

Fool!

To think Colorado, or anywhere, was safe from Sand.

Ben saw movement under the camp table. He felt his stomach tighten, his limbs get weak. He was expecting a stabbing roar of light in the darkness. The hot, searing pain of a bullet smashing through him.

A small dog trotted out from under the table. Ben flushed with relief. And shame.

It was some kind of a terrier. Grey, small and wiry, eyes black and shiny as marbles. The white that first caught his attention was a piece of paper tied around its neck. He came up to Ben and put his forepaws on his leg, raised himself up, cocked his head and seemed to smile a merry, friendly smile at Ben.

Axel, Ben thought. He reminds me of Axel. Strong, energetic and friendly.

He slipped the string over the dog's neck and bent to read the note in the early light of dawn.

Ben, it said. Thought you could use a little company. His name is Scots Highland King III. But he answers to Buddy or Bud. Good Luck, Axel

Ben smiled ruefully. REX promises me man power. Axel sends a little dog. I guess that just about sums it all up.

Ben smiled despite himself as the cheerful little dog dashed around the camp. Into everything. Chasing sleepy grasshoppers stirring up butterflies. Interested in everything Ben did. Like he was rediscovering the world one scent, one sight at a time. He made Ben forget for moments at a time the sense of impending doom that dogged him, trying to insinuate itself into every thought and to twist and deform every action.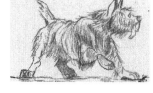

It seemed two paths stretched before him. He had to choose, something he'd sworn never to do again. So much for that.

In his wildest fantasy Ben couldn't see himself starting an organization to counter Dick Sand. Rex was impressive and what he said made Ben's thirst for revenge burn hot in him. In the cold light of day, however, Ben's old fears resurfaced. Hiding, running, trying to see Terry and warn her somehow   Even that seemed like more than he could do. His face burned with the old shame that was becoming so familiar. The choice he really wanted to make was to go away, avoid everything, just leave it all behind.

Ben had had time to think, to review his life, the destiny that had landed him here. It seemed upon reflection, that he'd never had any real personal options. He suspected his life was shaped by his parent's choices. By those who bullied him in school, and now by Deputy Dick Sand.

What would he have done .become if he'd only been allowed to find his own best way? If he hadn't been forced by the actions of others to use his giftedness as he had. To make the foolish choices to try to live white and to follow the Law? The silly, arrogant attitude that had put him in the trap he was in today. How might his native abilities have developed, in what directions might he have been led by them, if it wasn't that others always interfered. Made him adapt himself to their pressures and demands   Even now, left to himself, what would he, could he do?

He was just a pathetic puppet and Dick Sand held his strings.

You'll never know now, Ben. What you might have been. Can't you at least just run away? Don't you still have that choice, at least?

But Sand wasn't going to allow him that choice. Sand was trying his best to kill him. In the last analysis Ben's only real choice was whether to live or die. That simple choice was probably more than he could carry off, but at least his death might count for something if Terry was okay . Scared as he was, he could not just run away, leave Terry in Dick Sand's tender care, and wait for death to come for him in some isolated, lonely place.

When backed to the wall, even with life itself at stake, Ben found his old traits that made him make a fool of himself for Lester's sake, of sympathy and wanting to see others comforted and supported were still the hard-wired, "born with" essence of what he was. Even if death was the only outcome, at least his manner of dying could be his own choice ..

A dark sadness filtered through him like a black mist. How much his life had changed in such a short time .. He felt a huge sigh ripple through him. Nothing ahead of him seemed bright or hopeful ..

Bud came over and sat at his knee, placing one small paw on his leg in a ☐shake hands☐ gesture. Ben shook his paw and he backed off and did a circus back flip and scampered around the campsite. So full of life Ben smiled in spite of himself. He shut off the darkness, emptied his mind, turned on his Apache survival mode of thinking, re-patterned his body and decided it was time to move on.

Any path he chose led back to Utah. To Dick Sand's domain. To life or death.

No, Ben old boy. Don't try to sugar coat it. You know your own limitations very well now. Life isn't part of this equation any more .

****

Ben loaded up and moved to Montrose, Colorado, a larger town, and camped in a campground along the Gunnison River. After supper he made a trip back into town. He bought a Baby-on-Board sign for the back window of the car and a Garfield Cat doll to cling to the side window. Then he rummaged through the old clothes in a Salvation Army Thrift Store and found a old Harvard tee shirt about his size. A wide-brimmed hat and purple sun glasses made him look, he hoped, like a foreign college student touring the U.S. between semesters.

He bought some groceries, mostly canned goods and general camping materials like aluminum foil, paper plates and cups. His next stop was a sporting good store. He bought a battery powered lantern with a florescent tube to conserve energy and a small raft that could be inflated instantly from compressed air cylinders, a good, light Whelen tent-shelter, rope, a flotation vest that was inflatable by compressed air, survival meals and copies of survival and hunting magazines.

He also picked up a copy of Larry Dean Olsen's book "Outdoor Survival Skills". Olsen had been teaching classes in Utah for years. Utah had an excellent supply of wild foods.

Like Grandpa always said, when he was trying to get Ben to pay attention, that with survival skills and a knife you could walk out the door in the middle of winter and survive.

Ben smiled as he thought of Tony, his cousin and his friend. Tony had whispered to Ben behind Grandpa's back:

Sure. You can, use the knife to rob the Seven Eleven Store.

It was time for Ben to brush up on his training. This time he would pay better attention. There were no stores in the high Uinta Mountains.

He went to an electronics store and bought a CB radio, a Bear Cat scanner to listen to police radio bands, and a fuzz buster radar detection unit that would tell him when the police were in the area using radar. He bought a heavy 12 volt marine battery and a charger so he could run his equipment in camp.

He made up his bed back in the willows near the river this time. He'd have a better chance to escape if Sand found him. The silky sound of the water slipping by was not soothing to Ben, however. The thought of having to slide into the river to get away gave him a slick-sick cold sweat feeling.

Because he knew what a liar moving water was. Working as a flunky he had earned a trip down the Colorado two summers ago. The guide had allowed the patrons to ride the last rapids in their life preservers. Something had gone wrong. One woman got sucked so far under she could barely see daylight, far above her. People got scattered all over the river. Ben had been caught in the reverse current, carried back up river, only a few yards from shore, helpless, trapped in the force of the current and unable to swim the few feet to shore. Exactly like the undertow at an ocean beach.

He'd been carried up and then was driven down again, through rapids, swallowing water, feeling it burning his nose and lungs, feeling the sucking current jerking on his legs, trying to pull him under. He still had nightmares about it sometimes.

He was struggling in the whirlpool where the main current and the reverse current met, feeling himself being sucked inexorably down, when a worried tour guide got the raft over to him.

Growing up in the desert, but near the massive Chinle-Canyon Del Muerto wash complex, he'd seem families and homes swept away in spring floods or in the aftermath of the huge August thunderstorms. Ben had always distrusted big water.

Now he feared it.

But he would sleep near it. If it meant staying free he'd slip into it and try to float away on the raft.

But he wouldn't like it

He felt a shiver race up his back, his body jerked involuntarily. He turned away and went back to camp.

He sat up late that evening, idly stroking Bud while he read the outdoors

Warrior's Way

magazines, studied maps of Colorado and Utah, read an old army manual "Escape and Evasion".

Learning.

Using his scholar's mind and his study skills to learn anything he could that might help him survive against Sand and his crew of killers.

His 'combination' as REX called it.

Later, falling asleep, he saw Bud, on alert, sitting in the brush, between him and the firelight.

Watching. Guarding Ben.

The Black Prince he wasn't. He couldn't whip a big tom cat. But dogs as small as he must be survival specialists. Small dogs in a Rottweiler world. Just like Ben now had to be in his world. Where everyone but him had the poisoned hand.

Besides, as the little old ladies always said, it wasn't the size of the dog that scared off the burglars. It was the size of the bark.

Bud yipped sharply, then turned and gazed at Ben. Not his whole body, just laying his head back over his shoulder, cocked at a jaunty angle, mouth open. Looking like he was grinning merrily in the dark. Then he turned back to watching. Ben felt the hair stir a little along his scalp. Another mind reader? Ben fell into a troubled sleep, each time he awoke, however, Bud was there, on guard, through the night. It was a comfort and Ben felt himself relax and his dreams were not as ragged and scary as they had been.

****

Ben came awake with a start in the pre-dawn darkness when Bud's little feet hit his chest. Bud ran to the camp and back, inviting Ben to follow. When he got there Bud ran at the car, jumped up the side, and did a neat circus back flip.

Ben got the message.

He always loaded most of the camp gear before going to bed. Now he quickly threw in the raft and his bedding and he and Bud pulled out of the back road, onto the feeder for the freeway just as a sheriff's van, spotlight piercing the dark, started down the line through the campground.

Coincidence or not, Ben didn't want to be seen or remembered. He was a good way along the highway to Grand Junction by sunrise. He stopped in Delta at JB's for a big breakfast and then played tourist all the way to Grand Junction. He listened constantly to the CB and the scanner. He picked up lots of local gossip, nothing about himself. Making him all the more tense and suspicious. He was sure Sand wanted him quietly detained, to be picked up by Sand himself. So he could be quietly disposed of, another detail checked off of Sand's list. A detail and a life.

Besides, he was sure that some of the people hunting for him weren't police to begin with.

He stopped early at a Good Neighbor Sam campground down along the Colorado River. Being early, he was able to select a secluded campsite that backed up to the river. This time it was the Colorado itself that greeted him. Not as big as it was near Lake Powell where it tried to kill him.

Big enough. Deep and swift enough.

As he set up camp his eyes were drawn again and again to the twisting brown currents. The soft, liquid sound the river made tried to tell him lies. To calm his fears. To say it was peaceful, quiet, and still. Ben knew the lie. He'd felt the water's huge grip. Knew how reluctant it was to ever let you go once it clutched you in its powerful watery hands. How many drowning victims in the Colorado were never found.

But he set out the raft and other gear near the water where he made his bed. He's use it if he had to. He hated Dick Sand more than he feared the Colorado River. He felt a shuddering sigh ripple through him.

That was a lot of hate.

He fed Bud and warmed his supper over a cheery wood fire and then spent the long hours of the evening reading survival and hunting magazines. Weaving the facts and ideas into what he already knew. Thinking hard about what he'd have to do to stay out of Sand's grasp when he got back to Utah.

He had to contact Terry. See her. Explain. Relieve her mind of the burden Sand had made him put or her.

Tell her he loved her.

But his Indian instincts were strong. Sharpened by his study. Sand had all kinds of people and technology to use against him. Night vision glasses, helicopters, infra-red detectors, sound spikes, and so much more it made his head ache to think about it. If he wasn't cautious and wise, and very lucky, Sand would chase him around Utah like a jackrabbit in the desert until he drove him into a net and clubbed him to death. It would all be over then--for Ben. But not for the others.

Not for Terry.

His decision was made.

He spent the next day in Grand Junction. It was a fair-sized city full of the summer tourist crowd. People from all over the world were passing through, traveling between Utah's color country and Denver. Ben felt almost invisible in his little car and his Harvard tee shirt with his camcorder in his hand.

He had decided he would not rush back. He would be an Apache in this. Rule his spirit and prepare the territory he intended to operate in for his use. Looking at the little rental car Ben saw a donkey. He couldn't afford to go wolf hunting on a donkey. What he had to have was a mule. Sure footed. Enduring. Able to carry him over the foot paths and game trails he would have to travel to stay out of Sand's reach. He'd spent years on the reservation herding his grandpa's sheep from the seat of a dirt bike. Riding slick-rock like a goat, developing skills as he relieved the boredom. He knew exactly which bike could become his mule.

He went looking for mules at the bike shops. He finally found one that had a street package that included a very quiet muffler. It could be driven on the highway, but it was a full-blown trail bike. He weighed 220 pounds now and it had enough power to carry him and his gear. He selected a trailer that was normally pulled behind a big road bike and told the salesman he wanted it modified to fit behind his new bike.

Ben counted out enough cash to pay for half the deal.

"By tomorrow," he said. "Otherwise I take my business somewhere else. Noon tomorrow."

He left the salesman holding a handful of greenbacks, scratching his head. He went to a bakery and bought five 5 gallon plastic buckets with tight fitting lids. Then he went to a sporting goods store. He got five 2 gallon gas cans, five sets of emergency meals, five flashlights with batteries, fire starters, plastic sheeting, nylon rope, Swiss army knives and five wrist rockets sling shots with five boxes of 30 caliber steel shot. He bought small wire saws for trimming tree limbs and the most complete possible first aid kits. He might need one badly if he got too close to Sand and his wolves.

He didn't buy detailed maps or compasses. He had a natural sense of direction and he had traveled the Utah mountains enough that he would always know where he was. He did get five sets of compact rain gear and some space blankets. Waterproof match holders, flint, film cases and petroleum jelly for fire starting rounded out his purchases.

The thin, balding man behind the counter looked strangely at him. Paying way too much attention to Ben. Especially when he saw the writs rockets. Ben felt uncomfortable. Began to wish the bike was ready so he could leave in the dark. But he was stuck till tomorrow. He had to stay in Grand Junction, maybe give Sand a chance to catch up to him.

But he couldn't think of a simple story that would help this man forget him. So, uncomfortable, he did nothing. Above all he did not want to make a strong impression on anyone. Sand's dogs would be sniffing out his trail. He had to make it as hard as possible for them.

"New Scoutmaster, huh?" the clerk said.

Startled, Ben felt himself flush a little.

"Uh, yeah. Don't know much about the job yet."

"Well, you got enough for five patrols, all right. Make them get rabbits with the wrist rockets. That'll keep them busy."

"Yeah, I'll do that. Thanks."

Ben got his gear and left.

He toured the pawn shops till he found a Bear Magnum short limbed bow made for hunting in the brush. He wanted the old fashioned type without the gears and wheels. It was closest to the bow Grandpa had taught him to hunt with. And it wouldn't be likely to break down on him at the wrong moment.

He also got a dozen Bear razor broad head arrows and a dozen with interchangeable points, some with target points for practice, some with blunt heads for killing small game. They didn't penetrate, but killed by shock. They could break a knee cap, knock a man out. Fired at close range into the head from the 55 lb. bow they could kill.

Growing up Ben was expected to keep his family in small game. Rabbits, squirrels, very small, swift targets. He was good with a bow. Defending the sheep against coyotes and wild dogs had honed his skills, taught him to shoot to kill. The bow nestled into his hand like an old friend, half-forgotten friend.

By noon the next day Ben had checked his ATM, found the money from his road bike had been deposited, picked up and road tested the new bike and trailer, loaded his gear, dropped off the car at a local service station to be serviced and then picked up by the rental agency and he was on the road to Utah. The time it took the mechanic to service the car and call it in was Ben's head start time if Sand was on to him ..

He turned north at Loma, Colorado, went up over Douglas Pass, traveling slowly along with the tourist traffic, stopping often and breaking in the bike motor carefully. Everything from this point was a matter of life and death If he had to punish that engine he wanted it ready. In the best possible condition. On the drive up to Douglas Pass he babied it carefully. He stopped in Rangely for the night, still in Colorado, but only a few miles now from Utah. He would go into Utah through Vernal, along a state route, not a freeway. He would travel through the Ute Indian reservation, through Strawberry Valley, and on down to Heber. Along the way countless roads turned off into the High Uintas and to other remote wilderness areas.

He had many paths to choose from to get back into the mountains behind Warren Valley where Dick Sand lived.

As he went there he would set up his five gallon buckets full of supplies and he spare gas cans as way stations. Set them up very carefully. So only he could find them. So he could find them quickly, while being hunted for his life.

From this point on everything, every detail, was vitally important. Not that he expected to live. Just that he might stay alive long enough to do what he had vowed to do.

To talk to Terry .

Then, if he still could, to punish Dick Sand.

Chapter 19
Ben Talks To Terry

"Hello, Terry," Ben said.

"Who? Ben? Is that you? It is you! Your voice is different ..deeper." Terry sounded mystified, then her voice gushed out in a small explosion, tinged with emotions he couldn't read over the telephone. "Ben? Ben is that really you?" Then, more guarded, seeming to take control of herself with a definite effort, the words taking on what Ben heard as the same distant coolness he'd heard in her the last time she'd spoken to him, there on the curb, with Sand watching and tapping the video tape on his thigh. He jerked his mind away from the image.

"He's a liar, Terry. Everything he's told you about me is just a vicious lie."

"Dick has been very kind to me, Ben. After you left the way you did, so cold and withdrawn. He's helped a lot, personally, as a good friend. He's a dedicated and hardworking man, Ben. I don't think of him as a liar."

In the sudden silence Ben could hear the ghosting sound of other voices in the wire. People carrying on their lives, unknowing and uncaring about Ben and Terry and Dick Sand the liar.

The Murderer.

"He tried to kill me, Terry. Twice. Once he killed the wrong man, and the next time he killed the two men who failed to get me in southern Utah. He's been chasing me all over the four western states. He's a liar, Terry, and a killer, and probably a drug runner too."

"Sand hasn't been anywhere, Ben. He's been here with me, except for one day when he flew to Chinle to try to find you. He's not trying to kill you Ben. There's a warrant out for your arrest. For your involvement in the death of TJ."

Ben caught his breath, sharply, sending a stuttering whine over the line.

"Sand killed TJ, or had him killed, Terry. To cover up his drug-running operation."

Ben heard his voice rising a notch in pitch and in volume.

He knew enough about law to know what "your word against his" meant. That's exactly what Terry was hearing. And the terrible pain of thinking Ben had rejected her had her leaning toward Sand's versions of things. Ben felt a stab of agony, frustration, and boiling rage hit his stomach, burn like battery acid. When he spoke again he could hear the tightness of his voice, the hate that was torturing him.

"Sand is a liar. I feel like killing him for what he's done to us."

Terry's voice was so soft, the tone so distant, that Ben had the mental image of her having taken one step away from the phone, moving back, away from him.

"Don't say that, Ben. I can't stand hearing you talk like that. TJ-"

"I need to see you, Terry. I need to explain this, we need to talk it out. Sand did this to us. I love you. I need your friendship and your help. I need to help you .and Lester. You're in great danger."

"Dick didn't make you ride away without a word and leave me standing by the road alone.

Oh yes he did, Terry. He did just exactly that. The memory of the tape burned in his mind. He couldn't tell her over the phone. If I did would she believe me? I couldn't believe it myself ..

"I'll help you, Ben, if I can. If you'll give yourself up. Dick and I can meet you anywhere you say."

Ben saw himself, arrested, his hands manacled behind his back, Sand grinning that big Texas grin he hated so much. While Terry looked on. He shook his head. No way.

"I can't do that, Terry. Sand would have me killed within an hour after I surrender to him."

"I won't listen to you speak of him that way, Ben. You don't know what he's done, for me after you left me, and how many chances he's taken, to stop the filthy trade that killed TJ. That injures so many innocent people. He risks his life every day to stop people .. like you."

The words slammed into Ben. Terry's voice sounded very distant now. The Grand Canyon was back there, between them. Ben felt tears of frustration sting his eyes. He fought hard to keep them out of his voice.

"I guess I'll have to prove what I'm saying to you. I do love you. Please believe that."

"I believe what Dick said, Ben. That you would tell me anything, play on any emotion, dredge up any memories that would get you what you want. Why don't you give up, let the law take its course, clean up your life, and stop hurting .. stop killing children?"

Those cutting words, the icy tone, the surging emotion flowing through him, ripped open the dark space inside him, and it yawned open wide again. Ready to receive his soul.

What's the use? he heard the words echo hollowly in his mind.

Dick Sand has me beat again. The thought filtered through him like strychnine. Taking his breath. Tying his guts in knots. Killing his will. It left him feeling weak, inept, and unmanly, angry and vengeful. Awash in a boiling sea of emotion.

He was losing. Losing everything. Losing Terry.

He was a loser.

But deep in that darkness also smoldered the rage that Sand had kindled in him at Tibble Fork. It flared, flamed, and a grim and settled determination took hold of him. Altered this time. Focused, welded by he heat of his rage to his being like steel.

I may lose, Sand. But you won't win. Not if I have to kill you. If there's no other way, I'm going to take you with me when I go.

He saw REX again in his mind's eye. Huge, and full of anger. Ready to help Ben against Dick Sand.

"I've got to go, Terry. Please don't tell Sand I called. He doesn't know where I am I need some time to get proof that what I'm telling you is true. Be careful, Terry. Be very careful, please. Don't trust Sand ."

He tried to short circuit the rage in him and to speak to her as he used to, as a friend. He could tell instantly what a miserable failure that was. He was hearing himself as he thought Terry heard him. As a criminal trying to manipulate a friend. A despicable thing. Something Dick Sand would do. Was doing. To Terry.

But how could he help her see it?

"I can't promise that, Ben. You're a wanted criminal, perhaps involved in the death of a child. I can't hide you. Give yourself up, Ben. Don't hurt Dick Sand, please. If you ever cared for me, give yourself up and don't hurt the man I intend to marry. You've hurt me enough, Ben. Don't hurt me any more. Please?"

Her voice trailed of into a whisper, an appeal that tore out his heart.

Marry? Dick Sand?

Ben trembled. His mouth opened and nothing came out.

Terry and that monster?

But there was nothing to be said. Sand had done his work well. Still covering all the details. Insinuating himself between him and Terry.

Keeping Terry close where he could watch her?

Fear began to dominate the emotions Ben was drowning in. He was sure that Sand would eliminate her when she was no more use to him. Just as quickly, just as dispassionately, has he had TJ, or the men at Muley Point.

She was just another detail.

But what a dear detail she was to Ben!

"I'm sorry, Terry. I've got to go now." He heard the catch in her breath and realized that that was what he'd said that morning at WVCC. Sand had him on the run again, and again there was nothing he could say to her.

He set the phone gently back on its holder. The line went dead. Ben felt a little of himself die with it. He could feel his mind fraying at the edges. The unending emotional stress was wearing on him. Making him feel old, world weary. There seemed to be no end to it.

How did it come to this? How did I get here? What could I have done?

Grandpa Tsosie would saw everything leaves tracks. Even the Coyote men. You have to find tracks. Follow them back, find out what made them and why. Nothing happens by accident. Everything has its causes.

You caused this, Shony. You left the Navajo Way. You started thinking about yourself like you were a big shot. Like you were better than other Navajos. Like you could live the White Man's Way

This is all my fault Now I'm just making it worse

He thought back bitterly to his decision to see Terry at least once more, no matter what it cost, so that if the worst happened to him she would at least be able to make a life for herself knowing that he had loved her. If he died now he would leave her thinking he was nothing but a vicious criminal. What a stupid idea.

Sand had moved in and turned her against him. Created doubts and conflicts in her mind. Ben knew Sand would be tormenting her even as he held her in his net, helpless, vulnerable, innocent, and in terrible danger. Because Ben had heard in her voice that she was going to tell Sand he had called her. Sand would keep her alive only as long as she was bait for Ben.

Suddenly time was rushing past. Ben felt a driving need to do something, and do it fast. Most of all, not to get caught. That would kill him and probably Terry too.

He heard a car turn the corner and start up the block. A shock of adrenaline shot through him. What if it was Sand, trying his best to see that Ben didn't get any older. That he had a long rest on the bottom of some nearby reservoir. He was relieved to see it was only a small VW bug bringing a weary student home to the dorms.

Now he had Terry's life in his hands, the fear was breaking loose again, running deep and powerful in him, sucking at his strength like the rapids had choked off his air. Ben released his pent-up breath in a shuddering gasp. He should be far from here, not so close he could see Terry's front door.

But the rage was there too, the mixture of rage and fear making a horrible muddle of his emotions, overloading his mind. Scared as he was, teeth clenched, hands balled into fists so tight he could feel the fingernails digging into his palms, he vowed: So help me Sand, if you hurt her I'll kill you if it's that last thing I do.

He could see now that he couldn't just stand still and do nothing. Sand would win automatically, easily. His first plan lay in tatters at his feet.

Plan B was ..what?

He would get REX's help. He would go after Sand and his goons with all the power he could muster. I'll do anything, Ben thought, his body growing hard as the tension of his hate swept through him and he pulled himself upright and shrugged his shoulders, feeling the strength that was there now.

Then he saw Sand's cherry red sports car coming down the block toward him. He moved a little, to block more of his body from view, sliding behind the phone booth while he stared at his enemy. He heard Sand beep his horn and saw the door open on the passenger side. Then he saw Terry coming out of her apartment, hurrying down the steps, almost tripping in her haste to get to the car. She leaned in and said something.

Sand reached down and picked up a handset or a mobile phone. Terry jumped in the car, throwing Ben's furiously pumping brain into overload. He watched, fascinated, horrified, as Sand leaned over and kissed Terry lightly on the mouth. He was shaking his head, smiling, easy and relaxed. That rattled Ben. He should have been doing everything except calling out the National Guard.

Then Ben remembered that Terry didn't know where he'd called from. Sand didn't realize he was here, right next to him. His mind ticked over, despite the fury that scorched him. Terry was dressed for a picnic. Prince gazed out between them from the back seat, grinning at Ben through the windshield.

Ben felt the outrage burn up so bright, the winds of hate fan the fires so hot in him that fear evaporated like water on a red hot stove. His mind went icy cold.

Ben would tag along on this picnic. Maybe invite himself over for desert. He would make Sand confess to Terry. He wouldn't need REX's help or anyone else.

Sand started up and drove toward him. Ben stepped around the booth as they passed, keeping it between them and him in the twilight. But they were full of each other, talking animatedly, Terry gesturing as she spoke.

Only the Black Prince was aware that Ben was there. His head turned to hold Ben in his gaze as the car moved past him. He was grinning his devil grin, Ben saw him as laughing at him Amused, disdainful, deadly.

Ben raced to get back to his bike before he lost track of the jaunty red rich man's car.

****

"You don't have to worry about him any more, Sweet," Sand said softly. "We know where he is now. He's in Cortez, Colorado. They found his trail, found his rental car in the garage for service. When he comes for it they'll arrest him. They may find him even before that. They're looking through the campgrounds now." Sand squeezed her hand and gave her one of his best grins.

"Let's don't let anything spoil this evening. I got special plans for us."

Terry looked into Sand's eyes. She saw amusement, calculation, and maybe, just maybe, love. He's going to propose tonight, just like I thought. I won't let Ben spoil that for me.

She was furious with Ben that he would be so inconsiderate as to call her just at this moment when her life was about to take such an important turn. Angry that he would try to assassinate the character of this good man, to accuse him of doing what Ben himself was doing.

She firmly repressed the memories of her and Ben together. It left a huge vacuum in her emotional fiber, an unsettling dead spot in her life. Her feelings were

Warrior's Way

still in turmoil, but when she began to feel wrongly about Ben all she had to do was call up again what she'd felt the moment he'd coldly driven away, leaving all her dreams and plans and their friendship in little heaps of ash at her feet. How could he be so cruel as to just drive away

She fought down the surge of emotion, the loss. Not now, not here

She squeezed back and settled herself in for the luxurious ride up the canyon to Derky's Lake. She tried to imagine herself driving this powerful, smooth-running dream car after she and Dick were married.

Passing some of her former friends, waving gaily, seeing their looks of envy and disappointment. Her face burned a little as she thought of those 'friends' now. They had rallied around her when they learned what Ben had done, and then scattered like sheep before a lion when Sand showed interest in her. Sand had a rough reputation around school. And her friends were scandalized yet again when she took up with him. They reminded her of her upbringing. Not in words, but in long, sober, knowing looks when he was around. Yes, it would be nice to prove them wrong, to have something for herself to make up for what she lost with Ben.

" ..don't you think," she heard Dick say, realizing that she hadn't been listening, but thinking again of Ben. She pinched herself sharply where Dick couldn't see and put on a lazy smile as she turned to him.

"I'm sorry. This is so relaxing. I must have drifted away for a moment. I'm afraid I didn't hear what you said." She almost added "dear", but it got stuck sideways in her throat and she couldn't get it to come out of her mouth.

"I just said, I ought to let you drive this thing. I drive so much anyway that I get tired of it. Maybe on the way back later, what do you think."

"Oh Dick, I'd kill to drive a car like this."

"Not me, though, would you?"

He smiled, but she noticed a withdrawal of sorts inside him. That's right she thought, feeling foolish. The word kill would have a different meaning to a man like him.

"I just meant I'd love to drive, anytime."

Maybe drive home past Melanie's place, she thought, nestling down into a little glow of satisfaction.

****

They arrive at Derky's Lake campground, load their picnic gear into a rowboat and go across a narrow arm of the lake to a secluded little bay that has a sandy beach and high lava rock walls on each side. The back of the sheltered cove ends in brush and trees. Terry has no notion of what lays beyond. The cove gives the feeling of deep seclusion. Only from the beach can you see across the lake to the boat landing and the concession stands. Terry feels a fluttering sense of unease as they move up the cove a little, out of sight.

She tries to appear domestic, laying out the blanket and the picnic while Dick builds a small fire. Twilight will soon turn to full dark, and the early summer air will be cool. Cuddling weather. Again Terry feels a little unease, catches herself sighing. She may well have to match deed to word tonight. Dick will press her, undoubtedly. The next hours will be a watershed in her life. She gazes across the quiet water, feeling sorry for herself. Her prospects had changed. The life she'd hoped to live was no longer attainable. Now it all came down to a few hours, and fewer options.

Once she's lived them, one way or another, her life will take one road of two roads. She'd be alone or be bonded to Dick Sand heart and soul, having given all she had to give a man. The roads lead in opposite directions, never to converge again. You're going to be all grown up tonight, she thinks. Life will never be the same again. She wishes she knew what she will do.

"The fire will feel good soon, Sweet," Dick said, dropping down on the blanket, he leans back on his elbows and gazes up at Terry. The smile, friendly, the eyes? Calculating, measuring, weighing. She shivers involuntarily and moves to the fire to warm her hands. "Should have brought a pole to set out, we might catch a fish when the moon's up. They any catfish in this waterin' hole?"

He drops into that stupid Texas talk whenever he's feeling strong, in control, feeling self-satisfied and strong, she thought. Then he doesn't much care what anybody thinks of him. She's saved the trouble of finding an answer. The beeper Dick wears at his belt goes off.

"D ., darn," he says. "I meant to leave it in the car." He rolls over, gets to his feet in a fluid, powerful motion and heads for the boat. "You just relax, honey. I'll be right back. Whatever it is, someone else will handle it tonight. I got big plans and I ain't .I'm not going to change them."

Terry smiles, sits on the blanket, watches as Dick pushes off in the boat. Prince, never out of Dick's sight, leaps into the boat for the trip. Sand almost makes the boat plane as he pulls across the lake with long, powerful strokes. A man with a mission, Terry thinks. And I'm the objective. She sets down on the blanket, feeling a little like the princess in the castle tower, waiting to be saved by the knight in shining armor.

While she waits she wonders idly if knights of old had kill-trained Dobermans as a house pets the way hers did

Sand called the dispatch operator in Salt Lake and got the number of the Grand County Sheriff in Colorado. It took less than five minutes to get the bad news.

"Sorry, deputy. There's been a mistake."

"Mistake, what mistake? What are you talking about. You said you had Singer all but in custody. Just a matter of time, you said." He heard his voice taking on an edge, rising in pitch. He forced himself to remember that these were not his people he was talking to, just cooperating police agencies.

"If there's any fault in this, Mr. Sand, it isn't all ours." The coolness in the voice could be heard all the way from Colorado.

"I'm sure it's not, sir. I didn't mean to imply there was any fault. I just want this man badly. You understand. Sometimes we get our personal feelings involved in a case and it truly does cloud our judgment. The little boy was only 13, and I knew him quite well. If I'd had a little brother, he's the kind of kid I'd want it to be. Please excuse my bad manners."

That good enough for you? Sand thought. Have I said the right words? He knew how good he was. Part of it was that he could say anything at all, any sort of lie, and sound like he really meant it.

If it served his purpose. That's part of what got you where you are, Dick old boy, he thought.

"That's okay, Deputy. No offense taken. What happened was, the rental car hadn't been turned in. He left it at the service station because the rental agency asked him to so it could be serviced. It was one of them rent a wreck outfits, not a regular agency. We found that out only when they sent someone to pick it up. Unfortunately for him he was Hispanic, dark complected and all. I'm afraid we gave him quite a scare."

Sand heard the note of amusement in the distant voice.

"So you haven't a clue, is that it? About where he is now?"

"Well, there's more to this. We circulated the picture you faxed us. We haven't found anyone who has seen that man around here. Now we did find a bike shop where a guy walked in, ordered a street legal trail bike and a trailer. Paid cash. In another place we found a man had bought five sets of survival type gear, including five wrist rockets. That's what made the clerk remember him."

"But not the picture, is that it?"

"That's it, but it's not all." A note of satisfaction filtered down the wire from Colorado. "There's an apparent connection."

"Connection to what?" Sand felt himself chewing the inside of his lip. Irritated, he stopped abruptly.

"To the car and the other stuff. Though the man doesn't look like the picture, he was wearing an old Harvard tee shirt when he turned the car in. So we're pretty sure that guy was this Ben Singer. We know for sure that he was using Ben Singer's ID."

"Okay, so .?" Don't get impatient, Sand berated himself. You need these people.

"So, Mr. Sand, the man who picked up the bike, and the man who bought the survival equipment was wearing an old Harvard tee shirt too. General description matches. Chunky, Indian male. So broad he looks short until he gets close. Just over six feet tall. Spooky is the word one witness used. Intense, focused, something. Not your ordinary person."

"He may be using Singer's ID. But that's not Singer. He's just a hunk of flab. We called him the dough boy. Just a big, soft teddy bear of a guy. I had to get rough with him to stop him hurting one of our local blacks. He was hopeless as a fighter. Nope, somehow Singer has lost his ID. He was known to have bought wine. His dad was a wino who died in prison down in New Mexico .."

"Was that Frank Singer?" The voice was suddenly sharply interested.

"Yeah, I think so. Does it matter? He's dead."

"If I was you, deputy Sand, I'd get a confirmation on that. Make sure he's dead, I mean. We had him as a guest, briefly, about four years ago. Picked him up drunk in Cortez. Decided he didn't like the company. Kicked the door off of a police cruiser. Went through officers like a hay mowing machine. Broke both legs of one man. Walked off into McElmo wash. That leads through some rough country back to Utah. We got out posses with dogs, trackers, long-range rife shooters, you name it. Never caught sight of him. He popped up back at Navajo Mountain, but we couldn't get the locals to arrest him. Said they'd tried before, but couldn't do it. I heard they trapped him in Gallup. Caught him when he was dead drunk. Literally netted him with steel mesh nets, shackled him, and never took them off."

"I'm sure he's dead." Sand heard in his voice that he wasn't sure at all. Why hadn't he killed Ben and Lester that night and been done with it? Get a little fancy and suddenly you got big problems. Sand rubbed the ache in his belly.

"Won't hurt to check. Now that I think of it, that description sounds like him. Especially the spooky part. He might be using this Ben Singer's ID. Maybe Ben's his boy. And he's on your trail."

"Thanks. I appreciate your extra work on this. Hope we can help you out this well sometime."

"Take this seriously, deputy. Get yourself some help if you need it. Don't take chances. These people have been on this land a long time. When they set their mind to it they can be nasty. Real nasty. Remember the pioneers."

"Yeah, thanks. I'll do that. Better get on it right away. Oh, by the way, how long ago was this, when he was there? When he got the bike?"

"Three days ago, deputy. He could be anywhere by now."

The line went dead. The silence of the mountain fastness became almost a physical weight resting on him. He glanced around in the twilight. The shadows were getting deep, turning black.

What have I got here? Is daddy coming after me? I've got to know what I'm up against. What to prepare for. What assets to pull in. I've got everything I need. I just don't have it here. Right now. He hadn't planned on becoming the hunted. Mistake. Don't make any more. Take care of this now, once and for all ..

He fought down an impulse to get in the car and drive away, leaving Terry to find her own way back. You're getting sloppy, Dicky, he heard his father's voice say in his mind. Just down right foolish. Chasing a skirt. You never did that before

Taking vengeance on Ben Singer by ruining his girl for him. Not tending to business. Business before pleasure. That's always been your motto.

"Tend to business," he said aloud. He saw Prince prick up his ears at the sound of his voice, listening for sounds he knew.

"Let's go, boy," he said, motioning with his hand for Prince to precede him to the boat. "We'll get our business done, then we'll play."

As he rowed back to Terry he searched the surrounding brush and rocks. The cove looked like a trap more than a romantic hideaway now. He'd tell Terry they had to leave, that he had an emergency. That they'd have their special night another day, soon. "After I do some business."

Terry watches the boat coming back, bringing her knight, with the same mixed emotions she's had all night. A great drawing apart, a moving away, from this situation. And an equally firm determination to get something for herself, to make a try at having a life. Now the life she wanted most turned out to be a foolish dream. Like a princess in the tower. She would come down from the tower. She was sure of it. Almost.

"Took longer than you thought, I guess," she says, meeting him by the boat. "Is there a problem?" I hope, the coward in her says.

"Yes. Lost child. They're calling everyone in. Want me to bring Prince. I'm afraid we have to go back. Sorry. I know you were looking forward to this. We'll just have our special time together another day, Sweet." She sees the look again, calculating, almost predatory. He's the cat and I'm the bird, she thinks.

"I'll save my surprise for you for another time." The grin spreads all over his face. She thinks she sees it almost reach his eyes.

At this moment Prince goes on guard, lips drawn back from the huge white fangs, nose wrinkled, feet planted firmly in the sand.

Terry feels the hair rising on her neck, sees Dick staring past her, toward the brush at the back of the cove. She turns to look and there, in the twilight shadows stands a man. Short, square, dark. An Indian looking man with a bow fitted with a razor sharp broad head glinting redly in the sunset. Another arrow gripped in the bowhand, and the bow held crossways across the body, the bow parallel with the ground, the other hand holding the string, the arrow fixed tightly between the fingers. Held the way Indian warriors hold their bows in pictures of the old west.

He could be Mexican or South American. The chill in the air settles around her heart. Maybe he's here to kill Dick. The face is in shadow, the eyes dark holes in the mask of the face. He steps forward and Prince crouches, the growl in his throat doubles in volume. In the clearer light she can see that he wears an old, travel-stained Harvard tee shirt.

Chapter 20
Terry Shoots Ben

Ben steps out of the brush and sees Prince crouch lower, he hears dog the growl, sees the gleaming fangs, and doesn't care. The dog's bigger than a rabbit. He holds two arrows. He knows he can put one in the dog and before it hits, put the other in Sand.

Sand seems to know it too. He starts to shift his weight, to move behind Terry, his hand starts to creep around his back to the belt gun he wears centered on his spine.

"Do it, Sand. Go on and do it."

The voice rumbles in his chest. Propelled by the raging urge to kill Sand now, to end his evil, right here. Sand straightens up, drops his hands to his sides. Ben knows he can draw and fire from that position in less than two seconds. His nerves stay taut, his senses expanded, time slowed, everything around him part of his awareness. Another step.

Prince crouches deeper, his belly almost touching the sand, his muscles gather in knots and bunches, ready to launch him at Sand's command.

"It won't work, Sand. I shoot you first, no matter what, I'll get you first."

"Down, Prince." Ben hears the nerves in the voice. Sand is taut as piano wire inside.

"Who is he, Dick?" The voice querulous, almost squeaky.

"You don't recognize him, Sweet? He's our old friend. That's Ben."

Ben watches Sand watching him. Waiting for that two seconds, for the blink of an eye. He won't get it.

Terry starts to move forward, as though to see better the face of the apparition in front of her.

"Ben, can that be you, Ben? Are you here?"

Ben felt the slightest nod move his head, not enough to break his concentration.

"Get rid of it, Sand, left handed, and slow. Drop it in the boat and step away. If you want the dog, call him off, now."

He watches as Sand removes his small automatic. He isn't carrying the big 357. He's off duty. On a picnic. With my girl. Ben feels the steady burning of the hate in him. He steps forward again, stops a few feet away, motions Sand to move further away from Terry.

"Don't do this, Ben. I asked you on the phone not to do this. Give yourself up. We'll help if we can. But don't kill him . please?"

Sand looks a little sick, like he doesn't like to hear the word `kill' injected into the conversation. Prince gazes almost lovingly at Ben, mouth agape, fangs wet with the drool of anticipation. Barely restrained by Sand's command, fully expecting to be allowed to kill Ben. Just waiting for Sand to say that magic word. Just a leap, two bounds, and he's tearing out the throat. He's done it before, knows exactly what to do. He's kill-trained by murderers, not policemen.

"Tell her, Sand. What you've done."

Sand looks at him, at the broad head glinting in the declining light. He swallows. Takes a heaving breath.

"What do you want me to say, Ben?" Just a touch of quaver in the voice, the eyes? Still cold and dead, calculating, measuring, watching for that momentary chance. Ben feels the rage spill over the edge of his soul and start running down through him like hot lava down a hillside.

"What you did, you scum. You killed TJ, you tried to kill me, you killed the men who failed to get me, that you're a drug runner and a killer."

Ben sees Sand blink when he talks of the two who died. Sand is surprised he knows. Now, along with the watching, a little glint of fear appears in his eyes. Ben draws the bow a little tighter, the arrow centers unwaveringly on Sand's heart.

"Say it, Sand." Ben hears the finality in his voice, the deep rumble of it, how it burns with the rage burning inside him.

"Ben, don't, oh please don't." Terry screams. She stumbles forward, toward Ben, between him and Sand. Sand snaps his fingers, the dull pop igniting the rockets in the killer Doberman's legs. Prince is launched at his target, only a low growl now, like the sound of rocket engines in flight. Sand ducks sideways, looking always at Ben, but groping for the side of the boat and the gun.

Ben drops the bow, turns the right shoulder toward the dog, his hand hangs loosely, straight down. His throat offers an open target. Prince launches. His feet leave the ground. Ben whips his arm up with all his strength, the arm bent at an angle, the classic Karate defense for a blow to the head. He catches the dog airborne, smashes him just behind the forelegs, collapsing the chest. Hurtling the breathless dog upward, into the beginning of a backward somersault. He jerks his head back a little and hears the clashing chomping sound Prince's teeth make as they bite empty air.

Time flows in slow motion. Sand still hunches toward the boat, Terry falls to her hands and knees in the sand. Ben grabs the back legs of the dog, half-way up. locking strongly over to upper leg joint, gripping hard, his fingers biting deeply into hide and muscle and sinew. He makes the dog an extension of his arms as he steps toward Sand, swings the dog in a huge, fast arc so gravity keeps the body and the head extended, the jaws far away. Blood lust colors the edges of his vision, but Sand is centered in his gaze. He feels his mouth pulled into a snarl and hears a growl greater and deeper than any dog's, coming from inside him.

He sees the look in Sand's eyes as he brings the dog crashing around, the face of the dog aimed squarely at Sand's. Sand has to fall back, away from the boat, gets his arms up, takes most of the blow that way, but part of Prince's head makes it through and the fangs gash his face and the hard, bony head slaps him hard, high on the cheek bone and near the eye.

But missing the temple. Averting the death blow. Without pause Ben brings the dog around again, swings, not from the hips, but rotates his whole body, down to his knees in a huge movement that releases every ounce of strength in his body. Sees Sand's face go pale, his eyes lose luster, red spots on his cheeks. Awe and fear and hate in his eyes.

Ben accelerates the driving downward thrust of the club that was once an animal. The dog's head cracks against the bow of the boat, the neck shatters, the body goes limp. The blow this time glances off Sand's shoulder, spattering him with dog blood that is gushing from Prince's mouth and nose. Ben flails Sand with the dog, slashing and driving him away from the boat. But the dog's no longer enough.

Ben drops The Black Prince like a forgotten doll and moves at Sand, hands extended to choke him. Sand comes to his feet in a fluid, powerful motion, the grin in place, the body erect and ready. Ben feels a smashing blow hit his forehead. Finds its power absorbed by the massive muscles of his neck, moves on. He feels clumsy compared to Sand. He feeds his rage, lets it power his body, lock in his Isometric systems till his body is a rigid platform of bone and sinew and white hot rage, ready for his action muscles to go to work.

Sand grasps his wrists, trying to force his arms down. Ben twists, feels his arms rotate in Sand's grip, breaks free, feeling one of Sand's thumbs break or dislocate, walks through his defense and grabs Sand up close in a bear hug, burying his head near the armpit. Feels Sand's hands groping, unable to find a purchase, his body unable to position him to kick or throw Ben off.

Ben puts power, hate, fear, and pride into his arms and locks down around Sand's chest. Squeezing off the breath. But Sand's upper body is too strong. Like circus strongmen who break chains wrapped around their chests, Sand expands Ben's grip each time he breathes. Not good enough.

Sand isn't dying.

Ben sees Axel's instruction. Sand is long-bodied. He doesn't know how to deliberately energize his isotonic systems. He's not close coupled like Ben and his father. Will never be able to unleash the raw power that he can.

Ben drops his grip to Sand's belt line and unleashes every ounce of power he can send to his arms and shoulders. He feels Sands body give, hears joints pop. He looks up now, along Sand's chest. Sees Sand leaning back, an awful sound of strangling and agony coming from his gaping mouth. Ben feels his arms pushing at Ben, trying to break his grip. Pathetic. Goodby, Dick Sand. You killed me in agony in the cave shelter in Whitehouse Canyon.

Here, let me return the favor.

Ben shifts just a little, to get the small increment of leverage he needs to finish separating Sand's spine. He feels even through the anesthesia of rage, something hard and cold pressed against his temple. He looks and stares into the unblinking eye of Sand's little off-duty automatic. Behind it he sees Terry's face. Grim. Settled. Determined.

"Let him go, Ben. Now. I mean it Ben, let him go."

Ben hears the click of the hammer being pulled back and seated. He sees the pad of her trigger finger start to whiten as she begins putting pressure on the trigger. He

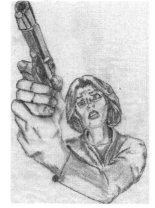

releases Sand, who drops, moaning, to the sand, both hands pressed into the small of his back. He breathes raggedly, shallowly to inhibit the waves of agony that roll over him when he moves.

Ben looks down at him. Knows exactly how he feels. With Sand's help, he has been there. He feels no pity whatever.

"That's what he did to me, Terry. At Tibble Fork the night before I left. He did worse to Lester. He deserves to die for what he's done to so many innocent people. To you and me."

Terry steps back, well out of Ben's reach. The gun stays steady. Terry has had police training with guns. If she wants to shoot she knows how. The look in her eyes, behind the fierce determination to stop him from hurting Sand, says she doesn't know what she wants right now. A dangerous mood for a woman, Ben decides.

He takes a step away, toward the brush. Out of easy range for a small automatic in the hands of a distraught woman.

"Don't let him go, Terry. You see how dangerous he is. You see what I told you is true. Every bit. Shoot him or make him get down on his belly. Don't let him get away."

Sand's voice is ragged, the look in his eye, triumphant. He has Ben's own girl pointing a gun at him, ready to pull the trigger. Ben takes another step back, stands on the edge of the bow, raises it up to meet his hand.

"If you pick up an arrow, Ben. I'll shoot. Don't try me. I will shoot to save Dick's life." Settled, determined. Ben believes what she says. Feels despair creeping in to extinguish the burning anger, great clouds of steam rise up, misting his eyes.

"Terry, you've got to believe me. Believe what he is. For " He almost says: For your own sake if not for mine. Not words to be planted in Sand's mind.

Another step back.

Sand starts try to get up, to get to Terry and take the gun.

"Stop, Ben. You've got to surrender. You are everything you accuse him of being. If you take another step I will be forced to shoot. Don't make me do that Ben, please don't make me do that."

A quaver, a moment of doubt. Ben takes a step back. The gun goes off with a shattering report in the small cove. Ben sees powder smoke rolling towards him, feels a pounding, burning blow along his scalp, above his ear. Turns and sprints to the brush, not looking back. She doesn't shoot again. In the brush he turns, sees Terry kneeling in the sand, shoulders heaving, hands over her face. He feels again the dark knot of anguish, loss, and frustration that he felt the day he left Terry with Sand and ran from Warren County.

Sees Sand crawling over to get the gun. Moving painfully. But alive. On top. Winning. Ben turns his face to the sky but suppresses the howl of anguish he feels. Then he races for the bike he left back in the willows. There are only two ways out of the canyon. Now the hunt is on. Ben Singer is the rabbit.

Again.

****

Terry lay in bed, watching lights dance on the ceiling as cars passed, as the night breeze stirred the curtains. Strange shapes formed themselves in the patterns of light and shadow in the room. crickets created their steady chirping racket outside the window. On the breeze that stirred the curtains she could detect the odors of the lake. Fishy, muddy banks, cattails and willows, mint and sagebrush all lent their odor to the cool night air.

It was another world, Natures world. It went on even when human worlds ended. Nature was cruel too. But at least based on predictable laws of instinct and science. Why couldn't human life be that way? She felt her stomach contract and rumble. Partly from hunger. She was eating less to be more like Dick's ideal woman. It was the least she could do for him since he planned to marry her and make her rich for life.

But much of the pain came from the memory of how different her life had become.

She had shot Ben! A man she had loved. Counted on, planned a life with. She had spilled his blood, she'd seen it on the bushes where he ran away. Perhaps she had killed him. Maybe he was lying somewhere out there in the dark--in pain. Growing weaker as the night passed.

She had to push that thought away. Put it at arm's length.

The man she had shot was a dangerous man. A murderer. Horrified, she saw again the murderous rage that had driven Ben as he fought with Dick. The madness in Ben's eyes when she had stopped him from killing Sand. The appeal she saw there. Let me finish this. Don't stop me now. Please, the eyes had said. Please let me kill this man

To kill a brave man, noble man like Dick Sand! She marveled again at how Ben had changed. So strong now. His body square and powerful. Not the soft, easy going man she had loved. Hard now. Hard outside. Hard inside. Filled with an anger that shocked and repelled her. How could a man who had dedicated his life to doing good, defending the weak, become such a beast in so short a time?

The answer was obvious. He couldn't. He had been that way all along. Down inside. Carefully concealed from her, had been this evil, criminal nature. He had deceived her all along.

She felt tears trickling down the side of her cheek. How could she have been fooled so completely? She had no confidence at all in her own judgments about people anymore. Ben and Lester. What a tragedy her life was. Thank goodness she had Dick to lean on. He could see her through this.

She saw the engagement ring on her finger glittering in the darkness, seeming almost to have an internal light of its own. Like the star that led Peter Pan and Wendy to Never-Never Land. It was a small beacon in the night. Reminding her of the secure future that awaited her with Dick Sand. He'd slipped it on her finger on the ride home as she sat, sobbing, torn by emotions too complex and entangled to express.

To see Sand and Ben fighting like wild animals.

To see the power Ben had now.

Frightening.

To shoot Ben.

A surge of fear washed through her. She had to get rid of these old emotions. She had loved a fantasy man. Now she had to put it behind her or the ghost of Ben Singer would insinuate itself between her and Dick. Make it impossible to give herself completely to him.

Her stomach rumbled again. Dieting and worrying didn't go well together. She though about going to the refrigerator. She put it firmly out of her mind. I have to have a life, she thought. I can't, I won't spend my life in mourning for a fantasy. I can respect Dick and given time I can come to love him too.

In her mind's eyes she saw Ben again, standing in dark silhouette against the western sky. The bow and the terrible arrow gripped in his hands, threatening Dick. She didn't even know it was Ben until she heard Sand call his name. He was that different. Frightening. At first she thought it was someone sent after Dick by the criminals he was fighting to bring to justice. She was right, of course. She just didn't realize that it was the man she once had given her heart.

She knew now he was not her kind of man. He had changed. Or rather, shown his true colors at last. No, she could never love such a person. The tears trickled again. She felt so sorry for herself. To have lost such a dream. Even though that's what it all had been. Just a dream. Never real.

She fell into a fitful sleep. Twice she awoke. Crying, shaking with fear, self-loathing. Remembering her dream. Starting with the feeling, the hardening conviction in her that she must stop Ben. That in the name of law and humanity she must shoot a man she once had loved. (Still loved the impish part of her mind said)

Warrior's Way

Feeling again the kick of the gun in her hand, hearing the sharp report of the automatic, seeing the cloud of gun smoke billow out to cover Ben. The startled look on his face, his hand flying to the side of his head, the sight of him running away, perhaps to die alone somewhere in the woods like a wounded animal.

She finally curled herself into a little ball of misery and waited out the rest of the night.

Sleepless.

Determined.

Feeling a hardening going on inside her as she shut down and locked away emotions that were worse than useless to her now. She vowed she'd become like the diamond. Brilliant. Glittering. And hard. Ever so hard and cold.

Chapter 21
Ben Travels In Time

Ben stared moodily into the fire. Yellow-orange wisps of flame licked up to consume the dry pine. Like his rage had burned up his reason when he saw Sand with Terry. He had thought it would be all over. That Sand would confess. Or be dead. That Terry would understand.

Certainly not that she would shoot him.

Shoot to kill.

Ben shook his head. A massive sigh rumbled through him. His head hung listlessly forward, every isometric system had let go. His body hung on its ligaments. As it had before he met Alex. His breath had sunk into his belly and his chest barely moved. It was uncomfortable, even painful now to sit that way.

It matched his mood perfectly.

Sand's trying to kill me, Alex lectures me but won't help. Rex says I□m a wimp if I don't go after Sand Granpa treats me like a non-person. Terry tries to kill me .. Lets see, what are people telling me about myself?

What options do I have left?

He sighed again. Just what he'd had all along. Sand was going to kill him. That was more certain than ever now. There would be a heavier search, more news coverage, more people trying to help Sand catch him. Terry would sign the complaint. Sand would play the hero and surround himself with lots of protection ..not all of them law officers. Ben Singer would be dead "resisting arrest", "attempting to escape". Killed all alone on some lonely mountain by a rifle shot he'd never hear, by a man he'd never see.

They had the poisoned hand. He had A dust mop of a dog, a dirty, travel worn bike, and an old bow. They don't have a chance. I'll get 'em all for sure ..for sure.

If rage were a weapon he'd be invincible.

He went over it again and again in his mind. He had nothing else to do, anyway. The shaking, red-visioned rage he'd felt scared him now. He would have killed Sand in another moment. And not have regretted it. How could one man generate such feelings in another man? How could such a killing rage be found in humans? He would have killed Sand and proven him guilty later. Ben knew now, that was in his mind when he clamped his arms around Sand for the last time.

Justifiable homicide. In the eyes of the law, perhaps. What of Ben's soul? What was the verdict there?

The jury was still out.

Ben made an effort to clear his mind, to shake off the gloom. He gazed out through the trees at an open patch of star-lit sky.

Empty sky. Empty, hopeless life. Being hunted gave life a whole new slant. Ben knew now what many early western outlaws learned. It's easy to stay out of sight if you don't mind rough living. If you don't mind having lots of time on your hands and just a dog for company. Everyone in 500 miles looking for you with guns. The one you love in the hands of your worst enemy.

Being powerless no matter how strong you are.

Ben was vastly more powerful now than Dick Sand. Due mostly to his genetic physical inheritance, the muscle, bone, sinew and metabolism he had inherited. Which was nothing by itself. He had supplied the determination and effort needed to raise his actual physical condition to nearly the level of his optimum genetic potential.

But Dick Sand still lived in a big house with servants. Ben lived in a camp on the north side of a slope, in deep timber and ate what he could catch plus some vitamins for a dietary supplement.

Dick Sand went on with his evil life. Ben Singer's life might as well be over.

Except that Ben Singer has a friend, a definite Ace in the hole. Named REX.

He pulled out a map, hunched over it, figuring the best was to get to Diamond Fork Canyon from where he was. Then he saw Bud prick up his ears and looked up to see Alex walking up the slope to the camp.

"Hi, Ben. You're looking good. Really filled out, haven't you."

Ben watched a little sourly as Bud turned himself inside out greeting Alex, bouncing around, wagging his whole body, trying to talk, it seemed, finally jumping up into his arms. He had never treated Ben that way, and since the fight with Sand at Derky's Lake, Bud had treated Ben with perfunctory courtesy at best.

"Hasn't done me a whole lot of good, so far." Ben heard the rough note of aggravation in his voice and instantly regretted it. He owed Alex a lot. No use punishing him because he couldn't do everything. Alex was not Ben's fairy godmother, he had no magic wand. But he had saved Ben's life so he could meet REX. That was certainly worth something.

"Sorry, Alex. I'm grouchy. Sit down and have some squirrel and rabbit stew."

"Thanks, Ben. I just ate. Anyway, I'm sort of here on business today."

He seemed to wrinkle his nose a little at the odor of the stew that wafted through camp.

Alex sat down, cross legged, comfortable and started talking again.

Mostly nonsense.

"Edmund Burke said it a long time ago, Ben. " Society cannot exist unless a controlling power upon will and appetite be placed somewhere, and the less of it there is within, the more there must be without. It is ordained in the eternal constitution of things, that men of intemperate minds cannot be free. Their passions forge their fetters."

Ben gazed off down the canyon. His mind filled with the sense of loss he felt. His emotions wrapped securely in a blanket of sullen anger at Dick Sand. Jealousy and anger and a hungering desire for revenge.

Alex shook his head in exasperation.

"You're not listening, Ben"

"What would I hear if I did, Alex? More prattle about some long lost Whitehouse Society? This is not a society, Alex. This is a jungle. In a jungle you need just one thing, overwhelming power. Sand has taught me that. Twice. I got the message. I know exactly what I have to do."

Ben looked a Alex, aware of the note of accusation that tinged his voice.

"I have people willing to help me do it."

Ben stood up, Alex still towered over him, but Ben was as broad in the chest and shoulders as Allex. He ignored the glitter in Alex's eyes.

"I can't take away from what you've done for me," He still couldn't bring himself to call the man "Alex". "But you said yourself you couldn't help with the rest of it. I have to go with the people who can. It's just that simple. I can't leave Terry in Sand's tender clutches........

"I won't."

"I told you once, Ben, that life is always simple for simpleton's. You're better than this. Find it in you. Don't shut your eyes and follow the wolves."

"The only answer to power is power, Alex. To organization, is to organize."

"No one said it wasn't, Ben. But organize for what. Power for what? To what ends?"

"To stop people like Sand with their own tools. Use them better. Drive them out of hiding. Do whatever you have to to stop their evil."

"Even become evil yourself."

Ben paused.

"Power used to accomplish a good end is not evil. You can make a better world. Make people do what they should, not whatever they want."

He heard Rex's voice in his mind as he spoke.

Alex shook his head, not looking Ben in the eyes now. Gazing off down through the timber.

"The only legitimate use of power, Ben, is to defend the rights of the powerless. You don't have to be evil to accomplish that. That's the Warrior's Way, Ben. The way of a true warrior."

"I'm not becoming evil. I'm doing what I have to do to stop an evil man. If I could give my life and stop him, I would do it. Right now. This minute."

"And if you could stop him by killing him you would. Right now. This minute."

The words hung heavy in the air between them. While Ben looked inside, honestly. Sifting through his feelings.

"Yes. I would."

"You aren't listening, Ben."

"You said that once already. I'm listening. I'm just not hearing anything. You said once you couldn't interfere with my choices.⊡

"I also told you we were committed to helping you see your choices more clearly, Ben. That was part of the agreement when you reached up and took the water. We aren't in the business of creating monsters, Ben."

"Is that a threat? Are you threatening me too now?"

Almost without thought, feeling defensive and letting it show in his voice, Ben turned so his right side faced Alex, his right arm hanging loose and ready for action.

There was the glitter in Alex's eyes again that made Ben nervous. Made him think of tigers and skeletons.

"You are listening but you aren't hearing because there are some important things that you know that you refuse to acknowledge and to include in your decision making. They're having no impact at all on your decisions. You haven⊡t integrated your new learning with what you knew, what you were before.

"You've lost your way. You're out of control, Ben. Ignorance and power does that to people. You can't detect wrong unless you have a model of what's right to compare it to. That's what willful ignorance and pride in your power does to you, Ben. You decide to just go ahead and pull the trigger. Just because you can. Never asking whether you should."

"This isn"t getting us anywhere. I won't accept that Sand can just kill people and walk away. I'm not turning the other cheek to someone like him."

"You're right, Ben. This isn't getting us anyplace. Your mind is closed up tight .. You need some more experience."

Alex's merry grin was flooding his face, lapping around clear back to his ears, wrinkling his forehead. He snapped his fingers as though he'd just thought of something important. But it must have been a signal instead. The world went out of focus and then faded around Ben .

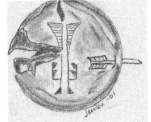

Ben and Alexron stood on a hillside. They were below the crest twenty yards or so. Looking out in what Ben took to be a southwesterly direction, since the sun was low on the horizon and it seemed too warm to be sunrise, Ben saw a peculiar landscape. He was used to mountains and red rock canyons. Here the land seemed older, more worn down. The area was spotted with hills that stood alone like gigantic, isolated haystacks and seemed to rise out of the mostly level countryside without any real plan or order.

Streams meandered through the area in the looping curves that said to Ben--old valleys. Not the lusty young mountain cataracts of the west. Some of the flat lands and part of the hills were covered with trees that were unfamiliar to him. The open areas alternated with stretches of brush and open meadowland.

He had no chance to notice more. His attention was riveted by the sounds that came from up on the hill. One sound was like a hum or a low wordless moan that must be coming from thousands of throats. Another was the clashing of metal on metal in a muted, continuous din that seemed like the metallic sound of a thousand blacksmiths pounding on red hot horseshoes.

Ben saw Alex move in the direction of the sounds and followed. He felt the hair at the back of his neck rise and a shiver convulsed him. As they walked the noise increased. And as they came to the crest of the hill Ben saw the source of the clamor.

Men with swords and shields fought along a line that seemed to extend the length of the hill. The ranks were several men deep with the front ranks slashing, stabbing and hacking at another group whose line also extended out of sight around the hill and whose numbers were vastly greater, whose ranks were much deeper.

Ben saw how ancient sword battles were fought. As men in the front ranks became exhausted others would replace them in the line and they would move to the last rank and sit, kneel and in some cases literally collapse on the ground. Some made feeble attempts stifle awful gaping wounds from which their life blood trickled or gushed. The air was bitter with the pungent smell of blood and of opened bodies. The noise was deafening. The shouting never diminished. It was mindless, enraged. The warriors on both sides fought in a blind frenzy of anger and hate.

Ben realized with a jolt that he knew what they were feeling. The warrior's frenzy. It's what he'd felt fighting with Sand.

Bloodlust.

Emotion run rampant. A willingness to suffer any hurt, ignore any pain, if you could inflict pain or death on your enemy.

It seemed that the ranks rotated about every five minutes, with individuals often dropping out on their own. These were the ones who collapsed when they reached the rear or who had terrible wounds to tend.

The uphill people had fewer numbers, the rotation went much faster. The resting time was much shorter and exhaustion weakened them and they were steadily, step by step, giving way, being driven back by the downhill side despite the obvious problems involved in fighting an uphill battle.

Then Ben noticed something else. He saw a real variation in the size of the warriors. In the center, on both sides of the line, stood men of almost gigantic proportions. Many of them must be of seven feet tall and massive in their armor. They looked like Axel or REX to Ben. But the armor was not the armor of English knights, but more of the ancient style he'd seen in books about Babylon, Assyria and even ancient Greece. Metal plates sewn on leather vests that hung halfway to the knees. And shaped metal that formed around the front of the leg and protected the shin and the knee. The swords were long and heavy and would wreak fearful damage whenever their crashing downward arc was not stopped by an equally powerful enemy. These men were the Abrams tanks of this fight.

No cannons here, no automatic weapons. No police force, national guard or United Nations to arbitrate disputes.

Conquer or die.

Simply conquer or die.

In other parts of the line Ben saw much smaller fighters. With a jolt he suddenly realized that he was looking at women, and even children in some cases. All in the armor of war. All desperately fighting the warriors before them. The smaller fighters were being cut down at a terrible rate and it seemed that the wings of the uphill group were being forced backwards faster than the center so that the huge men in the center would eventually be surrounded. But not until all the others had fallen. Absolutely no one attempted to run away. They all fought with a maniacal frenzy that said there was no place to hide, no place to run, and there was no tomorrow.

Then the sun sank below the horizon and suddenly it all stopped. Ben saw one of the warriors near the center, on the downhill side, raise his sword above his head and scribe a shimmering arc with it in the air. The ranks of the people fighting their way up hill suddenly stepped backward two paces, effectively breaking off the fighting. Ben noticed that this man was not much taller than Ben himself. But he was incredibly broad, blocky in build, and set upon two powerful legs that looked like young oak trees. He turned and the whole army turned also.

Not a single person from the uphill group stepped forward to offer to renew the fighting. The other group trooped down the hill. Only then did Ben see that there was a massive tent city out in the flats below the hill.

The "uphill" group promptly sat down where they were, their bodies bent over in fatigue, and it seemed to Ben, in despair. Only one man remained standing. He was from among the group of

large men, though by no means the largest. He moved quietly among the people, for they were just that, men, women, and a few children, though none younger than their early teens.

A word here, a touch there, a moment to bind up a wound, and then he moved on. Everyone acknowledged him, no one failed to respond to him as he passed among them. Soon he and several of the huge warriors were walking the perimeter, gazing down into the valley that was already alight with the cooking fires of their enemies. To Ben, in the twilight, it looked like a small modern city with the lights extending for more than a mile from the base of the hill.

Ben was startled by a long, shrill scream that seemed to come from the depths of a shattered soul. He looked downhill to see a woman cradling a dead child in her arms. A girl from the length of the hair that spilled over the woman's arm. Others were moving among the almost continuous heaps of dead that lay on the hillside. Soon the woman was joined by others who howled their anguish at the

Warrior's Way

darkening sky.

As Ben looked now he could see dark patches all over the hill extending down into the valley. Heaps of dead bodies. How many days had the fight lasted? How many had died? This was the death of a nation. Tens of thousands had died since this battle started. All killed in hand to hand fighting. Men, women, and even the children armed to struggle for their lives.

A battle to the death in war of extermination. Ben□s mind was stretched beyond its limits trying to take this thought in.

He saw the sky filling with circling pillars of vultures, still visible in the failing light, settling down like the darkness to begin their grisly work. So many, he thought. So very many, thousands at least. They said the battle of Gettysburg during the civil war was the greatest battle ever fought on this continent. Ben doubted it could be bigger than this.

He looked at Alex, who was looking at him, not at the carnage around them.

"Who are these people?" Ben said.

"They lived here once, 1500 years or so ago."

"Why are they fighting like this?"

"Pride", said Alex and he turned and walked away.

Ben was distracted by a new type of screaming from down the hillside. He turned to see that some of the "uphill" people were tormenting some of the "downhill" people who had been left for

dead, but were not. They seemed like maddened beasts, totally without human feelings. Ben had heard about this from others and knew that his own ancestors had had reputations for torturing

captives. He had been naturally sympathetic to the "uphill" people locked in their hopeless battle, now he began to wonder. Then, in the valley below he saw the "downhill" people burning those who could only be from the "uphill" group. So much hate, so much mindless cruelty. These people on both sides were barely human.

Ben felt a fire in his stomach. He knew their hate. The feelings he had felt while fighting Dick Sand welled up in him again. He knew exactly how they felt.

He was ashamed.

Ben caught up with Alex, and if he'd had enough nerve, he would have grabbed him by the arm and spun him around. But he was half afraid that Alex wouldn't be real. Besides, this was no time or place to make Alex any madder at him.

"What's wrong with these people? They act like they've lost every feeling that makes people human."

"Pride", said Alex. And he kept on walking toward the group of large warriors who were obviously planning the next day's battle.

Ben saw people dragging out bundles of clothing and utensils from nearby bushes and trees. It was obvious that they fully expected to be allowed to sleep and rest. Strange rules for a war of extermination. He could see no way that any of these people would be alive at sundown tomorrow.

He assumed that at dawn the forces in the valley would assemble and march up the hill again. He couldn't make himself believe that the battle would go on another full day. Why don't they run, he thought. Get away in the dark and hide. Then he reached the crest of the hill again and saw firelight, in all directions, as far as he could see. Not as closely spaced as immediately below the hill, but covering all the surrounding countryside.

Run where?

You can run, but you can't hide.

The fires of vengeance burned hotter than the campfires. They would consume the "uphill" people tomorrow.

"I'd give my life if I could stop him. Right here. Right now." Ben heard his words in his mind.

"And if you could kill him you would. Right here, right now. Wouldn't you," Ben heard Alex say.

"Yes. Yes I would."

"Because you got your pride hurt. Dick Sand rubbed your nose in the dirt. That's all you're thinking about, no mater what you say about helping others.....doing good. Humility says: I'm not better than you. Pride says: you're no better than I am."

He nearly ran over Alex, who had stopped near the huge warriors who stood slumping, exhausted, yet somehow still angry, as they talked among themselves, speaking a language that meant nothing to Ben. Then, avoiding Alex's gaze, which was making him feel very uncomfortable, he saw two of the large men break off from the group and walk over the crest of the hill, away from the battle zone. They looked supremely weary. It was more than physical. Mind and spirit were worn to the breaking point. Whatever they were doing must be important to them.

Ben wondered what could be so important to two men who had only until sunrise to live.

Alex followed and as Ben turned to go with them his question about what's for supper for these people was partially answered. Some obviously had some grain and other supplies in small amounts. Too many were simply passing among the dead with knives in their hands and deadness in their eyes and in their movements.

Ben scurried after Alex and the warriors. His skin crawled. He felt bile rising in his throat, leaving a slick-sick feeling in his stomach.

On top of everything else, these people are cannibals.

Alex moved down the hill. Ben followed. This was no time to get separated. Ben had no desire to be around here alone when the fighting started up again.

"What's going to happen tomorrow?"

"You mean what happened 1500 years ago."

"Uh, yeah, that too, I guess."

"The Father dies leading his people. The son spends twenty years as a fugitive, returning from time to time to write a book they hope will preserve the story of their people.

"That's how it works on the American continent. Extermination. In Europe, in the rest of the world, societies blend and go on. Here, people serve the God of this land or are swept off. Room is made to bring others here. America is a promised land Ben, not like other places.

"Each time a society here degenerates into barbarism the land is emptied, with only a few of the original inhabitants left. Native Americans learned that the hard way. Those that are left, like you, can participate in the building of a new and better society. That's what the Whitehouse represents. That hope."

"Individuals are given knowledge, and lessons in character development.

Tested and tried. Then are added upon as they live their lives. In the end, they surpass the selfish, the criminal, the lazy. These kind are not so much punished as they are simply left unenlarged, untaught, undeveloped, while others move on. In time, those who listen and learn are superior in every way to those who will not. That's the great danger you're in now. That you will follow Dick Sand. Become like him. Adopt his methods.

Alex stopped and looked at Ben directly. His eyes glittered again.

"You saw the leader of the others?"

"You mean the one who waved the sword?"

"That's right. He look familiar to you?"

"Didn't get that much of a look at him."

Ben felt his eyes slide away from Alex's direct, glittering stare again. He mentally hunched himself against what he expected to be another lecture. A lecture that pointed out his inability to learn from the instruction he was getting. He wasn't prepared for what happened. Suddenly he was seeing his father again, lifting the car, his shirt ripping with the effort, the massive muscles of his back standing out in sharp definition.....

And then they were back in their own camp. That is, Ben was. Alex was gone. Ben was alone again with Bud. As he built his fire and warmed his supper Ben thought again of his mother's words. A warrior without a cause to fight for. A man out of step with his times. More like a fish out of water, Ben thought. Suffocating in an alien environment. And pride. Ben wondered how pride could be a nation-destroying personality characteristic.

Later he fell asleep thinking about Dick Sand. About what he did, how he talked, and how he moved, and how he treated people. Like he was a king. And people had best know that up front and treat him with respect. Or else. And now Ben knew what "Or else" could mean. Those who'd crossed Sand had been dispatched quickly, efficiently, but also, as in TJ's case, and Lester's for that matter, with an overwhelming cruelty. To maximize the suffering. To serve as a lingering example of what it meant to displease Dick Sand, even when no one could know it was him who did it. Ancient Assyrian kings had tortured thousands to show what displeasing them meant. How as Sand any different?

Could Ben Singer do that? Was that what REX had in mind for Ben?

Did Alex mean for Ben to understand that his father was a direct descendant of the warrior who led the "downhill" people in the fighting? What did this say about Ben himself? He'd never spent much time thinking about the past. Suddenly he was overwhelmed by the thoughts that flooded his mind. The vision of countless lives that had been lived by those who had passed on the gift of life to him. One generation at a time until it came down to him.

Do I owe them anything? He felt himself flush red when he thought about his desire to die and to end that unbroken chain of life. How many of those people had suffered and wanted to die, but did not. They must still be alive somewhere. Still organizes as real human beings, not distilled down into something evil and dangerous like a ch'iindii. If they weren't what was Alex doing? What purpose did all this tutoring serve otherwise? Ben felt no sense of specialness, but he felt a growing sense of obligation and of mission. Something to be done. For the good of mankind.

A passage from a book he'd read came to mind. He'd puzzled over the questions many times himself:

-----The Hopi Questions
Where did I come from?
Why was I born?
Where am I going?
What am I?

Martin Cruz Smith, Nightwing, (1977), Ballantine Books, NY.
Every time Alex showed up it turned out the same....Nothing was solved. He only had more questions. And he was tired, with the soul weariness he seen in the huge warriors. He certainly had things in common with them. Tomorrow could easily be the last day of his life. If Dick Sand had his way.

Wearily he went to bed, Bud stood guard again, at least giving Ben a small sense of safety as he lay brooding in the darkness.

When Ben woke up, early, a bad taste in his mouth, his mind troubled by what he'd seen and by a night of bad dreams. He saw the early morning light glinting off of something metallic, lying on the ground near the trail bike. Curious, he got up to investigate.

What he found was a sword. Not ornate, but large and serviceable. The kind of sword you would trust your life to in battle. The scabbard was slightly dented in places, worn from years of steady use. But it had done its job well, protected shaft of silver-white steel within it.. When Ben pulled the sword free the movement was easy and free, coming out with a snicking sound that sent a little chill along his shoulders and down his spine. Like it had a mild charge of static electricity that had been passed through him by the act of drawing the sword.

The sword itself was gleaming. Not polished because many sharpenings had given it's surface the texture of Hopi silver work. Like it had been burnished by fine emery paper, the way master auto body workers polished their repair jobs before painting them. It gave the blade the touch of velvet to his hand. The edge was sharp, but also thickly massed near the edge, to support the blow, the bite of the sword. It could be used to parry massive blows from a similar weapon without losing its edge, without breaking under the strain. It was the weapon of a man such as he had seen fighting on the hillside.

He'd never seen anything quite like it. He thought at once of the blade in William Wallace's hands in the movie Braveheart, but this was not quite like that. The edges were pecularly thickened just before the edge itself, almost like a battle axe. It was a consumate warrior's weapon, not for show, not to be seen in a parade. A weapon to keep it's owner alive in intimate, personal, onon-on-one battle to the death....Like he'd seen on the hillside... Yes, that was it. It looked like the blade the war captain had twirled above his head to stop the battle on the hillside.......1 500 years ago...

He raised it to the morning sun and scribed a shimmering arc in the air and thought of the man who looked like him. Then he noticed the inscription. Near the hilt, it looked like the letters had been raised by some sort of acid process that took a little of the surrounding metal away. It raised the letters, made them stand out plainly. He read:

The Sword of Light and Truth.

As he slipped it back into the scabbard he saw Bud's beady black eyes boring into him from across the clearing.

"Alex, Right?"

Bud opened his mouth in his panting dog smile. Then he did his famous back flip and went off to terrorize the local squirrels and field mice. As he fixed his breakfast Ben's eyes were drawn repeatedly to the sword. It was an anachronism in today's world of automatic weapons. In it's day it had been the ultimate weapon for personal defense in combat.

What of Light and Truth he heard Alex's voice say in his mind: Are enlightenment and truth anachronisms too?

Ben looked inside himself and found he had no answer.

Maybe this was the day of Ignorance and Pride.

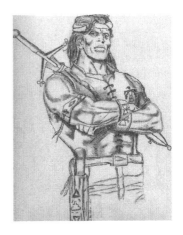

Chapter 22
Ben Recruits Lester

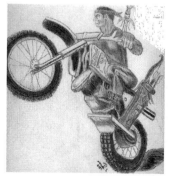

Ben had drifted down out of the mountains at nightfall. Moving like a dark wind, the darkness in him blacker than the moonless night in which he traveled. The sword nestled in a sling across his back, ready for instant use, though the thought of facing a police shot gun made it seem silly. There was something reassuring about it, a connection with the people he'd seen struggling for their lives .

Like me .

He'd mostly given up thinking about them. Whatever lesson Axel tried to teach him just didn't take. There was no time for delay, to re-think everything, to sit around pushing abstract ideals around in his mind like pieces to a puzzle, to find a way to fit them into his plans .his life.

There just wasn't time.

The radio police channels were full of the news. He was wanted for attempted murder of a police officer (Dick Sand of course, guilty there, for sure). Suspicion of murder in the deaths of two as yet unidentified men at Muley Point in southern Utah. (Sand covering his tracks, making sure Ben was hunted by every lawman in the four state region.) Armed. Extremely dangerous.

The fun just never stopped...

He heard Rex's voice in his mind. Start with one, then you two can get another and soon you will have a group of men to sustain you

Worth a shot. If that first one was Lester. Lester knew a lot that Ben needed to know. If Lester wanted to help get Sand .good. If not, well, Lester knew a lot of stuff Ben needed to know. So one way or another, Lester and Ben were going to have a talk.

Ben couldn't get past the idea that Lester had known what Sand was like and he'd led Ben to Tibble Fork that night and had sworn he would tell everyone it was him and Ben in the video. Ben had been Lester's friend, humiliating himself to keep Sand from beating and kicking Lester any more. Was Lester Ben's friend? Or had he sold Ben out?

Time to find out. Look out Lester, I'm on your trail ..

Every nerve was raw, tuned to his surroundings. He could make only one mistake, one small slip, and Sand would have him. But he had to keep trying. Lester knew plenty. Ben had to talk to him. Make him tell what he knew.

Ben slipped out of the irrigation canal and went over the fence onto the asphalt pavement. Warrenville was a large city. But it was sprawled along State street for miles. The river from Deer Creek Dam ran through part of the town and a series of major and minor irrigation canals, many of them overgrown with willows and grass, laced the town from one end to the other. Ben was never more than a block away from good cover. He had a path in and out of the city whenever he needed it. In many places the city backed right up against the eleven thousand foot high mountains. A ten minute drive from any part of it would get you to the wilderness.

The Utes had used the area for wintering grounds for centuries. Good land close to the mountain refuges they needed when they were attacked. Ben knew a lot about that now, and he used every advantage he had to escape Sand's dragnet.

He searched every shadow, peered into every car to see if Sand had lookouts watching Lester. To see if Lester was bait in a trap with Ben Singer's name on it. Maybe by moving quickly Ben would be ahead of Sand. But it was only a matter of time before Lester was bait.

He fought down the icy feeling in his stomach. He'd have to chance it now. He couldn't wait any longer.

Ben spotted Lester's car in the parking lot of the Miracle Bowl bowling alley on State street. Lester still worked there. A good place to meet people, to do business for Sand's organization. Ben felt a burning anger rising in him again, to match the desperation. He'd decided Lester was Sand's stooge. Voluntary or not. Lester knew what Sand was doing. That's what Ben wanted. To know too. That, and to have Lester tell Terry what Sand was.

Lester was in a position to do both of them for Ben. If he wanted to. Ben felt his hands clench into tight balls of bone and sinew and muscle. You're my only hope, Lester, You should have told me about all this before we went to Tibble Fork. You let me walk into a trap, Les. I thought you were my friend.

He moved in the shadows between the building and the wholesale lighting warehouse next door. Then he settled in beside the dumpster, near the chain link fence that divided the business section from the residential area behind. He spent the next hour waiting for Lester, carefully watching for signs of a trap. Hoping Sand would not know the lesson of the big deer. Of the Apache. Keep your enemy in sight. Stay close. Watch for a weakness. Be there.

The radio net said Ben was being sought all over the western United States. Maybe that meant that Sand thought he would run away. Maybe Ben's phone call to the bike shop in Cortez, telling the man he was coming for his money, had given Sand something to do for awhile.

Ben's head ached and he gently explored the scabbing wound in his scalp. He'd cleaned it and dressed it with Neosporin and covered it with bandana cloth. Tied in a dark band around his head. Like the Apache wore. Maybe he ought to paint his face too. Scare Lester a little more. Make him just a little more afraid of Ben Singer than he is of Dick Sand. Show him he's not safe from Ben anywhere, no matter what Sand tells him.

REX and Sand know the score, Ben thought. Get one on your side, then another, then build your organization from there. That's what REX had said. That must be what Sand has done.

But I can "turn" Lester, as the spies say, Ben thought. I can make him a double agent. Working for Sand but spying for me. First he'll tell me what he knows about how Sand's business works. Then he's going to tell Terry. That'll be a good beginning. We'll just see how it goes from there.

Ben saw Lester leave the bowling alley and start toward his car, which was parked in the employee area, on the side of the building. Ben was there when Lester arrived, ghosting up behind him as he fiddled with the door lock. When the door started to open Ben took Lester by the arm and jerked him around, pinning him up against the door. Hard.

"Don't do it, Les."

"Who ? Ben?" Peering into Ben's face, looking at the size of the man he faced. Opening his mouth and sucking in a deep breath.

"Yelling won't help," Ben whispered harshly. "Just shut your mouth and listen. We're going for a ride. You seen Dick Sand lately? How he looks? What I did to him?"

Lester nodded, then looked at the ground.

"I need your help, Les. Badly. You're the only hope I have. Don't back me into a corner where I have to do something desperate. Where I have to choose between you and Terry. It doesn't have to be that way."

"Sand will know, Ben. He knows everything. His eyes and ears are everywhere."

"One of them's black now, you may have noticed. And two are gone forever. Sand isn't superman. He just thought he was. Get in, Lester. You're driving."

Ben got in the back seat and hunkered down. Lester pulled out onto State and turned left, off the bench, down into the main part of town.

"Drive around some neighborhoods, Les. So we can talk."

"So you can tell me what to do."

"Don't make it rough, Les. What I want is simple. Just give it to me. I want to know what you know about what Sand does and how he does it. Give me the clues I need so I can start to unravel his little scheme. That's all I need from you."

"At the moment. Until you think of something else."

"You let me walk into it, Lester. At Tibble Fork. You could have said something, you know. I tried to help you that night the only way I could. Now you're going to help me."

After 30 minutes of easy cruising Ben knew Sand was drug running, setting up a major supply operation, had some kind of a new wrinkle to bypass the security between Mexico and Utah, maybe clear into Canada. He had a blank check from his bosses to set it up. He had corrupted people in the right places or removed them and put in his own. Whatever he was doing was ready to go, to start delivering the goods.

So much time and effort, Ben thought. Then TJ decides to tell what he knows about Sand. That involves Ben, and Sand handles him like just another detail. That's all it would have been, too, Ben admitted ruefully. If Axel had not stepped in to tip the scales the other way. There was nothing wrong with Sand's planning and execution. But somebody, somewhere, didn't like him and was willing to help Ben stop him. At least two somebodies.

REX and Axel.

Ben could not picture them working together. Their motives and philosophies were diametrically opposed. But I can use them both. If I can't find someone right off REX will know some people.

Lights from an approaching vehicle brought Ben back to reality.

"Okay Les. Thanks. That's all you know? Honest Injun?"

Lester didn't even smile at Ben's attempt at humor. But he nodded his head. His hands gripping the wheel. A look on his face like he'd just heard that a close friend had died.

"Sand will find out that I told you this, Ben. He's not just vicious like you've become. He's intelligent and very evil."

Ben felt his anger build. Vicious? Not a word he would have chosen to describe himself. What's going on in Lester's mind? Dedicated, determined, and right. Those were much better words more like Ben saw himself, despite what others might think or say.

"He won't find out from me, Les. I'll find ways to confirm what you've said so Sand will think I learned it for myself. He knows he's mine now. I can beat him anytime I want to. And Prince isn't around any more to make him feel safe. Don't worry about him too much, Les. I'm going to take care of him for you."

"Who's going to take care of you?" Lester's voice was almost lost in the noise of traffic. He glanced at Ben in the rearview mirror and his face was a black copy of a Greek tragedy mask, the corners of his mouth pulled down, his eyes full of pain.

"Not you, Les. So remember that. What we were was friends. Maybe we will be again. After Sand gets what he's got coming. But I'm going to get him, he's not going to get me. Not unless we go out together."

Lester had no answer. He's good at that. Just goes off somewhere and leaves you all alone.

"We're going to do one more thing tonight, Les. Then I'll let you go."

"Why am I not surprised?" Lester said bitterly. He was looking around, peering through the darkness. Maybe wishing he could see a police car.

"You're going to tell Terry what Sand is."

"I won't do it. You might as well kill me." Lester stared straight ahead, out into the dark.

"I don't want to kill, you Lester. You've got to help me with her. She believes Sand, now. Not me."

"She shot you."

Ben touched his head lightly. Seeing the smoke rolling toward him again, the noise, and the sudden burning pain.

"Yeah."

"She won't believe me."

"It will be a beginning. That's enough."

"Providing you don't care what your beginning costs. You're going to get more people killed, Ben. Innocent people. Some who mean a lot to me."

"Like you?"

No, Ben." Lester sighed, weary maybe. "I'm not innocent. Not anymore. But I know some who are."

"I'll do the best I can, Les. But to stop people like Sand, you can't always be sure. It's like cutting out a cancer. Sometimes you have to take a little healthy flesh along with it."

"She won't believe me. She'll tell Sand everything I'd try to tell her. Sand has her in his pocket, Ben. If he thinks she's going to get away, when she's no good as bait for you, he'll get rid of her."

"I won't let that happen."

"You can't stop him. You're an amateur bad guy. Sand is for real."

"We'll see. In the meantime, we're going to see Terry."

"I told you, I told you.." Lester squirmed in the seat, leaned his head forward, forehead pressed to the steering wheel. "I won't do it. Not if you kill me, no matter what you do. I told you, she won't believe me. Why can't you listen?"

Lester finally turned and looked at Ben. Tears glistened in his eyes. Misery and shame melted his face, seemed to make all his features flow downward into a mask of despair.

"Dick Sand takes care of details, Ben. He took care of this one days ago. She's seen the tape. She despises me. She despises both of us now."

Ben felt his anger wither up in him. Dry up and become dust. Leaving the taste of ashes in his mouth. Sand again. Everywhere I go, Dick Sand has been there first. His capacity for hurting other people seemed infinite. Never stopped, never rested, never had a human feeling for the suffering he caused.

"Telling her wouldn't do any good. It would make Sand madder and he'd hurt some more innocent people. Go away, Ben. Just let it go. You can't beat him. He can't be beaten."

Ben felt an explosion of emotion in him. He was fed up with hearing how great Dick Sand was, and how inept Ben Singer was.

"Yes he can. I have people who are willing to help me. We'll get him. I promise you, we'll get him."

Lester turned away and looked out through the windshield, into the darkness that seemed twice as thick as it was.

"Sure Ben. You get him."

"Drive back to the bowling alley, Les. I'll get out there."

Ben heard the note of doubt in his voice. Knew that Lester heard it too. It would be hard, with every lawman in four states hunting him. But there was a way. Ben didn't know what it was. But he knew someone who did. REX would help. He'd give REX whatever it was that he wanted. And REX would give him the only thing he wanted. Victory over Dick Sand.

Vengeance.

He thought about it all the way back over the ridge, riding the motor bike up the hiking trails to avoid the sheriff's patrols on the canyon roads, returning to a lonely camp in a clump of tall pins just under the snowline.

Funny. Nothing seemed to go right any more. When he got to camp Bud was gone. Without his little furry guardian he only dozed fitfully through the night, dreaming again and again of Terry walking down the aisle with Dick Sand. It was so pretty, so many flowers, that you could almost forget the wedding was being held in a funeral parlor ..

****

Sometime after mid-night he jerked wide awake. He could feel it. He wasn't alone. Someone was watching him. Ben grabbed the sword, pulling it smoothly across his knees, ready to throw off the scabbard and bring it into play.

Then, across the fire, at the edge of the trees, a huge form emerged from the shadows and moved toward him.

REX

"So, Ben Singer. You have been given a sword, we see. A small gift from a small man, no doubt."

The voice, like a sound from the grave, tinged with scorn.

REX came only as far as the edge of the camp and made no move to sit down.

"What have you learned, Ben Singer? Have you found virtue and gentleness good weapons against Dick Sand?"

"I beat Sand. I killed his dog. I would have killed him ."

"But a woman stopped you."

Disappointment dripped from the words. Ben's manhood hung in the balance.

"I love her .I-"

"Love is not a warrior's weapon, Ben Singer. As you have learned. There is no love whatsoever in Dick Sand. It is foreign to his mind. Never enters his thoughts. He is beyond that softness. Thus Sand has beaten you at every turn, despite your strength of body."

"I uh "

"It is your own mind that defeats you. Will you lose everything? Or will you change your tiresome, womanish way of thinking and become a man other men will follow?"

Stung, Ben felt a hardening in his voice and anger warming his mind.

"I'll do whatever I have to do to stop Dick Sand."

"Yes. You have already demonstrated that you are ready to kill in support of your goals. Otherwise I would not have come back."

"Tell me what I need to do. How to find the people I need."

"You must first have treasure, Ben Singer. Always treasure attracts the kinds of men you need. Sand pays well those who serve him. Have you treasure, Ben Singer?'

"No. I don't have any money, at least not the kind you're talking about."

"Then you must obtain it. If you goal is right you are justified. Take it from those who have it. Any way you can, any way you must."

Ben was lost in thought for a moment. This was a new aspect of his task. One he hadn't appreciated before. But of course, it was logical. It made all kinds of sense. He could buy guns and men to use them against Dick Sand's guns and men. But how was he going to get treasure....money?

"Dick Sand has great treasure, Ben Singer. And he is getting more. Soon he will be too powerful to be stopped by you. Take his treasure. When you are ready camp near the head of the place you call Hobble Canyon and we will speak again. Fail to do this and you will be left to yourself. We do not invest time in losers, Ben Singer. The time has come for your actions to follow your words."

REX turned and walked back into the dark. Ben didn't bother to follow him this time, he knew he was gone. But he stayed awake the rest of the night, thinking. When Bud came back ..reappeared? ..to stand guard he finally laid down for some rest, a partial plan at least in his mind. Dick Sand's treasure was guarded by Dick Sand's Wolves.

Ben would go wolf hunting

****

Dawn three days later found Ben above Dick Sands alpine cabin near Sundance. He had been haunting the area for two long days. Dodging hikers, avoiding police patrols, watching out for Sand's wolves, the security men Sand had called in to watch his house.

He was across from the compound, slightly higher, and buried in thick brush just behind the crest of a shoulder of the mountain that extended for miles, eventually coming down off the mountain on the backside of Deer Creek reservoir, or leading into Heber, or leading back over the divide and clear up to the mountain fastness that formed the wilderness above Park City or that led down the canyons into a number of Warren Valley towns.

That was the point. Just as a big buck would lay near the top of a ridge, sniffing the air rising up to him, listening for sounds coming from behind, using his eyes everywhere. If he was disturbed, he could go in several directions. So could Ben. Only Ben could travel half a state in any direction if he needed to.

Bud was back with him, coming from nowhere to jump on the bike when Ben was packed and ready to leave the other camp. Ben wished he could predict when he would be around and when he wouldn't. The only thing he'd noticed so far was that when he was angry, violence prone, vengeance ridden, the dog backed off. As though he were afraid of those emotions. Or that he just didn't want to be around them. Today, Ben was unarmed, depending on stealth. Bud was underfoot every time he moved. Always alert, perky and friendly. Letting Ben know he wasn't alone. Reminding him always of Axel.   Not always a comfortable feeling.

Ben jerked his mind back to business. Sand came out of the cabin and climbed into the suburban. Like he owned the world.   Ben saw exhaust smoke blossom briefly from the tailpipe as he started up the engine. But he didn't drive off right away. Ben went through the channels on his hand held CB rig, and listened to the scanner. If Sand was talking it was on something that Ben couldn't track.

Then he heard Sand's voice on the scanner. Talking to the dispatcher somewhere. He couldn't hear the other part of the conversation. Sand must know by now exactly what Ben had bought in Grand Junction. What kind of electronic ears Ben had. On this channel he was all business. There were long pauses, times when Ben nearly stopped listening. Then Sand would come on again.

Ben fumed as he waited. Sand knew he was just as safe as if he were home in his mother's arms. If Ben killed him now Terry and everyone else would call it murder. Ben had to get evidence against him. First he needed some idea of how Sand was operating. In the meantime he could fume. Wait. Watch. Listen. Visit Sand when he wasn't home. When his housekeeper left. When only the two guys back in the woods above the cabin were left. Nobody was protecting them from Ben. Just the fact that he didn't know if they were cops or robbers.

Ben had no desire to hurt policemen who were doing their duty. If they were Sand's dirty cops that was something else. Even then, hurting cops would only re-enforce Ben's outlaw image. Deepen his reputation for viciousness and violence. No, he didn't want to hurt anyone. But he had to get in Sand's house. Find a clue.

Do something.

Sand pulled away. Down the road, then right, down the Deer Creek Canyon road that branched to go to Warren Valley or to Heber. No way to tell which.

Ben saw no movement in the place where the watchers waited. It was time to do something. Ben could grow old waiting for Sand to make a mistake. The only one he'd made that Ben knew about was when he underestimated what Ben was doing. But that was not a mistake so much as a failure to plan for something like what happened to Ben in Whitehouse Canyon. Who could have planned for that?

Ben opened a small box and removed one purchase Sand didn't know about. A set of electronic ears that hunters could use to magnify sounds out in the woods. Much of it looked like a walkman, headphones and all. In a little while tourists and locals would be hiking the trails around Sundance. Ben would be one of them. Being careful not to let the watchers get a good look at his face. Surely they had better optics than he did. Probably including army see-in-the-dark stuff. Ben would come around in daylight, right out in plain sight. Trust to a little luck and some skill. See if he could collect a conversation. Find out who he was up against. Learn what he could about Sand.

Maybe take a high speed, long range bullet between the eyes if he wasn't as clever as he thought he was. But not sitting around anymore.

Doing something.

By noon Ben was across a small gulch from his target. Tall grass and many weeds and small brush clumps had hidden his approach. This area held a ski resort because winter snows were deep. That meant summer plant growth was lush.

He aimed his little device in the direction of Bud's ears. The little dog had scouted, returned, circled, and finally pinpointed the men for Ben. He'd earned his dog food for this day.

Ben turned up the volume till there was a steady hiss of static. Nearby locusts almost hurt his ears. He would catch any words spoken near him. He could hear the distant sounds of hikers, almost understand what they were saying. He hoped the watcher's would have lunch and visit a little. He was not disappointed. He

began to pick up sounds, then a word here and there. He risked moving a little closer. He concentrated until his head began to ache. Something. Give me something to go on. Please. A crack in Sand's perfect defenses. Anything.

What Ben got was beer hall language and bedroom subjects. He seldom heard a sentence, but the gist of the words was obvious. The watchers were not talking business. They seemed to be constantly turning their heads, the voices faded, came back, faded again. Frustrated, Ben began to consider going after them. Even though it meant risking everything.

Then he heard the word `Mules'. Nothing to do with barrooms and bedrooms. He strained to hear as the voice faded away and was replaced by background noise. `Dog' came through. Maybe they were talking about him killing Prince.

Something .something ..`trail'. Then they were talking about campgrounds and campsites that Ben didn't recognize. They weren't around here.

Then the voices stopped. The silence was profound. Bud looked at Ben, then trotted back the way they had come. It was time to go. Ben withdrew carefully, then re-entered the trail and strolled along between two groups of tourists who were bent on hiking up over the Mount Timpanogos trail. Eleven thousand plus feet high. Ben had never made the trip. Before this he was not into physical exercise. Since then he had been a little busy for tourist travel.

Idly he watched the group ahead. They obviously planned to camp overnight at the cabin high on the mountain. They'd enjoy the trip more if they had pack animals to carry their gear. There were people around who rented Lamas for mountain hikes. Old timers had just used donkeys and mules to haul the excess weight of their camp and prospecting gear .

BAM! It hit him like a physical blow. Actually, like a blinding flash of light. In reality, what it was was a small sign along the trail. "You are hiking on the Utah portion of the Great Western Trail. Maps are available at the National Forest office at Timponogos Cave National Monument."

Could that be it? That trail was supposed to become a finished hiking trail, some places allowing motor vehicles, trail bikes, horses, from Canada to Mexico. Most of the Utah trail was done. Ben knew that much from an article he'd seen in the Daily Herald one Sunday.

Ben could imagine the scenario. Hikers along the trail carrying drugs in their packs. `Mules', paid to hike the trail. Always in rough country. A million places to hide the goods if you needed to. Drop off points, meeting places, supply points. These mountains were riddled with three hundred years of Spanish mining ventures using Indian slave labor. Just the old mines alone would offer infinite hiding, stopping, re-supply points. And Utah was about halfway along the way, Salt Lake City was known as the "crossroads of the west" with major freeways connecting the nation in all directions.

Perfect. Warren County was a spot of deep wilderness just where they needed one. Dick Sand, careful planner that he was, could throw a rock from the front porch of his cabin and hit a hiker on the Great Western Trail.

Ben loped off to get the bike. Daylight or not, he'd make the 15 mile run down the American Fork canyon and get a map. The canyon was tight and winding and brush grown. He had a good chance of getting away if he was spotted. Bud hopped on for the ride, taking a little of the tension out of Ben's shoulders as they thundered up over the crest and started down the canyon.

I've got you Sand. The exultant emotion that thrummed through him was not joy, not even satisfaction. It was glee. Tinged with anger and vengeance and unbounded hate. I've got you at last. When they came to a sharp turn and had to slow down to pass a car full of teenagers Bud jumped off the bike and disappeared into the brush. Leaving Ben to go on alone. He viciously fought down the twinge of anxiety he felt. Bud, Axel, whoever .was not going to stop him now. Not now that success was his. If he could bring it off.

Ben had a whole new set of problems to solve. Knowing in his gut what Sand was doing and proving it was two different things. Especially when any law enforcement people he tried to contact would try to arrest him.

Unless they were Sand's people of course.

They would kill him.

Utah roads and mountains and parks were bursting with summer tourists. People of many nationalities were in the state, making the job of hiding just a little easier. Actually, only making the hunters look at many more prospects. Ben didn't look like anyone else. He was square, blocky, thick in the chest and in the waist. He had to eat regularly and well. His body burned fabulous amounts of energy now as he kept his isometric systems locked on 24 hours a day.

His body was getting heavier as he added bone and muscle. The more he weighed the more muscle it took to carry him around. He weighed about 220 pounds now. All the fat was long gone. He knew he'd added much more than 20 pounds of muscle. Much of his former body weight had been fat. It had turned to muscle too and he could feel it when he moved. He should have been ponderous, bulky, under coordinated. But the muscle carried him like it carried the great cats.

He had the physical foundation to excel in any sport that suited his body type. Wrestling especially. Any power sport. He had the `natural build' as the coach would say. All he needed was the practice to develop the physical skills he needed. And he found that his strength, stamina and agility made him pretty good at whatever he tried, whether he knew the `skills of the sport' or not.

All that was great. But it wasn't getting him into the winner's circle. Sand still had him being hunted by every lawman in the west. Terry and Lester were still within easy reach of Sand. Terry still despised Ben, and loved him, and was tormented, Ben was sure, by those feelings. He had to believe that she had mixed feelings. That he could still reach her with the truth. What haunted his nights and drove him through the days was the fear that she would marry Sand .

Or worse, that he would see her stroll out of his cabin one morning, arm in arm with that monster. That she would give herself to him. That's what moved Ben down the canyon to Timponogos and drove him back up again to camp and that kept him at his work, studying the map, until it was too dark to see. He didn't dare use a light at night or build a fire. He cooked his food on canned heat and went to bed when it got dark.

He saw Bud across from him, lying down, head on paws, looking at Ben like he was deciding whether to go or stay.

"Stay, Bud." Ben's voice was a whisper in the dusk. "I'm on to Sand now. But I'm all alone. Till I get some help I need you around so I can rest. So I can keep going. Don't leave now, please."

Bud got up and walked away. But in a few minutes Ben could see him, just the tip of his ears sticking out of the brush, his face pointed toward Sand's cabin and the watchers. Fine, Ben thought, here I am pleading with a dog. What would REX think of that? What will he think? Ben expected to see him soon. Now he had something to work with. Something that would interest others. Ben had already thought of stealing drugs from the mules. But to sell them or give them away to get people to help him get Sand? To become a drug dealer, to become all that Terry believed he was? Could he afford to care?

Ben hoped he wouldn't have to do that. But he was too well aware of sting operations that sent on for months where the flow of drugs continued destroying lives until the lawmen got the higher ups. A trade off. Catch-22 situation. Not something Ben felt comfortable with. Maybe Lester was right after all. Maybe Ben Singer was only a junior apprentice bad guy.

Ben shook off the thought. Time enough later, when REX was helping. But he knew that if it was the only way to get Sand, to Save Terry. To take revenge. Well

"Sometimes to cut out the cancer you have to take some of the clean flesh with it." He'd said that to Lester. Had he meant it?

Much better would be to catch a courier carrying the drug money. That would be a double blow. Cut Sand's cash flow and use the money to fight him. That's what the DEA did when it caught the crooks. Took everything. Cars, boats, planes, houses, bank accounts.

Ben only knew that he had to do something. Die trying. But die moving. He fell asleep, troubled again by dreams of Sand and Terry. Tinged with the awful fear of failing again and losing her forever.

****

"You boys out there?" Sand's voice was full of sleep, and a lazy, easy going warmth. Why not? He was the one sleeping in his own bed every night. Not Herschel and Virgil.

"Yeah Dick. We're right here. In the woods just a couple of boy scouts lookin' to earn our Eagle .."

"Good, good. Just checking in. I'll get back with you after breakfast."

"Breakfast, Virg. Mr. Sand, he's going to have his breakfast now."

"He don't seem to catch the irony does he, Herschel. Us sitting out here in the cold nothin' hot to eat in a week ."

"He really don't care about anyone but himself. He figures cause he pays us we're just doing our job and don't deserve no extra thanks or respect. I doubt he thanks his suburban when it gets him home, either."

"And this has nothing to do with the business. This is just cause that Ben Singer guy scared the bejeebers out of him."

"He never did say what happened, just showed up looking beat and without his killer dog."

"That's what impressed me, Hershcel. Singer musta killed the dog and beat Sand too. Whew. That would take some doin'."

"Yup. And here we sit, surrounded by all this brush and poison ivy and such and we're supposed to be guarding Sand against this guy."

"Who's guarding us, Virg? Who's got our back?"

"Why Ben Singer, Hersch. Ben Singer's got our back .if he wants it bad enough."
Herschel looked off into the brush, then back at Virgil.

"You know, I'm glad we talked to Montero's boy. This is getting way beyond okay. We didn't sign up for this .how come we're doing it?"

"Cause we're suicidal. That's why. We don't want to go on living .."

"I do. I want to live. I ain't done livin' yet by a long shot ."

"Then why you hanging around this pine studded jungle, Old Buddy. There be Indians out there."

"Lets tell Sand to stay away for a day or two while we re-supply and then let's get us out of here."

"Words to live by, Virgil. Words to live by."

Just then a small, friendly little dog popped out of the brush, nearly scaring the men to death .
****

Ben heard Sand's Wolves on his `ears'. He was moving quietly through the brush, hearing their voices in the distance when he lifted the earphone, taking his direction from that. Bud was doing his job.

"Cute little mutt, ain't he. Commere dog. You want somethin'? Looky what we got here."

"Here, boy, here boy."

"Lookit him jump, Virgil. Just like a circus dog. Right over backwards."

Ben was so close now there was only a screen of brush between him and the two men. They wore Camoflauge clothes, carelessly. Like hunters in the second week of camp.

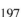

Bud saw Ben start to move forward, coming out of the brush. If either man turned his head Ben would be spotted instantly. Each man had an automatic rifle close at hand. One looked like an AR-16. The other looked to be Check or Russian made. Both looked deadly to Ben. Bud did a double backflip and then dashed in just close enough for one of the men to reach out to grab him. He sidestepped neatly and nipped him sharply on the hand, growling ferociously. Like a dog three times his size.

"Ow. He bit me the little ." The voice trailed off as both men saw a bulky shadow fall between them. They turned in unison and looked at Ben, then at each other and then at their rifles, which suddenly seemed to be a long ways away.

"Do it, guys, if you want "

Both men dived for the guns, one doing a somersault over the rifle and coming up with it in firing position just in time to be smashed into the dirt by the body of the other one. Ben had simply grabbed him by the clothes and flung him like a large rock. He followed close behind, smashing his hands into the face of each man in turn. Not full force, but he felt cartilage and bone shift and heard some teeth break. He ripped the rifles from their hands and smashed the trigger housings against the trees.

"Enough?"

Both men nodded.

"I need you to take a message to Sand for me. Tell him I know what he's .."

"Sand who? The one called Virgil said, full or innocent guile.

Ben lifted him up by the heavy coat, not clear off the ground, but mostly. Enough.

"Oh, yeah. That Dick Sand." There was a little blood trickling out of his mouth. Ben handed him his handkerchief then let him drop back to the ground, watching the other one at the same time. No moves toward hidden weapons.

"My turf, guys. I don't like garbage in my neighborhood. I'll only tell you nice once. Just this once.

"Go away. Don't come back. Tell Dick Sand if he wants to find me I'm hunting mules along the Great Western Trail."

The two men looked at each other, a little green in the face. Neither was going to tell Dick Sand that they had given Ben what he needed to know.

Virgil tried to smile past his broken teeth but only managed to look like a clown with a blood-red mouth. Ben saw in his eyes that he was not amused. A coiled rattler gazed back at Ben. Annoyed, wary, deeply offended by his defeat.

Dangerous.

Not cops. These were the genuine bad guys. Ben felt his hair crawl a little. Should he have alerted Dick Sand that he knew what he was doing? Would it give him something to worry about, or was it only waving a red flag in front of an already enraged bull?

Should Ben let these men just walk away? Was this the time to start killing people?

Seeing something in his face they didn't like, the two men hurriedly gathered their gear and started moving down the hill. Ben kept their night vision goggles. When their backs were turned he stepped back into the screen of brush. Virgil produced an automatic from somewhere, stopped, and gazed back up the hillside. Ben put an arrow between his feet, slashing his pantleg, cutting the sole of his shoe. Nailing it to the ground. Before the little puff of dust kicked up by the arrow had settled the men were out of sight, crashing and cursing as they hurried through the brush. Away from Benjamin Franklin Singer. The mountain was his. Dick Sand himself wouldn't venture here again without an army behind him.

Ben turned and slipped back up the hill toward his camp. Like the big bucks, using the brush and the hollows and arroyos to hide his body from the searing impact of long-range bullets. Virgil and his buddy were probably not the only people out there in the mountains looking for him.

Chapter 23
Terry Makes Plans

Ben took advantage of a busy early summer Saturday when the mountains seemed to have more people that the valleys. Everyone was out to enjoy the day. Hikers, horseback riders, fishermen, rubber-neckers and bikers. Especially trail bikers. Especially motor-powered trail bikers. The mountains echoed to the roars of the biker's engines. In the wide-brimmed hat and non-descript clothes Ben felt invisible. After carefully concealing his equipment and the sword Ben left Bud in charge and rode the bike to town. He rode directly to the Smith's Food King on center and State and lost himself in the crowds inside.

He ate a hot meal, relishing the food even as he watched people around him to be sure there was no one he knew. Watching for that little glint in the eyes that meant he'd been recognized. He was far from his regular haunts in Warrenville and saw no one from his former life.

He took seconds on Chinese food, then strolled the aisles picking up canned goods that he could use. On the way out he bought the Saturday edition of the Daily Herald. What he saw there on the society page made him fight to hold down his food.

Richard Leland Sand and Terry Renee Richardson announce their engagement to be married.

The picture leaped from the page and burned itself into the retina of his eyes and hung there like a sun spot. Blinding him to his surroundings. Weakening his knees. Turning his insides to ice water.

Sand and Terry.

Terry leaning on his shoulder. Sand trying to look human, and nearly succeeding. Except for the grin. Ben knew the grin. It reeked of self satisfaction. Reminded Ben of Tibble Fork. The awful smile. The inhuman cruelty. The uncaring eyes. It was all there for Ben to see. Sand couldn't hide it from him.

Ben burned rubber getting up Center and down off the bench and into the river bottoms. He realized then that he could have lost it all just by getting stopped for speeding and recklessness. Lucky the police were all up in the hills chasing the weekenders.

Ben spent the day on the riverbank. Moving occasionally when people were around too long. Waiting for dark. Then he went looking for Lester.

"Don't worry, Mr. Montero," Dick Sand said. "I have things under control here."

There was a pause while he listened. He rubbed a damp palm on his shirt front then touched his cheekbone. It still hurt sometimes and seemed to burn whenever he thought of Ben Singer.

"No sir, I don't have a major problem. Who! Who told you that?"

Pause

"I know you do. I'm not saying you don't have a right to double check any of your people. I just don't want you to get a wrong idea about my work, that's all. I'm takin' all the necessary steps."

Pause

"He got lucky, is all. Sucker punched me. Anyway, doesn't matter. This is not a personal vendetta. Not just him and me. He's in the way. I'm using company assets to get him out of the way. Business, strictly business on my part."

Pause

"Soon, Mr. Montero. Very soon now. I have his most personal possession in my pocket. He's crazy now. Bound to make an amateur's mistake. I've given him a time deadline of two weeks."

Pause

"Not at all, sir. The operation is moving on schedule. We already have product in our warehouse ready to be transhipped north and west. The eastern loop was never meant to begin this year anyway . Yes sir, right on schedule."

Pause

"You know me better than that. I never take anything lightly. I handled him right right from the start. Two nincompoops failed to do their job. I fired them on the spot. And, Mr. Montero, I already had backup systems in place to be sure he couldn't run to the reservation and stay. He didn't. He's back here."

Pause

"That's not how I see it, sir. His attack on me is a fine measure of the pressure I've put on him. He's a loose cannon. Alone, his own girl friend helps me against him and his best friend is one of my operatives. No, I'm sorry to contradict your informants, sir. But it's just not as bad as they say it is."

Pause

"I don't have to hear that. I've been with you a long time. You know my work and you know I know the stakes. You don't have to threaten me."

Pause

"Sorry. Yes. We'll call it a reality check then. We both know the rules of the game. Ben Singer does not. He won't live long enough to learn them. His streak of beginners luck is wearing out."

Pause

"No, much better than that. I'm going to marry her. That's right. We announced our engagement yesterday. That will bring him out. Every lawman in four states is looking for him and I have company assets in the game that he can't know anything about. All he has to do is stick his head out of the woods and the game is over. He won't be able to stay in there and keep his girl from marrying me. Yes. Now you see it my way."

Pause

"That's right, then I'll quietly clean up the loose ends. No. No. Can you picture me being married? To a Utah farm girl?" Sand laughs, gleefully and long. "I'll tell you some new farmer's daughter jokes when I get to Tucson again."

Pause

"Yes sir. Goodbye Mr. Montero."

Sand threw the phone into its cradle.

"Yes Mr. Montero. No Mr. Montero. Sorry Mr.Montero. I hate it when you call me Dickey-boy Mr. Montero. Soon I'm going to have enough money and people to burn you. Personally. Like I'm going to burn Singer."

On the way down from Nebo he dialed another number.

"Any activity?" he said.

"What old guy? You say he followed her home? Who was he? What do you mean he disappeared. People don't disappear. You doin' your job or not, Herschel? Somebody put a kink in Montero's tail. Wasn't you, was it?"

Pause

"Okay, okay. This is no time to get crossways of each other "

"How many you got watching her."

"Is two enough? You absolutely sure? You can have what you want, make sure you get what you need." He didn't bother to hide the irritation Montero had generated in him.

"I'll tell you your business so long as I'm responsible for what you do, Herschel. If you don't like that I'll drive over there and explain it again to you in person. Black belt or no. Black beret or no."

Pause.

"Yeah, right. Okay. I'm touchy. No, forget it. I'm behind you. But this is such a sweet deal. It means so much to us. Lets be sure we get it right. We're on the edge of a river of money, my friend. I've already aimed a little of it our way. You'll find a deposit to your account tomorrow. Spread it around. Make everyone happy. Give them a taste of what's in store for us all if they stop Singer."

Pause.

"Oh. I didn't know that, see. That's why I was edgy. Night vision? Electronic security. And of course we got Rhetta right there in the apartment with her. She□ll tell me everything that happens. I see why you don't need as many people. Yeah. Any more would set off the security systems themselves stumbling over each other."

Pause.

"Good ..Good. He's going to move soon. There's no question that he will. He's a do-gooder to the soul Ignore the muscles . I don't know. His daddy was that way. He just went away and grew up quick. But he can't get away from what's inside him. He's weak. He'll move. He'll come. He has to."

Pause

"No. Lester will tell me if he contacts him .No, this time you don't understand. I have Lester's soul in my pocket. I own it Just as sure as you are you've got your end covered."

Pause.

"You don't need to know everything. That's how I work. You do your share, you get your share. I run the show to suit myself."

Pause.

"Glad you see it my way. Get to me the second you get a reading. Don't try to take him alive. But if by any chance you do save him for me. I'll buy him from you. Coin of the Realm, Herschel. Coin of the Realm. I'd love to have him for awhile. I'd know just what to do ..Cause I think about it all the time." Sand touched his cheekbone, rubbed the soreness a little.

Pause.

"Well, look at it this way, when he's dead we still have his gal and his pal Sure, you do that. You give it some thought. Later."

Sand hung up, his good humor restored a little by thinking about catching Ben alive. Of having Terry and Lester around either way. There were some good times in his immediate future. To celebrate his new found treasure in the hills of Utah, where the Spanish mined silver and gold for 300 years with Indian slave labor.

As he thought about it, in a way Sand's customers were his slaves. Their chains the chemicals in their blood. But they worked like slaves to get him the money that was making him rich. Too bad the Spaniards didn't know about it. They'd done it all the hard way.

"I could have shown them Caballeros a wrinkle or two," he said. Then he drove down the grade whistling tunelessly a Texas range rider's version of `Get Along Little

Warrior's Way

Doggy'.
****

Ben found Lester doing his laundry at the coin-op on Sate about fourth south. He parked in back, went in the front, took Lester by the arm and frog-marched him out the back door before the other customers realized what was happening. Ben stood in front of Lester, his back to the dark, looking over Lester's shoulder back into the Laundromat and along the side of the building toward the street.

"Terry's getting married," he said, not hiding the pain he felt.

Lester nodded.

"That's what I hear." He sounded far away again. Gone somewhere in his mind. Ben had to get him back.

"We have to stop her, Les, stop him. You've got to help me."

Lester looked at the ground. He shook his head, but said nothing. Ben slapped him, knocked him back against the building. Lester stood there, his hand on his face, still looking at the ground. Ben wound up to hit him again. Lester looked up, his eyes glittering moistly in the dark.

"I'll tell you how to stop him, man." The words came out in an almost breathless rush. "Surrender to him. He won't marry Terry then. Save her yourself, Superman."

"He'd kill her ten minutes after he killed me. Then he'd come after you. You know that. Don't talk nonsense to me. I don't have time for it. I don't have to put up with it."

"Sure, Ben. If you don't like somebody you can whip 'em good. Great. So what do you do for an encore. After you whip them good? What else do you do, Superjerk?"

Ben doubled a fist, swung hard at Lester's midsection, but stopped the blow before it landed. He pushed his fist forcefully in under Lester's rib cage and heard the air squeaking out of his lungs. Lester looked him straight in the eye. Not blinking, not trying to move away.

"Tell me how you do it, Lester. I really want to know. Maybe there's something I can use. How do you let people die? Or suffer. When you have the power to do something about it? Tell me, Les, I want to know."

Lester looked down at his shoes.

"No, Les." Ben moved his hand and lifted his chin, made him look in his eyes. The way Sand did to him that awful night at Tibble Fork.

"You know what Sand will do. To me .To Terry." Ben felt the strain in his voice that came from speaking past the massive lump in his throat. "She's going to marry that monster! You've got to help us, Les. Don't let him do this to us. What have we done to deserve this from you?"

Ben saw tears leaking from Lester's eyes, running down his cheeks, dripping in great dark spots on his shirt.

"I tried to help you that night, Les. You must know I did. I did what Sand wanted, to keep him from hurting you. I shamed myself as a man, Les. I shamed myself to death. I went away to die. I couldn't leave you to Sand. Now I need to know how you do it. How can you go on living in the world knowing that two people who were your friends are being destroyed by an inhuman fiend?"

Lester slumped against the building, suddenly limp and soft. Ben saw him gazing over his shoulder, at the brightly lit homes on the bench across the river. He was gazing like Ben had gazed that night at Tibble Fork. When he had looked out at the valley, so far away. He had felt so terribly alone.

"Okay, Ben. That's enough. I'll do what I can." A sigh seemed to start at his toes and travel a trembling path up through a hollow emptiness inside him to emerge like the final breath of an old man. "I'll tell Terry. In a way she might accept. That may turn her against Sand. But she'll still be in his pocket. I can't do anything about that. She'll be in danger still, and if she lets on, Sand will kill her. She's being watched every minute. Don't try to see her."

"I won't, Les." Ben tried to keep the joy out of his voice. "Thanks, Les. I mean it. I can get help. I'll start right now. We'll work out the rest somehow. But we have to make a start. We have to try. We can't just let him win."

The edge of rage tinged his voice and Lester looked at him.

"Yeah, Ben. Like you said, it's a beginning. So long as you don't mind paying a price to get started. You'll work out the rest, I have no doubt."

Lester pushed away from the wall, turned his back on Ben, and ambled back into the Laundromat like a murderer walking his last mile. Cheer up, Les, Ben almost said aloud. Cheer up. Sand will kill us if we don't try, so what do we have to lose? At least we can fight back.

Ben spun on his heel, jumped on the bike and skimmed across the river canyon to a hiking trail up rock canyon. In twenty minutes of hard riding he was on the road that led to Hobble Creek and on from there to Diamond Fork. He lost himself in the homebound crowds, went over the hill and broke camp. In an hour he and Bud were on their way to Strawberry Valley. He would not approach Diamond Fork from the west. He'd come back to it from the east, over the Strawberry Ridge, the way the Spaniards Dominguez and Escalante had come. Through heavy brush, with miles of wilderness at his back. This was no time to take chances.

****

Back in his apartment Lester wrote a long letter, put it in an envelope, then in another envelope addressed to Terry's roommate, dropped it in the mail drop near the office a thick packet addressed to Ben in care of his grandfather in Chinle, made a phone call to Dick Sand's answering service, left a message and walked out of the building, got into his car, and drove away.

****

Ben spent a day and two nights camped at the head of Diamond Fork Canyon. Listening to the water run. Sleeping during the day, staying awake nights, staring into the dark, looking for the hulking figure of REX to appear at the edge of the firelight.

Brooding. Each moment that passed a moment lost. The time speeding away. Terry's life, his life, passing like sand through the hourglass of eternity. Time was running out. Lives were running out. Ben's life. Terry's. Lester's.

Ben knew he'd never let the wedding take place without trying to kill Sand first. Sand knew that, counted on it. Planned for it. The closer the time came, the less room to maneuver Ben would have. The easier a time Sand would have with him.

Thinking. Puzzling. Reviewing events. Seeking connections in what Axel had said. What REX had said. Trying to find a way out.

REX was a simple straight forward man of power. Axel was abstraction itself. Talking principles, showing Ben a picture so big he couldn't understand the parts, see the details. See the point. Useless.

What good was seeing the destruction of an entire people. And the degradation of another people to barbarism? Of extinct societies that painted white houses on rock and spoke of peaceful societies? Of words on an old sword like light and truth.

How could he get close enough to Dick Sand to use the sword on him? What good was anything Axel said or did?

None. Zip. REX at least had experience, knew a way. Maybe he had an organization too. In place, ready to move in. That was great. But what did Ben have that they could possibly want? What price could he pay that would interest such men?

Such profound mysteries. Either way it was an enigma. Any way, time was running out.

Ben was so preoccupied with running around inside his head like a rat in a maze, desperately seeking a way out before the cat caught up, that he almost missed spotting the trap closing on him.

Hearing a vehicle, he looked down the hill to the Hobble Creek-Squaw Peak road to see a sheriff's department van pull up and unload several men and some dogs. They were upwards of a mile away. Because he'd been cautious and come into the area from the long way around, he had left no scent in the valley for them to find.

More vehicles appeared from the Highway 6 road that led up Diamond Fork from Spanish Fork Canyon. Without seeing them he knew that the Strawberry Reservoir road would be closed off too. Men would be going up Highway 6 and cutting back into the mountains around Strawberry Ridge at two different places, one just under Soldier Summit, cutting off a run to the east. The net was cast large, but it was drawn around the fugitive. When it tightened he would be trapped, caught, arrested. Murdered.

He felt the steady smoldering anger in him flame up into rage. Like he'd felt when he had Sand in his death hug. Like a cornered beast must feel. Desperate. Lives in his hands. He had to live, escape, stay free. Where was REX? Why hadn't he come? Ben couldn't wait to find out. Sand's organization had kept the appointment instead.

Ben dropped back behind the ridge, down to the campsite. He'd come in over game trails. He'd have to go out the same way. Hide in the timber, move carefully out in the open. Wary of helicopters. If he was spotted they would close the net in a matter of minutes. When the dogs found the camp he had to be far away.

He loaded what he could take, made no attempt to hide the rest. Speed and distance were his allies. He couldn't hide the camp from the dogs. He could spend that time running. He motioned to Bud to lead out. He started the motor on the bike, trusting in the quietness of the bike and the blocking of the ridge to hide him. In moments he was gone, twisting down the trail, slipping through brush, skirting along hillsides, out of sight, but able to see. The deer knew this game. The game of life and death. Ben would follow their lead and follow their trails. South. To jump the highway and break out into the wilderness that ran all the way to Arizona. Some of it the old Outlaw Trail the Wild Bunch, Butch Cassidy and the Sundance Kid, had used a hundred years ago. But most of it the trails of animals that were hunted, killed on sight. Ben was like that now.

They had the poisoned hand and he did not.

Chapter 24
Ben Singer Calls On His Clan

"He rides that bike like it was a goat. Where he can't ride it he carries it, where he can he rides almost flat out."

Pause

"Sure, Dick, Sure. Anywhere on the Colorado Plateau. 2/3 of the state. Five national parks. Canyonlands. Badlands We're doing that, Dick. Flying the bird, using infra-red, checking everything. We've scared half the bikers in the State of Utah. Not to mention mules."

Pause

"You've got a blind spot where Singer is concerned, Dick. You underestimated him. I think you still are .He's Indian. He knows stuff he doesn't know he knows. But that's not all of it. He's a master at using the land against us. That camp on Strawberry Ridge? He came up the backside, through country where they tried to track the bear that drug off the little girl. They got lost in there. He went through it like he was on the freeway."

Pause

"We know he was southbound. Jumped the highway below Soldier Summit. Must have gone up the old railroad bed or something. Topped out on the crest. The Scenic Highway cuts through all the old Ute hiding places, clear down the state. He can drop off on any of a dozen roads and circle back. Or he can go south."

Pause

"Roadblocks and patrols are in place for now, yes. But you got to get the picture on this, Dick. He rides the game trails. His bike is super quiet. He moves like game moves. He sneaks like a four point buck, but he's as dangerous as a grizzly."

Pause

"No, don't get me wrong. He's not Superchief. He's desperate. If we don't get him you know he'll be coming for you before the wedding. Ready to die to get you. That's what worries us. Assassins that are willing to die can be hard to stop. So we need to the keep the pressure on. But that's a problem. Law people we talked to say they've got other priorities. Singer's not a murderer after all. He just wants to be. He's only wanted for questioning in the death of the boy. They know now he didn't push Blinky and Two Step off Muley point. They're backing off on us."

Long Pause.

"Yeah. I get you. Whatever you want. You can handle that end. If you know how to get them mad at him again then go for it. We can use the help ..Yeah. Gotcha."

Herschel set the phone back in its cradle and looked at Virgil.

"'Bout time we pulled the plug on this, Virg."

"Sand's gone round the bend. Making Montero mad, wasting manpower and money on this."

"Pulling in people we don't know, making threats, not putting the money out like he should."

"Tomorrow, no later, we give him till tomorrow then we do something."

"Yeah. You bet. We do something. Maybe Singer could use us, you think?"

"Maybe. Tell you what, Hersch. You find him and I"ll ask him."

Time to check Sand's "fiance". Singer was slick enough that he just might be there. If there was a pattern to his actions it was that he never ran far. Was never far from you. He didn't act like a fugitive so much as he did like a predator. Herschel shivered a little. What he'd done to Sand was impressive. He'd also put the run on Virgil and him. Some very hard men. Sand was having to swear out charges of assault against him to get the law after him in full force. Dick would rather eat dirt than have to admit someone had killed his scary dog and beaten him to his knees the way Singer had. Singer had better hope Sand never caught him alive. On the other hand, Singer had some temper himself.

The girl? Herschel shuddered a little. Knowing Sand's mind the way he did. Bad times ahead for her, for certain.

As for Ben, hope he never rises out of the huckleberry bushes and wants to shake hands with me.

Virgil got the Land Rover turned around and headed back down Hobble Creek, back into Warren Valley.

****

Ben was still going south, half the state away, using back roads, the Skyline Drive highway, game trails. Whatever kept him headed south through the high plateau country. He'd work his way past Fish Lake, down to Boulder then, about dark, he could burn the road to Escalante, down to the road that led to Page, and be back in Monument Valley by daylight. He could be in Chinle late in the afternoon. Even taking the back way through Bluff. Gas and food were problems only after Escalante. He had stopped at one of his survival sites for gas and something to eat.

He was relieved again that his Indian instincts hadn't allowed him to rush back to Utah. Had forced himself to prepare a backup for emergencies.

Not getting help from REX was an emergency of the worst order. He puzzled about that as he rode. REX had either thrown in with Dick Sand or had been with him all along. In which case he had set Ben up from the beginning. To get rid of him. In order to help Sand? Ben tried, but couldn't make a firm connection to the two of them. Not enough information. He'd have to ask Axel about it if he ever had the chance.

But not now. He was out of time, out of options, almost out of hope. All he could think to do was to go home. To ask Grandpa and his clan for help. That was his last hope. He couldn't recruit crooks, so family would have to do.

As he traveled he struggled on trying to make sense of what was happening. To find out what he was supposed to do with what Axel had given him. Bud rode along, comfortably curled in Ben's lap on a towel pad over the gas tank. Too bad he couldn't talk. Ben was desperate enough that he was finally even willing to take advice from a talking dog.

"Come on, Axel," he said aloud. As much to hear a human voice as anything. "You went to a lot of trouble over me. Now I'm ready to do something. You going to let me fail?"

There was no answer in the keening wind that whipped past him.

Ben came into Bluff, Utah early in the morning. He stopped at the Buckhorn Cafe to eat and clean up. He worried that the local deputy might be an early riser. But this backwater little pioneer town was far from the Great Western Trail Sand was using. Chances were good that he was an honest man. Somebody further north, along the Cortez Highway, around Monticello, was in Sand's pocket. He or they had killed the two men chasing Ben at Muley Point.

Down here the chances were good that Ben was far from the hunt and that the deputy worked evenings around the bars to keep the Navajos and the Utes from tangling. Otherwise it was just a quiet little Mormon town on the banks of the San Juan River.

From there he could go four or five ways, three of them into the reservation. A running start of even three minutes was all he needed. So, weary, hungry, confused, anxious, angry, he decided to eat well and then rest a little under the bridge, over on the reservation side, among the willows.

He cleaned up in the rest room behind the cafe. As he came out he say the twin towers of rock balanced delicately on the canyon rim above. They were called the Navajo Twins.

The hero twins, Monster Slayer and Born-for-Water. Sons of Changing Woman, probably the most benevolent of Navajo deities. She was often thought of as representing the changing of the seasons. Their father was Sun Bearer. He carried the sun disk across the sky each day. They had made a perilous journey to visit their father. They had been remolded, made into beautiful, perfect specimens of human beings. Then they went to their father to ask for help.

Where's my father when I need him?

The twins had been born when the Earth Surface People were being progressively destroyed by monsters that lived in the land. One, a giant bird, swooped, picked a hapless victim and dropped him or her into its nest where it was consumed by its children.

Shiprock was said to be the tip of its wing sticking up out of the ground where it had crashed when Monster Slayer killed it. There was Kicking Monster that lived on the edge of the canyons. She sneaked up behind you and kicked you over the cliff to be eaten by her children.

Ye'ii Tsoh was a giant who ate everyone and everything in sight. His blood had formed the lava rock escarpment down toward Albuquerque. Whenever Monster Slayer was out killing monsters his twin, Born For Water was home, chanting and staying `holy' (charged with supernatural power) so that Monster Slayer could not be defeated.

Finally there was only Sickness, Old Age, Hunger, and Death left. When he cornered them they convinced him he must leave them alone so people could appreciate health, youth, a fully belly, and so the earth would not fill up with people so there was no room for any more.

Ben was sure he would not have let Dick Sand go. Here was one monster who needed to be destroyed.

Ben ate ham and eggs and french toast and drank milk till he could hold no more.

When he paid his bill the cashier, a lady about his mother's age, smiled at him and handed him a blue paperback book.

"I just feel you might like this. It's a story, among other things, of your people a long time ago. If you don't want it, maybe you can give it to someone else."

Ben wasn't going to argue or be rude or do anything else to make her remember him. He took the book, thanked her, and drove away. He searched as he rode and soon saw the sheriff's car next to an old two story stone pioneer house. The garden and flower bed were well tended, green, and healthily looking. The place was neat and clean. Typical of many Mormons Ben knew. He saw a man, bent over, back to Ben, moving a hoe among the tomato plants.   Ben relaxed a little and stopped at the gas and go to top of his gas tank and check the bike. He set the book on the light pedestal, fully intending to `forget' it. He had no time for reading. Wasn't planning on starting any book that he might not live long enough to finish.

But when he slid wearily back onto the bike seat and called Bud, the little dog jumped up on the pedestal, took the book in his mouth and jumped into Ben's lap. Shoving the book into his

face. Black beady eyes fixed on Ben. Tail wagging furiously. A dog doing his best to say something. Ben took the book, slipped it into his jacket, and drove to the willows under the bridge. The river was running fast and deep, the spring runoff now reaching this part of the river. Ben stopped well back off the bank, feeling a creeping sense of unease when he saw the muddy current racing along. Here it looked just like the Colorado. The river that had tried to kill him.

He settled down to rest, pulled the book out to get rid of its bulk against his chest, and dropped it in the sand. It fell open and Ben glanced idly at the page.

There was a picture of a battlefield full of dead, vultures sailing overhead, and two men, huge men--dressed for war.   One was on his back, gravely wounded, pointing out over a multitude of bodies. Men, women and children, all dressed for war.

Ben took a jolt of adrenaline that stood his neck hairs up and washed the sleep from his mind. Those with Axel, on the hill. Where men, women, and children were destroying each other, wiping out a whole nation. What's going on here? Ben saw Bud looking at him, mouth agape, head cocked to one side. Laughing?

Ben looked at the title. The Book Of Mormon.

He saw another picture of a great warrior with a magnificent sword being attacked by what looked like robbers. Almost without thinking Ben caressed the hilt of the sword that now hung on its straps across his back. Axel, what's going on?

He heard a noise and instantly went on the alert .listening .

A vehicle pulled to the center of the bridge and stopped. Ben could see emergency lights and a whip antenna and parts of running lights and the black metal top. It was, probably, the Sheriff's van that had pushed the truck off Muley Point. Looking, stopped on the Utah side, not crossing to the reservation. Probably glassing the willows. Checking things out, just in case.

Sand was tireless. So were his people. But not the regular law enforcement folks. They were weeding their gardens. Tough, Dick. You can't keep me on the top of your priority list. I'm not wanted badly enough, Ben thought.

He eased back only a little. He had already taken care to conceal himself, to hide his tracks coming in, that just came naturally to him. Bud was looking hard at the van. But not moving. Not panicky. Not yet. It would get sticky only if a Navajo Police vehicle pulled up on this side. Then it could get bad real fast. Ben strained his ears but could hear nothing but the whispering water. He hated the thought of having to dive into the river to escape. Spring floods rolled rocks, old car bodies, uprooted trees, almost anything, along the river bottom. It would be next to impossible to avoid being smashed and battered and driven under by the force of the moving water.

He pulled his mind away with an effort of will. This was no time to be distracted. He waited it out. The Navajo Police show up or they don't. Either way, I don't move just yet.

But he got ready to move. Put the book carefully inside his coat. Looked for a route that would get him into the reservation without making him come up on the road. Because if he was the deputy he would do just what he was doing. Put the scare into someone and then pull up on the bluff where you could see clear into Arizona and see what moved.

When he heard the van start, Ben started the bike. When the van turned to go back Ben took off through the willows, headed downstream along the bank very fast, but being sure to screen his tracks from view from across the river. It would take two or three minutes for the van to top out on the bluff. Ben took two minutes to get to the mouth of Chinle wash where it joined the river a hundred yards downstream from the bridge. It was fifteen feet deep here, over a hundred miles from Chinle Arizona, winding, and running with six inches of water. That made the bottom firm because the sand wasn't dry and powdery.

He had traveled with Grandpa up Chinle wash to their orchard in all seasons. And damp sand was the best. He had to watch for rocks, debris, holes, bank cave ins, a whole host of minor threats. The water was too deep to run really fast. But it beat a bullet in the back. Or being delivered to Dick Sand alive.

He was tempted to go after the deputy. If he only had the time. He could bring him back on the reservation side and treat him to a leisurely Apache picnic. Where he would be offered various selections of his body parts, lightly roasted over a slow fire, until he decided to get talkative. Ben tried to see himself doing such a thing. To save Terry. If there was no other choice. If it would stop Sand. Would he could he do it?

Part of Ben was revolted by the idea of using Sand's methods. He still felt deeply ashamed of having hit Lester. Desperation was making him do desperate things, trying to help save himself and Terry and Lester and others from a real monster.

Trying so hard he was becoming a monster himself . So hard to know what to do .

That was the difference, if there was one. When it came time to kill someone Ben would have to feel like he did when he went after Sand.

REX says a good end justifies any means of getting there. War, death, theft, deception. Everything I went to school to learn to counter

For men like Dick Sand it came as second nature. Just a part of doing business. Nothing to lose sleep over. Ben saw again the dead eyes of Sand as he'd seen them at Tibble Fork. Whatever had been human in Sand was gone now. Buried too deeply to be seen, perhaps too deeply to be found. Axel thought Ben was headed the same way. Becoming the same type of person. So did Lester. Terry? What she thought was even worse.

Despite the qualms of conscience, Ben found himself growing angry again. Sand deserved to die. He was doing everything he could to destroy Ben and Terry, and who knew how many others? Stopping him could not be called murder. It was no more than killing a rabid coyote.

He became aware of the book pressing against his ribs. The words. Blood and revenge. That was Dick Sand. And because of people like him, people like Ben Singer had to be that way too.

Ben popped up out of the wash after it worked its way around behind the comb ridge escarpment. He never did see a Navajo Police car. He took that as his cue to stop and rest near the upper reaches of Whitehouse Canyon, where it started as little more than an arroyo. He dropped into it, far from any habitation, built a fire, ate as much as he could force down, and fell back try to get some sleep.

Going home was a chancy, desperate proposition. He might get the help he needed. In the Navajo way they owed it to him. But the way things were he could just as well leave there with Dick Sand and his people and 8 or 9 Navajo Apaches on his trail. If that happened, he knew he'd be lucky to even see Warren Valley again.

No, he couldn't afford to arrive at Grandpa's hogan in a tired or weakened condition. He'd need all his strength and will to persuade his clan brothers to join him in a raid against Dick Sand. He fell asleep thinking about revenge and the journey of the Warrior Twins to see their father. To get the weapons and the support they needed to destroy the Monsters that endangered all life on earth. Surely none of them were more evil than Dick Sand. Unfortunately, the Monsters were half-brothers to the twins. Same father, different mother.

It had not been easy to get their father to agree to help them kill his own children, no matter how bad they were. It might be just as hard for Ben to convince Grandfather Tsosie to give his clan resources to Ben, the half-Navajo Mountain Navajo. So he could kill a monster named Dick Sand.

Ben got into Chinle just at dusk and started up the road to Grandpa's camp, hoping he hadn't moved up into the canyon for the summer. It was early yet, the peaches wouldn't be getting ripe and the squash and corn would be just getting a good start. But Ben felt he's used up most of his luck in the past 6 weeks. So he wasn't expecting much.

Especially not to see six or seven vehicles, mostly late model Chevrolet 4x4 short bed pickups in various colors. The whole Tsosie clan seemed to be home. Ben wondered why. Realizing it would be possible to put his case to everyone at once. Would that be good? Or very, very bad? There was lots of strain in every extended Navajo family. Strain that had to be glossed over, swallowed, set aside. Cooperation for the good of the family, so it survived, was the only acceptable standard. Not all of Ben's uncles and cousins liked him. Many envied his success in the Anglo world. Or they had. Now they'd be gloating.

Ben felt his cheeks burning a little. He uncapped the rage that seethed always just inside him and warmed himself at its fire. The fire that had burned Dick Sand. He was a dangerous man in a dangerous setting. He might find his family rallying around him. Or he might find himself an outcast, a no-one. A non-person left to shift for himself, to die alone. But he had to try.

He smiled wryly inside. Some bad guy you are, he thought. You're still what you were that night at Tibble Fork. Soft. Too sympathetic. Unable to leave Terry to her fate. Trying to find someway to help.

No wonder REX didn't come.

Ben left Bud sitting on the bike, looking a little nervous. There were some big camp dogs around somewhere, and turkeys were often meaner than the dogs. Maybe he doesn't know that. Bud looked at him, solemnly, then returned to watching the dark corners of the house.

There was a fire in the shade alongside the hogan. Cottonwood posts with cross bars and fresh cottonwood limbs on top made a pleasant out door `summer porch'. Cooking out there in the summer left the hogan a cool spot in the desert heat.

Ben stepped around the east side of the hogan, past the doorway, and stood in the broad entrance to the shade. Grandpa and his clan brothers all sat across the fire, along the west side, in the places of honor. Some sat cross-legged on sheep pelts others on small benches or five gallon buckets turned upside down. No one seemed surprised to see him. No one spoke. There was no room for Ben on that side of the fire so he stepped into the shade and stood just inside the door, not showing his outline against the fire to anyone who might be out there in the dark.

Ben took the measure of these men from the new pinnacle of his strength. He stood with his feet parted shoulder width apart and folded his arms against his chest. Alone or in a group, he could defeat them all. He knew that and he knew that they knew that too.

He felt his voice rumble up out of his chest as he spoke. This time he would choose the language they would speak.

"Hello, Grandfather," he said in Navajo. "I've come back."

Chapter 25
Sing, Ben, Sing

Thoughts buzzed in Ben's head like angry wasps. So much depended on what he said and did. So many lives rested in his hands. His options all gone. Sand closing in. REX no longer a hope. Probably an additional enemy. Each worry bit him again and again, as wasps do, not losing their stingers like bees, able to inflict searing pain again and again.

And beneath it all, Ben's fundamental fear that he was not of these people. That he was a mongrel, a step-child at best. The awesome, awful son of his father. He felt a wave of weakness wash over him. What could he say? To get them to help him kill this `witch' Dick Sand that was destroying so many lives?

Like Monster Slayer, he had come home to get the power to slay the drug monster. How?

Grandpa's voice broke the heavy silence that had settled over the shade house.

"You've been remade, I see. Have you been to see your father?" Grandpa asked.

His were beady, hard and glittering. His laugh dry and brittle. Not a shadow of awe or fear in him.

Navajos love double meanings. The men smiled a little at this. Watchful grins around the mouths. Not reaching to the eyes.

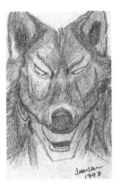

"You one of the Hero Twins, Ben?" This from Tony, Ben's cousin who sat near the door.

"More like a billy goat twin. Where's your brother, the big billy goat gruff?" Uncle Charley spoke this time.

Obviously Grandpa had told them about Ben's fight with Sand. They didn't know yet about his second meeting with Sand .. He felt his face start to burn. Shaming was the most powerful form of discipline and punishment the Navajo used. It sounded like they were getting warmed up to drive Ben away. Ben suddenly felt his anger break through. They could respect him. Or they could fear him. But they would not humiliate him.

Ben stepped sideways and grabbed Tony by the front of his coat, left-handed, and picked him up, holding him at eye level with his feet just off the dirt floor of the shade house. Tony looked back at him, faint amusement in his eyes, the old grin touching his lips, only a faint shadow of fear crossed his face. He and Ben had been friends longer than either could remember. Tony acted like he knew he really had nothing to fear from the huge Ben Singer that confronted him today. They had teased each other endlessly over the years. Ben realized, through the anger that put a red haze over his mind, that he would have been a little put off if Tony had not teased him tonight. It was just a little like old times. A glimmer of hope stirred near his heart.

The anger winked out for the moment. He set Tony back on his feet. No one looked at him. The teasing was over. Ben shook his head like a great bear that has taken a wound, but can't understand where the bullet came from.

There was a stubborn, sullen silence in the shade. The fire popped and crackled as it consumed the dry cedar wood. A foot scuffed the ground, a stool creaked a little. But no one spoke and no one looked at Ben.

"I don't understand this," he said, hearing true wonder in his voice. "This man has ruined my life, lied to my friends, tried to kill me. He's driven me from the woman I love, from school. He made me go off alone to die in Whitehouse Canyon."

Ben saw the sudden stir that went through the men. He felt a sudden drawing back in them. He knew what that meant to them. But he didn't stop.

"Then he came in a dream as a Navajo Wolf and killed me."

Heads turned and looks were exchanged. The sense of isolation increased.

"I'm trying to stop him. I'm willing to die myself to stop him. And you won't even look at me or listen to me. Are you such weakling men of peace that you close your eyes now to barbarians like this? The man is like a witch. Full of evil and power and dangerous as a rabid coyote."

"So are you, Ben," Grandpa said quietly. "What you bring us here is death to us. Can't you see that? You want us to fight Billy Goat's people for you. That trail they use is far from here. But it goes right past the place where your mother works down in Flagstaff.

"If we start a war we can't go hide in Tseyi' any more like we did in the old days, up in the canyon walls. These men here have to scatter out and work. Right in Billy Goat's cities. They can get us alone, one by one where we can't support each other.

"What makes you think this man doesn't know right where your mother is? That he won't take her and use her against you? Have you thought of that? Or has your rage made corn meal mush of your brains?"

Ben hadn't thought that far ahead. He scarcely noted how much Grandpa seemed to know about Dick Sand's affairs. He felt a stab of pain in his stomach. His mother. In Dick Sand's hands.

"You ready to destroy your clan brothers and sisters and your own mother to protect them whites?"

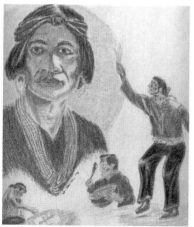

Are you a witch? The implication hung in the air like unventilated smoke--smothering Ben. One who has to kill a brother or sister to be accepted? Ben saw the question was fair. He'd been so desperate, so angry, so anxious for blood and revenge, that he'd given no thought to his family. He was ready to use them as REX advised. Make them serve. His cause was more than just. They were the ones to help him reward Sand properly.

But they weren't. They were ordinary people. Like the ordinary people Monster Slayer was trying to help.

Grandpa's eyes bored into his. He was not afraid of any power Ben might bring here with him. Grandpa knew the Beautyway ceremony and believed it was proof against any evil. Ben's uncles and cousins seemed to have no such assurance.

"You've had a vision, haven't you. Maybe more than one."

"More than that, Grandfather. I was taught how to get the strength of my father. I was given instruction by two people. I saw ancient battles fought far to the east of here, and I found the words of that day written in a modern book the Mormons have. Somehow they got it out of the ground and read it. More than that, one of the men gave me a weapon."

He saw a quick exchange of glances. Monster Slayer had also been given special weapons to use against the monster. Some of his uncles began to look a little scared. This was like a ghost story, only at the end you bring in a real ghost so nobody can pretend it's just a story.

Ben went out to the bike and brought back the sword. When he pulled it from the scabbard it flashed in the firelight and reflected in the eyes of his listeners. When he offered it to Grandfather he held up his hands and signed: Ch'iindii.

Without bringing it near enough to threaten anyone with contamination Ben showed the etching near the hilt: Light and Truth.

"But it all makes no sense. Axel saved my life, taught me to be strong and then said he couldn't help me against Dick Sand. He could only help me see my choices more clearly." Ben shook his head again. "Nothing he said has helped me at all. I don't know why he went to the trouble. In twelve days I will kill Sand or he will marry the one I love. There's no time to sit around making clearer choices about anything."

"I always said them Navajo Mountain people was witches," Ben's uncle Charley whispered.

"That's only part it Shida'i," Ben said to him. Another time in Colorado this man, bigger than Hulk Hogan, came in the night. Told me to do something. Said he knew how to help, that my`fathers' knew about me and wanted me to do something, if I was any kind of man. Told me to meet him up on Diamond Fork. When I was there he didn't show up. Just Dick Sand and all his people. I couldn't understand it. I didn't have time to do anything. I ran and then came here. It was my last chance.

"I didn't want to do this. But I have no choice. I can't let that monster win." Ben looked quietly at the floor. At least he'd had a chance to tell his story.

In the quiet Grandfather told about getting the tape. About almost believing it. About burning it. About Billy Goat coming around when he was cleaning his gun.

Ben felt a strange sense of poignant, emotion-shredded peace. He could die now. Knowing that his family knew what he'd been doing. That though it was strange and spiritually very dangerous. It was not evil. Not against family. Not like Ye'ii Tsoh. Just dumb and bumbling. Just trying to be of help.

He realized now that he could never ask them for help. Put them in danger. He had to go back and kill Sand. He could face that if he only knew that Terry knew the truth. He had to hope Lester had kept his word.

He had to go. He couldn't hurt these people or endanger his mother. He was just too dangerous because of his `visions' and his uncontrollable rage and his fear. Just as he prepared to step out into the darkness he heard Grandpa's voice again. He recognized the lecturing, sing-song tone he had always used when instructing his grandsons.

"Your problem in living by the good part in the face of great evil is just the same, my grandson. You speak to the good with your lips, to do good for others is in your plans. But the faith, the knowing of the power of it, to save you is not there. You are dead to it, as your father was dead to it. That's what this Axel is trying to tell you. That there is a power that helps people do right things, the right way.

For us Navajos it can be found in the Beautyway. You can't see it. Thus you must make your way along the path of other fools. Moles. Whose life and works are in the dark.

"As you are you have no right to expect to live your life in the light, nor even to be able to find it. Those who choose to walk in darkness are lost, though they think themselves to be in the Way.

"That's why you and Billy Goat are twins. It's just that you think you are Monster Slayer.

"But you aren't."

Ben felt bile rising in his throat. The anger and resentment came close behind. Terry would marry that Monster. He had taken everything from Ben. All anybody did was prattle about right and wrong. Nobody was showing him how to beat Sand. He felt the choking emotion restricting his throat. Felt his hands clench, his isometric systems pull him up tight and strong. Settled. Determined.

"I will kill that man."

"And what will you accomplish?"

"At least he will be gone."

"Then some of his people will seek vengeance and blood and they will kill some of us. That is how the cycle always starts. That's how it started with us and the Spaniards, then us and the Mexicans. It always ends only when one side or the other is all dead."

"You don't see him as he is, as a part of this world, or nature, as a bilaa' 'ashdlaa'ii who was formed by forces in the real world. You see him only as a thing to be destroyed, removed like a festering cactus spine in your hand. Not as a human being.

"Since you can't see him right you can't figure out how to respond to the threat he represents. You distill him out of the world and concentrate his evil in him until you can no longer see him any other way. That is the only way, Ben, that you can get angry enough to murder him. When you do, you will take yourself far out of harmony with your world. Far from the Pollen Path of the Blessingway. You'll push yourself as far away from the center as you push him.

"Evil does not stand alone, by itself, my grandson, outside of everything. Evil is embedded in the way people act. You cannot distill out evil and destroy it. Monster Slayer knew that. Good and evil? It's all just in what people do to other people and to themselves at a certain time and place.

"And when we do evil to someone else, well then we also do evil to ourselves. We're off the Beautyway Path ourselves if we can do that.

"Everything that is true about people is true about all the people. Every bila' 'ashdlaa'ii. The Dine, the Kiis'aanii, the Naakai, the Bilagaana even.

"Everybody, all the 'atsi' yishtlizii (browned skin people-Indians) all call themselves THE PEOPLE. Meaning the most important people, the first created people. But mostly, it means they are the keepers of the right way, the true path.

"The Dine are supposed to be the people who know about and who keep the right way. The Zuni claim it's them. So do the Hopi. The Jews say they are. The Mormons say they are. The idea has been around for a long time.

"But if the Dine run off, like you, and do things just any old way then who's going to show the world how to do it right? Or teach them that it can be done right by just ordinary human beings? Where will things go then?

Warrior's Way

"You've given that man all power over you, Ben. He shapes your days. He directs your thoughts. He owns you. The *haske* you feel inside for him is the chain that binds you to him. You are his slave. You live for him, work for him, maybe you're going to die for him."

Grandpa stirred the fire with a stick and seemed to shrink a little, like Old Age had come up to him just then and hugged him with her bony arms.

"You fight him, that's one end of the stick. Then you run away from him, that's just the other end of the stick. He's still pulling the strings on you, making you move. You got to let go of the stick and just walk away."

"I don't see how I can do that, Grandpa. I could try, but I'd only be lying to myself." Ben gazed into the fire, shaking his head slightly from side to side.

"You're right about one thing, Shony, that's for sure. You don't see how it can be done. I can't make you see it. I can't give the blind their sight."

"How am I supposed to kill Dick Sand with my faith? Or stop his evil just because I believe that harmony is the way to live?"

"You cannot know, Ben, because you neither have faith nor believe. Those ideas mean that you are connected to the world outside yourself where the supreme powers support such things. You are all alone. You live inside yourself, with your pain and with your self-centeredness.

"There's rot in you Ben. The smell of decay. Of great unharmony. Of selfish living of indignant rage at those who thwart you. That's what makes you a part of the problem. A Twin to Billy Goat.

"No balance

"No perspective

"No philosophy of living. You are empty now, Ben. You'd better fill up that hole in you before something evil creeps in to fill it. Maybe its already too late, I don't know. I hope not."

He stared into the fire and then looked steadily, rudely, into Ben's eyes. "Be careful you don't become like Ye'iitsoh, Ben."

The giant monster. The epitome of ruthlessness and rudeness. Who took what he wanted and destroyed everyone who got in his way.

"I've got to be a man, grandpa."

"You didn't say `man'. You said `warrior'. That's an Indian idea, not a Dine idea. Navajos and our cousins the Apache, we don't see it like the plains Indians. We don't see a need to fight one on one to prove something. We never did. When we fight we gang up if we can, we fight to win and we kill if we must."

"Where's the manhood in that, grandpa?"

"Where's all them Indians? The Navajos is the only tribe that's growing. The others are all dying out because they can't adapt what they know to the new world they live in. Dinosaurs is what they are. What are you, Ben?"

Ben felt an emotional jolt when he heard grandpa say that. It had two meanings, one was: What clan are you? A wrong answer could make you an enemy.

Ben searched his mind for answers. Grandpa was just talking in circles, saying Ben shouldn't act alone, then telling him he had no right to call on his family, to put their lives in danger.

Ben shook his head again. What he should do is let Sand have his way. Do what he wanted. Win. Go on winning.

What's the sense in that?

Where was Ben going to get help? Every man's hand was turned against him. There was no solution anywhere that he could see. If the "powers" like Axel couldn't help, what on earth was Ben supposed to do? REX wasn't going to help. Ben couldn't bring himself to be ruthless enough to kill, to use others, to force people to help.

What else was there? With time running out, with Dick Sand getting ready to marry Terry to force Ben out into the open. What options were left?

What choice did Ben have?

Sadness settled on him. Wound itself through his mind, tendrils seeped along his nerves, filtered into his muscles,. He felt his shoulders slumping, his isometric systems letting go.

He faced the certainty of death. The great uncertainty was whether or not he could stop Dick Sand before he died. Either way, the end of Ben's life was there, in front of his eyes, in the firelight of the quiet little shade house. Outside the world loomed large, unknowing and uncaring. What warmth Ben had known here, from these caring people, was gone now. Forever beyond his reach. Overhead the cold and glittering stars went unheedingly on their way. What was one life to them? To anyone?

He could see parts of the Milky Way shining through the branches that formed the roof of the shade. The Spirit Path, as some Native Americans taught. Perhaps the Beautyway, the straight way marked out as the Pollen Path, for the Navajo. Ben felt far from it. Then he heard Grandpa's voice, but Axel's words:

"Choices are always simple to simpletons, my Grandson. Look inside yourself for a way to trust in and to serve the power that supports good. The voice is quiet and small. But it's there for every man to hear if he will.

"Hagoonee', Shichai."

Without a word Ben left the shade. There was nothing left to say and his emotions were so deep that he could not have trusted his voice if he'd tried to speak.

He started back just at dawn, the early light casting the arroyos and canyons in blackness. Ben felt he had seen his people for the last time. It was hard to leave so majestic a place, knowing you could never return. He rode slowly down off the ridge, coasting along the highway like the ghost he soon would be. Seeing the little night animals scurrying across the road, headed home to sleep away the day. Their little minds content. Not knowing that Rattlesnake could come into their den as they slept and eat them alive.

Better they don't know, Ben thought. It's no good knowing when you're going to die. Better when it comes as a surprise.

He looked down at Bud on his lap. Content now it was daylight and they were away from the camp.

"Sorry, Axel," Ben said aloud. "I guess what you did was delay my death a little. Maybe for a good cause. But I won't have a use for the dog or the sword or the book."

He speeded up passing through Chinle. Seemed like he never went through here anymore that he wasn't crying a little about something.

****

"Maybe better he doesn't know we're helping him. He's such a greenhorn Hero Twin he'd go round like Ye'ii Tsoh. Five hunnert pound gorilla. Call Billy Goat up and tell him to surrender."

There was a little laughter, but it was soft and solemn.

He held up the package for Ben that Lester had sent. "These are pictures taken

Warrior's Way

by the little boy that Billy Goat killed."

"Who's that nephew of your wife's. The one couldn't do nothing else so he joined the FBI? I doubt the Billy Goat got to him. Tell him what's up, give him the pictures, get us some people to work with.

"Jim Tso and his wife work for the forest service over around Kanab. They should be right on top of it. Let's see what they can do. Tell them to just watch. This white man's a killer and we don't want him mad at Indians. He'd come after us straight off if he gets wise before the FBI saddles up.

Grandpa smiled a wicked little smile.

"I guess Tony and Freddy will be getting back to that sheepherdin' job at Fariview, huh? Might be able to keep Ben in sight a little. Billy Goats kid's want him real bad. Maybe you can set up a coyote hole for him in case he needs it. Maybe catch some mules if things look right.

"But stay out of it boys. These are mean people. I don't think we can keep Ben alive. He's going to have to do that himself. I know if I was Billy Goat I wouldn't want a wolf like that hunting for me.... If he's not dead right off Tony you can tell him what we're doin'... so long as he knows it's mostly just to defend ourselves.

"One thing we know for sure—Ben didn't start this fight. For a while there, looking at his dad, we thought we might have ourselves a fighter in the family.....What we got right now is a rogue warrior as likely to hurt us as help us...."

Grandpa threw his pointing stick on the floor and, sunwise, they filed out the door into the starlight night.

****

Terry left school early, headed home, skipping three classes, yearning for the solitude she'd find in her room while Rhetta was gone. The ring ..Dick's ring, hung heavy on her finger. Gold, white gold---was it platinum?----and a massive stone that caught the early morning sun and cast a glittering rainbow of colors on her hand. She put her hand in her pocket, afraid to take the ring off for fear of losing it and but uncomfortable with its glamour.

The bride price. What Sand thought she was worth .or else he was just showing off his money. A huge, heavy sigh pushed past her throat and seemed to carry with it the last shattered bits of her former life. It was over. All hope had died when she pulled the trigger of Sand's gun. When she tried to kill Ben. For what he had become? Or because he threatened her future with Sand, her only hope of obtaining a life for herself?

She didn't know. It was like her mind was hiding from her. But looking back, she saw plainly now when it had ended. When Ben rode away. Whatever his reason, his coldness still chilled her. He could have said something

"Terry?"

Terry almost ran into a huge man standing in the sidewalk. How did she miss seeing him? She noted instantly that he was bigger than Dick Sand. Bigger than anyone she'd ever seen outside the football stadium. Her antenna went up.

She had an impression of maturity, earnestness, good humor, and tension. His companion, a little dog, jumped up on Terry's pant leg and did a back flip, then scampered off a few feet and sat down, grinning at her. Somehow the dog took away the fear she would normally feel during such a confrontation, when she was alone and vulnerable.

"You are Terry, aren't you? I don't mean to make you uncomfortable. You can call me Axel, and this is Bud and we have an important message for you extremely important. Could we talk for a few minutes? Please?"

"I um I need to get home, Mr. Axel. I .have a lot of class work to catch up on." She noticed his suit. Modern and stylish like professional athletes might wear. What on earth could he have to say to her?

"Knowing what you've been through, I'm not surprised that you're behind in your lessons."

"What I've been through ..how do you know about that?"

"That's one of the things I want to tell you, Terry. But I can't do it standing here like an ecclesiatical missionary. It's very private, and just for you ..and it's literally a matter of life and death .."

Terry started looking around. For help. For a line of safe retreat.

"I don't feel comfortable, Mr. Axel. I-"

"First, let me assure you that he's still alive. You only burned the edge of his ear." Terry was hit with a tidal wave of emotion. Her voice was thick with it.

"Ben. You're talking about Ben, aren't you."

"Yes, Terry. I've come to give you some important information. For your own safety, and his."

"Who are you, Mr. Axel?"

"Just call me Axel. I'm the one who found Ben in Whitehouse Canyon where he had gone to die, actually. I've managed, at least temporarily, to get him stabilized. But as you saw at Derky's Lake, he's a very angry young man. Anger clouds the intellect and can lead to disastrous decisions. I'm afraid Ben has already made some."

"To commit murder. To work as a drug runner-"

'No, Terry, that's why I need to speak with you, actually. Ben is doing none of those things but if we can't help him I'm afraid he will cross the river, as we call it, by committing a crime that will forever separate him from us. Sadly, he's ready to do it to protect you.'

"I don't understand any of this. You aren't making any sense at all."

Axel sighed.

"No, I suppose I'm not. But if you won't speak with me somewhere besides on this public sidewalk, I doubt that I ever can."

So suddenly she surprised herself Terry turned and started walking toward her apartment. Logic said this was madness. But her heart led the way. Something she sensed in this man, in what he was saying, pushed her with a power that amazed her.

'We can talk in my apartment, but I can't give you much time. My roommate, Rhetta, will be home soon."

"Ah yes. Rhetta the roommate from the dark side ."

Terry's head snapped around and she studied Axel again. *This is so unreal. I must be crazy to be doing this*

Axel smiled a cheerful, knowing smile and the little dog pranced importantly along beside her.

When they were seated in Terry's living room Axel wasted no time.

"What hurts the worst, Terry? What causes the greatest pain about what happened between you and Ben?"

"I don't know...." She knew very well.

"It was the way Ben rode away. So coldly. Without offering you anything to cling to , to hope for, without apologizing, or even acknowledging your existence and importance in his life."

Terry felt the tears start, misting her eyes. She brushed them away. No other answer was needed.

"Let's just start there, Terry. Time is so very short that I'm afraid I will need to be very direct, perhaps even seem a little short with you. But we believe you can work your way through all this to proper conclusions. Ben is very lucky to have you and he needs you desperately right now-"

"He has a strange way of showing it." Terry felt a lot of heat in her voice. Enough to boil off any tears that might be lurking in her eyes.

"Let's start with the day he left. Here's the backstory on that "

Axel directed her attention to the TV across from them. Suddenly Terry was looking at the events in Tibble Fork. She saw the beating Ben took trying to help Lester and then the awful, shameful thing he did in dancing and howling like a Hollywood Indian. She couldn't believe what Dick Sand was capable of. She felt sick to her stomach.

Then she saw Sand drag Ben to the back of the van, she saw some of the video tape, heard Ben and Lester, saw Ben sign away his scholarship. Heard Sand tell Ben to be gone by daylight

She was thunderstruck. She looked at Axel, preparing to say something, when he motioned her attention back to the screen. It was daylight, she saw herself through Ben's eyes, but now she knew why his movements were so cold and stiff. He had been beaten, he must have been in terrible pain .. she saw him start to set up the bike, to get off and come to her and then she saw Dick Sand, tapping the video tape in his hand against his left palm. She saw Ben stiffen and heard again those awful words.

"I'm sorry, Terry. I've got to go ."

Then he rode away. The screen went blank, leaving her with a thousand questions and a million emotional shards striving to reassemble themselves into a perception of her world that she could feel and understand.

"They tried to kill him in Mona that night and sent men to kill him as he went home to Chinle when they learned that he didn't die in the campground in the rainstorm. Dick Sand sent a copy of the tape to Ben's grandfather. Ben couldn't bring himself to stay there, he had nowhere to go so he went back to Whitehouse Canyon and decided not to ever come back out. That's where I found him."

"Who are you, Axel? Are you an angel or something?"

"I think of myself as a good friend to good people. Why don't we leave it at that, for now?"

"But-"

"Terry, we've got to help Ben-"

"Get Dick Sand, you mean, for the awful things he's done ."

"No, Terry that's precisely not it. Ben was given knowledge that helped him acquire the great strength he now has. He was offered other counsel concerning how best to use that strength that he has rejected. As you well know from the incident at Derky's Lake, in his present state of mind he's quite capable of becoming like Dick Sand by killing Dick Sand. If he does that, no matter what good he thinks he's serving, he will cross over to the other side of the river and cannot ever return. Rather than have that happen we may be forced to allow his original decision to leave this world to stand ."

"Whaaa ..what are you saying? That you'll let him die? You can't do that . that would be so outrageously unfair ."

"As I've tried to help Ben see, Terry, life is not a playground. It's a battleground. Between good and evil. We can choose, for the power is given us. But a higher power assigns the consequences of our choices.'

"I know all that. I"ve been taught that all my life. But-"

"That's one of the reasons why I said that we need your help. That Ben is lucky to have you in his life."

Terry was suddenly awash with complex feelings. Rellief. Hope. Awful fear....to complex to understand all at once. But one message came through it all, clear and strong.

"Ben loves me. He did this for me."

"He did, and he does and he stands ready to die for you. That's a lot of love, Terry. A lot of caring and concern. He's a good man who has lost his way in difficult circumstances."

"We've got to stop this. He can't be allowed to .to ."

"You're right. I'm glad you see how important this is-"

Terry heard a key in the door. Sheer terror shot through her. *Rhetta*. What's she doing here? She's supposed to be in class.

Terry was awash with anger and fear. Rhetta was the last person on earth she wanted to have see Axel in her apartment ..

"Terry? You there, honey? Someone said a strange man followed you home. Are you alright? Should I call the police? TERRY! Oh, why won't this door open. What's wrong with this key?"

Axel stood up.

"I think we'll continue this later. Please be aware that you must not allow Dick Sand to learn of any of this. Your life and Ben's are in jeopardy. May Bud and I use your restroom?"

Without waiting for an answer, Axel and the small dog disappeared into the bathroom and closed the door. Then the lock clicked and Rehtta rushed in, her eyes glittering, searching for the scandal she obviously hoped to find.

Terry nervously got up and got a drink in the kitchen, hoping to distract Rhetta. Her roommate moved quickly from room to room and seemed disappointed when she didn't find a man under Terry's bed. Hands on hips she stared around and then her eyes locked onto the bathroom door. She stared at Terry, studied the flush of red Terry felt seeping up from her neck to her face, and scurried to the door. With a brief, triumphant glance at Terry she whipped open the door.......and gazed, incredulous, at an empty bathroom.

With a sudden flood of relief Terry realized.....

"Axel" was gone ..

Chapter 26
Lester Takes A Leap

Who am I? The Hopi question

Ben sat tucked in below a ridge near Fish Lake, a high volcanic depression ringed by high mountains, filled with a deep, cold fresh water lake full of mackinaw, splake, rainbow trout, brookies ..craggy outcroppings of grey rock that sheltered the tall pines that Osprey Eagles used to raise their young. A special place to the ancient Fremont Indians, just as precious now too many Utahns. The peace and tranquility and beauty of it made a massive effort to penetrate the pall of gloom that hung around Ben as he sat watching a three or four mile section of the Great Western Trail that wound along far below.

He always thought he was a fierce and dedicated defender of --what? The law? Then why was it that his victims were most often people who had offended him, personally, in some way? Honesty forced him to admit that much of his work was aimed at doing to people essentially what Dick Sand did. He used the law. Dick Sand used his fists.

When all this started, though he didn't know it at the time, he was going after Dick Sand. He'd thought it was only nameless, faceless dealers in drugs and death. A worthy cause, in a way. But deadly and dangerous in ways Ben took too lightly. As a direct result of this TJ was gone forever. Dick Sand was not nameless and faceless, not an abstract idea. Sand had responded. Overwhelmingly. He would never have even noticed Ben Singer if Ben hadn't innocently? started it all.

I rattled the wrong chain that time

Life is a battleground, not a playground Ben, Axel said in his mind.

Guess who's losing the battle? Not Dick Sand

Sooner or later good intentions have got to be replaced by expert knowledge.'

Oh Lord, protect us from the people with good intentions.'

Ben squirmed uncomfortably.

How many more will die? Ben, Terry, and Lester were all stuck square in the middle of a nest of killers. Ben was wondering if he could do anything for any of them.

His thoughts traveled always in the same circle. Always coming back to the same point.

Kill Dick Sand.

Kill Dick Sand. If you can   There's no other way that might succeed in the time Ben had left. Certainly Sand was doing all this with Terry just to flush Ben out, to bring him in close. So he could kill him first. Ben would have to operate knowing up front that he was walking into a trap. His only hope was that he could stay alive just long enough to stop Sand from ever hurting anyone else again.

Ben detected a subtle shift in his attitude. He wasn't thinking so much about the insult Sand had given him, the shaming, the unmanliness he'd made Ben feel. That was still there. But coming to the forefront of his mind was a feeling that to save Terry he would surrender the rest of his life.

Didn't that count for something?

Next time you see Dick Sand ask him

Everyone said he was practically married to Dick Sand himself. That Sand shaped his thoughts and his actions. On reflection Ben could see it was true. Ben looked into the boiling rage in him. Really looked, standing back a little mentally. He was not the rage. He was something else. He tried to look at it dispassionately.

It was pride. Injured pride. Humiliated pride. Ben thought of himself as something special. Dick Sand had dismantled his image of himself in a few intense, physical moments. Ben, in a flash of understanding, caught a meaning in this. Sand was so outrageously unfair, not a shadow of humanness in him that his actions had produced a skyrocketing reaction in Ben. That's what uncontrolled force did. It created rage, outrage, a thirst for vengeance and revenge. To save that wounded pride, the self-image that said: He can't do this to me.

REX was a man who knew how to take vengeance for such an insult. So was Sand, who responded with overwhelming cruelty to any threat. People so motivated would create wars of extermination as they murdered and were murdered in turn, by those caught up in the ebb and flow of violence and revenge. Ben was ready to do that. When he swung the dog down onto Sand he'd had every intention of killing him. He still remembered the keen disappointment he felt when the dog hit the boat first and struck Sand only a glancing blow.

Ben had used everything he could get, Axel's instruction, Lester's cooperation, anything and everything to get back at Dick Sand. A personal vendetta.

"Be a warrior, not just a strongman, Ben," he heard Axel say. Strongmen hurt people who offend them. What do warriors do? The best of them fight to defend themselves and others from the ruthless outlaws who know no mercy, show no humanity..

"The only legitimate use of power is to defend the rights of the powerless."

"Help you see your choices more clearly."

Ben sank deep into thought in the quiet of the warm afternoon. Can I choose not to respond to what Dick Sand did to me? Could my pride take that? How. How else can I look at this?

"You must see Sand as he is, a bilaa' `ashdlaa'ii, just like the rest of us. Not a devil. Not a unique creation made just to torment you," Ben heard Grandfather saying.

"Just a man who does evil things to people," Ben said aloud.

Ben took another step back mentally. Away from his personal feelings about Dick Sand. He tried to see what he was seeing when he and Axel were on the hill after the battle. Pride could lead to the destruction of an entire people. Or of any individual. What Sand did, carried to its logical conclusion, was exactly what had brought that ancient nation to self-destruction.

Ben shuddered as he felt again the raging anger he'd seen that day. Bloodlust. No human feelings. No compassion. No mercy. Vengeance and revenge for his loss of manhood. Just what he had felt toward Dick Sand.

So...... What? Let Sand have his way? Ben had always held to a saying of his own: For evil to triumph it is only necessary for good men to do nothing. Doing nothing around a man like Dick Sand was a formula for slavery, persecution and death. In a real way, this situation was only an extension of what his life plan had been all along. He had planned to use the law to defend the weak. Sand had sidetracked him. Blindsided him. Made it personal

No, that wasn't true.

Ben had blinded himself. He had taken this whole thing very personally. Lost his perspective. Lost his way. Foundered in rage and hate and had almost killed a man with his own hands. Ben felt his cheeks burn.

Warrior's Way

Where's the honor in that?

"We must triumph over evil," he heard in his mind. "But not for vengeance or revenge. Not for reasons of personal satisfaction or gain. But because it is our duty to do so. Our duty to those who cannot fight for themselves. Our duty to the young, the old, the helpless. To our society. So people can live together in peace. Like the Whitehouse Society."

Axel had said that clear back in Whitehouse Canyon ..why wasn't I listening?

Ben felt his mind tick over as the pieces fit together.

So, if Ben stopped his personal vendetta, to revenge his shattered pride, but still had to do something about what Sand was doing to others, what should he do. It still took power to control such a man. More power, more resources than Ben had.

He got up and fetched the sword from the bike, drawing it in the late evening sunlight. It gleamed, almost with a light of its own.

Light and Truth.

Evil men try to do their work in the dark. To hide what they do from the outrage and indignation of ordinary people. From those who exercise the executive power of the ordinary people. From the righteous indignation of the majority. The law abiding, middle of the road people.

"Drag him into the light," Ben heard himself whisper. "Let people know the truth of what he's doing. Expose him!"

****

Ben was back in hiding above Sand's cabin before daylight the next day. It took him only an hour or so to relocate the watchers. It took less than that to learn from the police radio net that Lester was missing. He'd been gone for two days. He must have disappeared right after Ben talked to him. Right after I beat him up. His cheeks burned at the memory.

He couldn't have seen me as being any different than Dick Sand.

The news broadcast said his car had been found abandoned in American Fork Canyon where the road forked to go to Tibble Fork or up to Derky's Lake. He was wanted for questioning, which told Ben that Sand wanted him back badly. Ben also heard that a `hiker' was missing and feared dead. Motive? Probably robbery. Weapon? A blood stained arrow was found nearby .. Ben Singer was now wanted on a murder warrant. Not hard to figure that out. Trace the purchase of the Bear bow and the arrows to Ben. Terry would have to confirm that he's had a bow when she last saw him.

Who was the poor hiker? One of Sand's mules?

Or was nobody dead. Just Sand inventing evidence of a crime...

Sand was drawing the net tighter around Ben. Raising the stakes in the game. Keeping the pressure on. Cutting off options. Getting him back at the top of the police priority list. He was playing his half of the game like a master. Now he was squeezing Ben. Forcing him to move, to expose himself. And encouraging the law officers to shoot him on sight

For now Ben had to find Lester just to save his life. Of that he was sure. Something had gone wrong after he left Lester. Was there a connection between Sand showing up at Diamond Fork and Lester's disappearance?

Ben had to see Terry. By now she should know the truth, assuming she heard it from Lester. Would she accept it? If not she would turn Ben over to Sand. Or to the nearest police officer. If she did accept what Lester said as true, then her life was in terrible danger as long as she was close to Sand. Ben had to know which it was before he would know whether to proceed to try to expose Sand or if he would be forced to try to kill him outright and at best die with him.   To save Terry from him.

Ben crossed the ridge on foot,-Bud scouting ahead,-that led to an overlook of the canyon where Lester disappeared. There was some rugged country in there. High mountain trails leading over the top, even down into the Salt Lake Valley. Lester could be anywhere. Like Ben he'd be almost impossible to find, unless he wanted to be found.

The falls at Derky's were running full now that the snow was coming off in the High Uintas, many miles away. The valleys echoed to the subdued thunder of the falling water. Ben felt a little pang of fear along his spine. What a fearful force that falling water represented. Worse than any Colorado River rapid had ever been.

From the timber below the crest he glassed the area, slowly, patiently, like a big game hunter looking for a trophy deer. Bud's whining alerted him and he looked down in time to see a white WCCC truck pull into the parking lot by the falls. Terry got out of the truck. She was alone.

His heart began beating hard. He looked along the road. No traffic. Where were her shadows? He should have spent more time watching. But he couldn't. He didn't know why she was there or when she would leave. He cautiously started working his way down the hill, using Bud's senses as well as his own, hoping against hope that he could get to the truck before she drove away.

When she came back to the truck after a short search of the park, probably looking for Lester too, Bud was sitting by the front wheel of the truck. Looking irresistible. Cuddly. He never looked that way around Ben. Never turned on the charm. When he saw Terry stop and bend over to speak to him and scratched his ears he decided to forgive him.

She said something he heard, but didn☐t understand.

☐Hey little guy. Where☐s you boss? Is he around here somewhere?☐

He moved from the brush, around the back of the truck, scooped Terry up with an arm around her waist and a hand over her mouth, and was back in the brush before she could start to struggle. He placed her on her feet in a little bare place in the willows.

"Please don't scream, Terry. I need to talk to you about Lester. He's in great danger. I think I did it to him and I've got to try to help him. I won't hold you against your will. Sand has you watched all the time. His men could be here any second. If they see me they'll shoot me."

He sounded rushed, breathless, untruthful to himself. Even as he talked he was feasting his eyes on Terry. Trying to see in her eyes what her feelings were telling her about him.

"I don't mind dying, Terry, so long as I know that you know the truth. That I've never stopped loving you. That I've never betrayed the love you gave me in any way, with anyone else. I can only hope that Lester has told you something that will help you give me the benefit of the doubt till I can prove myself to you."

Terry looked at him like a beginning fortune teller trying to see images in a crystal ball. She hugged herself as though it was very cold in her lonely world.

"I've talked to Axel, Ben. He came to see me at school and brought Bud with him. He showed me what happened at Tibble Fork the night before you left   I saw what Dick did to you, what you did for Lester, part of the tape he used against you . I saw it all. Now I know why you just rode away. I'm so sorry, Ben for all you've been through."

"I brought I on myself, trying to play secret agent with TJ. I must have scared Dick Sand pretty good, considering what he did."

Ben started to move closer, Terry took a step back. The coldness was still there .. Ben wasn't at all sure why.

"You're so different, Ben. I don't know you anymore. I don't know what to feel about you.. When you tried to kill Dick I saw a side of you that revolted me. I feel like you've become something fearful and ugly. Axel is very worried about you too, you know."

"Yeah, he's made that pretty plain."

"I got Lester's letter. I was hoping to talk to him. To find out if he was telling the truth or if you made him write it."

She handed him the note. In a nutshell, Sand would have his sister kidnapped and sold into slavery and prostitution. And Lester would get progress reports on video tape from time to time showing how her life was going. He said that Sand had simply enslaved him when he learned Lester was vulnerable and that he might be useful. Lester had never been able to break that bondage. But now he would, for his families sake. At Derky's Falls today.

Ben could only shake his head. Wondering how Lester had been able to function at all under such pressure. Such daily misery and fear. No wonder he'd given Ben no warning of what was coming that night at Tibble Fork. Ben had no doubt whatsoever that Sand would do what he said. And enjoy it. He felt a sick feeling. How close he had come to being just like Dick Sand.

To letting that monster make a monster of him. He felt a shiver go through him, despite the warmth of the day. Like the cold breath of death itself. For surely men like Dick Sand were dead to all human feelings. Every good person would despise them and seek to destroy them. Like the book said. It was so true. And Ben had been well on his way to becoming just like that.

And REX had been willing to help him! Ben had no time at the moment to think that thought through. But it opened another feeling of unease in him.

"I know now how far off base I've been, Terry. I was out for vengeance and revenge for what Dick Sand did to me personally. I was letting my hate for him make me into what he is. I'm over that now. I want to help the helpless, just as I always have. Only now it means using whatever force I have to use to stop him. He's a monster and it's the duty of good people to try and stop people like him. But to do it legally. To shine the light of truth on him and to let the will of good people take its course. I don't want his life, Terry. Not any more."

Ben didn't say he was willing to die to stop Sand. There was enough talking of living and dying just now. Terry didn☐t do anything to show she believed him, either.

"We've got to find Lester, Terry." Ben's voice echoed his concern. "Before Sand does. Do you have any idea where he is?"

In answer Terry dissolved into a tearful, hiccoughing bundle of sweetness and vulnerability. She melted into Ben's arms, pressed her head into his chest, still hugging herself miserably. Ben folded his arms all around her, pinning her arms inside his. Holding her gently, feeling his eyes burn with tears of gratitude and relief and love, and comfort. Just like a woman .full of feeling and a magic, non-logical, but beautiful way of saying, showing how they cared. A giving of self, a surrender, a melding that had to be one of the most powerful forces on earth. A woman☐s love.

"I love you. I didn't know how much until I lost you. Saw you with Dick Sand. I've had a hard time, Terry, reacting to what Sand was doing to me. To you. To us. I was a little crazy for a while. I know that now. But I'm not crazy anymore. I want to bring Sand to justice. Not kill him myself. But I will kill him anyway to prevent him from ruining your life. Even if I have to die to do it. I love you that much, Terry... "

His voice rang with his conviction, his care and concern. He thought Terry must be able to feel it too.

"Just like a man ."

Terry looked up at him through misty eyes and struggled to free a hand and arm so she could rub the heel of her hand awkwardly across her eyes. She sniffled and smiled beautifully. Like the sunrise of a new day after a dark and story night. Snoopy could appreciate the moment.

Then Ben saw the ring sparkling on her finger and in a flash Dick Sand was back. Moving between them. Separating Terry from Ben. For Ben realized that in winning her back, if he had, he had placed her in terrible, terrible danger. He could still lose her so easily. At any moment. He could die himself. She would not survive him long.

'You"ve got to be careful, Terry. Sand"s more dangerous that a rattler. He"s only staying close to you to draw me out. If he gets me he won"t need you any more, nor Lester I'm afraid of what will happen to you. I know how ruthless he is."

"I can handle Dick Sand. Don't worry about me," Terry said. She looked down at the ground again. Her voice sounded thin, unsure.

"Come with me now, Terry." Ben grabbed her hand, held it in both of his, ached to have her look up into his eyes. "We can hide from him till I get the evidence I need. I have some people helping me." If you count Axel as people. And as help. Bud at least was some help. Ben couldn't get an optimistic tone into his voice. It sounded hollow, pleading, unsure.

Terry looked up and then past him and he saw her eyes widen, the pupils dilate a little. He felt himself flinch. His body expecting the burning impact of a bullet. He knew now how it felt to be shot.

"There his is," Terry whispered. "Lester."

Ben turned. High above them, near the falls overlook, stood Lester. Dejection showed plainly in his body language. Dejection and resignation.

"Oh Ben, he's going to jump. Help him, stop him."

" Stay by the truck. I'll go talk to him."

Ben sprinted off through the willows, staying out of sight, planning to go up the edge of the sight-seeing trail, making less of a target of himself. But going much closer to the thundering flow of water. Feeling the ground shake under him. Smelling the wet rock, dank moss smell in the air. He gazed for a moment into the boiling currents below, where the falls plunged back into the riverbed.

Deadly water.

Not trying to hide its deadliness.

Shouting it to the world. At Ben.

Come, let me kill you, it said in its vicious water spirit voice. The water leaped and boiled, as if in anticipation of clutching Ben with its watery fingers.

Ben shut off his mind and climbed rapidly to the top.

"Hey! Lester! I've been talking to Terry. We know what your problem is. About your sister. I'm sorry man." Ben saw himself hitting Lester out in the dark behind the Laundromat.

"I ..I'm sorry, Les. I didn't know."

"You didn't care," Lester said. He glanced briefly at Ben, eyes full of misery. Misery and something else. Something that made Ben very uneasy. A look like he must have had in his eyes when he rode down into Whitehouse Canyon.

Lester turned back. Looking down into the greenish-black water boiling past his feet. He inched a little closer to the edge.

"Lester, wait. Don't do this. I was crazy. I know that now. I'm sorry I slapped you, Les. That I accused you of not being my friend. Let me help you now.

Lester looked at him again.

"That's what you were always trying to do. You just aren't all that good at it, Ben, that☐s all. You had good intentions. But you were right. You tried to help me that night at Tibble Fork. Now I've tried to help you with Terry. We're even, Ben. Now I've got to think of my sister."

Ben saw Terry, still by the truck, gazing up with her hands shielding her eyes. No other traffic. Where were Sand's dogs? The rabbit was here. Why weren't they?

"Sand knows. I called him and told him on his message service. I promised him he wouldn't have to hurt my family to keep me in line. To keep my mouth shut. That I wouldn't be able to help him or hurt him anymore."

Lester turned back to the falls, his body leaning now toward the edge. When Ben took a step toward him Lester held up his hand.

"I'd like to do this on my own, Ben. Not have you make me jump. Just stay where you are."

"Lester, don't do this. You don't have to. We can hide, you and Terry until we get the evidence we need against Sand."

"Sure, Ben. Sand, if he doesn't know for sure I'm dead, will have my sister taken today. Then when you get Sand we can get him to tell us where she is. She'll want to come home again for sure."

He seemed to shrink, to withdraw inside himself. Ben knew exactly what was happening. Lester was finding death easier to face than life. Oh yeah, Ben knew all about that, thanks to Dick Sand.

But Ben was stopped again. He had done this to Lester. Not Dick Sand. He had backed Lester into a corner. He had killed him. Not by slapping him. By calling him a faithless friend. Now Ben could see just how faithful he was. Willing to die to help Ben and Terry. To protect his family.

"Wait, Lester. There has to be a way."

"Sand's on his way here by now, Ben. He'll be here any minute. I wanted him to be sure he knew I did what I said I'd do. So he wouldn't have to worry about me. Wouldn't have to hurt my sister or my family. I'm sorry, Ben. I have no options left.

"Goodbye, Ben."

Ben watched in horror as Lester stepped off into empty space and disappeared into the roaring cascade of water going over the falls. He was gone. Ben had killed him. Axel had given Ben new choices. Ben had only succeeded in robbing Lester of his. Ben felt salt in the spray that got into his mouth. The salt of tears. Of regret. He couldn't bring himself to turn and look at Terry. To face her again.

He felt a howl of outrage and anguish echo in his head. Nothing he did worked!

What good was his strength? Everyone he tried to help suffered. Died. He looked down into the parking lot. Terry was standing there, thunderstruck, a hand pressed to her mouth.

Would he kill her too? Trying to help her?

For a moment he was powerfully tempted to step into the raging water himself.

Chapter 27
Ben Singer To The Rescue?

Ben peered down into the greenish foam-flecked water that hissed and roiled below him. Dark shapes shifted and moved in the depths like images in a cracked crystal ball. One of those shapes was Lester, caught in the swirling currents below the falls, being pulled to the falls by the powerful reverse current at the surface that moved upstream to fill the "hole" that was being pounded into the river by the tons of falling water. Only to be sucked under at the falls by the descending current created as the massive weight of the water plunging down the falls drove deep into the pool and created the deathtrap known as a suckhole.

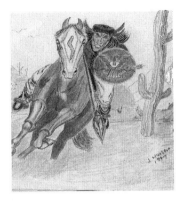

Deep underwater his body would be pushed out by the force of the falling water, being scraped against submerged rocks and battered by trapped driftwood and other debris. Only to be caught up by the reverse current to be returned again to the falls. The water a giant cat, toying with a sodden mouse and petulantly refusing to end its game and let go of what was left of Lester.

Ben fought an almost irresistible urge to leap after Lester. To try to pull him from the turbulent currents. Foolish thought. His legs felt weak, a sharp pain went from his chest to just inside his eyes and began to throb there, a steady drumbeat of terror.

The Colorado had taught him well.

This waterfall, though it was only three or four stories high, was running full. As strongly as it ever ran, the river banks brim full, the tons of water thundering and crashing wildly against unyielding black lava rocks. It was wilder than any Colorado River rapids.

Ben rubbed his sweating hands on his pant legs. Gazing into that turmoil of tortured water Ben could see his own future.

If he jumped in after Lester he'd be dead in five minutes. Just like Lester was dead. Only fools would say he was brave after he was dead. But this was real. Dead was dead. The end of everything he'd planned for. The end of the new hope that had sprung up in him as he held Terry in his arms.

Funny, mere weeks ago he had gone away to die. Now everything in him screamed for him to go on living. Not to dive into that raging pool to try and recover a dead body.

Ben knew too well the ponderous hydraulic forces at work in the seething cauldron below him. He knew no human was strong enough to buck those currents or to go anywhere they didn't want to take him.

Weren't some lives more important than others? Didn't they have committees to decide that some people would get their blood cleaned by scarce dialyses machines while other people were allowed to turn yellow and die? They decided by looking at the candidates to see who would have the most useful and productive lives.

Ben's life was important. He knew things. Valuable things that other people needed. He had new insights and commitments to use his gifts to bring justice, not vengeance, to his work. He knew about Sand, too. Dick Sand was evil. Sand must be stopped. If Ben killed himself now it would be the greatest gift anyone could give to that evil man. To remove Sands's worst enemy, to take away his fear. To make him confident again. And to let him go on wasting lives, helping other human beings destroy themselves so that Dick Sand could grow rich like a Navajo Witch, by killing others. Gain even more influence and power to murder the humanity if not the bodies of many, many TJs. Sand would do it, too, sure as sunrise, if someone didn't stop him.

If Ben Singer didn't stop him.

Lester was dead.

Let Lester be dead.

Ben started to move back up the slope, away from the water.

Ben Singer was alive.

Ben Singer was strong.

Alive and strong, Ben Singer could bring Dick Sand to justice for TJ and Lester. For Ben Singer's humiliation.

And when people knew the facts? Well then Ben Singer would be a hero. And no one then would look down on him because he didn't throw away his life trying to fish a dead body out of a suck-hole.

No one except maybe Ben Singer.

He saw movement in the corner of his eye. Terry was there, waving, shouting and pointing at the falls. Ben again searched the water through the mist and could see nothing that looked like Lester. Looking back at Terry he raised his arms from his sides in an elaborate shrug. Terry signed for falling water, showing it cascading over her left hand, which was held rigidly on edge before her and then gave the sign for under or behind and then for look.

Ben clambered down the mist-slick rocks, using massive amounts of strength to grasp handholds in the crevices or at the base of the stunted bushes clinging to the broken walls of the cliff. In a few moments he could see a little of the space behind the waterfall through a gap created as the rushing water roared off into space and began its plunging descent.

He peered, scrubbed the wind-borne mist from his eyes, and looked again into the mottled landscape of light and dark, shadow and filtered sunshine that danced and faded and grew brighter again in step with the changing translucency of the falling sheets of water.

Suddenly a large, narrow shadow, like a plunging arrow, traveled down the wall at the back of the cave-like hollow at the back of the falls and just where the shadow's point entered the water Ben saw Lester, huddled on the rocks just above the boiling cauldron of water under the falls. In the same fraction of a second Ben saw, outside, going down the falls, a tree, maybe thirty feet tall, branches green, bark a shaggy dark brown and the top rounded in shape. He recognized it as a Pinion pine from somewhere upstream where the banks had given way under it.

Ben looked back at Lester. He couldn't see him well, though he was less than thirty yards away. But Ben saw him stand and shakily climb up a few feet above the water with gross, exaggerated body movements as though he was being absolutely sure that he wouldn't slip back into the water. He saw Lester turn then, to look at his surroundings and when he looked up Ben risked a fall waving and shouting. But he could barely hear his own voice above the sounds of the water. Then he saw Lester looking steadily at him, peering as if trying to decide if he was a friend or an enemy.

Ben brought his hand up and forward, palm out in the sign for peace, then brought it down and laid it on his heart like he was saying the pledge of allegiance to the flag.

Lester didn't know much about Indian sign language, but anyone who had seen a traditional cowboy and Indian movie would know the meaning-friend. And Lester would know that it was Ben even if he couldn't make out the figure up on the rocks because he'd seen Terry and Ben talking many times in their private language.

Ben saw Lester's head turning again, this way and that, getting acquainted with his prison, where he might be serving a short life sentence. He couldn't walk around the back of the falls now as so many did in low water times. The rubble pile at the back of the cave was gone, underwater many feet now. And the powerful reverse current being generated by the falling of tons of water was as powerful as a rip tide on the ocean. Absolutely beyond the power of even the most powerful swimmer. If Lester slipped into the water and tried to swim across the back of the cave the surging current would carry him back to the falls where the falling water would pound him under again.

How on earth had Lester survived the jump?

How must he feel.

Still alive.

How long before him simply slipped back into the water to finish what he'd started. Not long at all, Ben was sure. Nothing had been solved in Lester's mind. Ben had to get to him fast.   The question was, how?

Ben looked out at the pool on the downstream side of the waterfall. He felt a jolt of fear as he saw the tree, caught in the suckhole, being pounded under at the falls. It should be far down river by now. He watched until it emerged at the bottom of the pool. It scared him to see that the tree was invisible as it was pulled down stream by the vicious underwater rip tide at the bottom of the pool.

Then, like a stricken giant he saw the tree surface, rolling slightly, the branches reaching up briefly like the arms of a drowning man reaching toward safety, and watched as it began drifting inexorably back upstream toward the falls, being swept along against the pull of gravity by the awful power of the reverse current that had carried Ben against his will to the head of the rapids, and sent him down again. The falling water was hitting the bottom of the pool with a force that was shaking the ground Ben stood on.

Literally, he was looking at two massive suckholes, operating back to back, in opposite directions, with the pounding waterfall making a ponderous, moving curtain of water between them. If Lester by some miracle could break the force of the suckhole behind the falls he would be smashed by the falling water only to be gripped by the other suckhole that was even now pounding the tree down to the depths for another round of cat and mouse.

He looked back at Lester, who had finished looking around him. Lester raised his arms partway up from his sides, then let them fall in a jerky, despairing motion. Hopeless, they said. Absolutely hopeless. Ben felt himself nodding in agreement.

Because Lester was still in the middle of the river.

Lester knew as well as Ben that the rocks that gave him temporary shelter were only a part of the massive rib of rock that ran to the top of the cliff and ended in a large pile of black stone that divided the falls into the two parts that gave it its name, the Twin Falls.

Even if he could drag himself somehow through the pounding curtain of water without being swept back into the suck-hole, he would only find himself on a narrow, wet pile of boulders and rubble that was isolated by the two rain-thickened columns of roaring water.

And where that rubble pile sank back into the pool the water was being pushed upward by the forces of the joining of the waters of the suck-holes into the huge haystack of water that boaters feared so much in river running.

At best, the water was a surging, mounding hillock of churning foam and debris. But from time to time, hydraulic pressures under the water increased beyond all the tolerable laws of pressures on liquids, the water would fountain into the air, leaping and splashing back again. Trying to escape the tormenting forces by leaping into the air.

Lester wasn't dead. Ben felt a spreading sense of sickness in his stomach. Lester was alive. But he was trapped between the twin water falls. Could Ben leave him there?

Will he? Will Sand let him? If Sand could drive him back into the water to drown, would he? Would Terry be able to stop Sand from eliminating one witness permanently in such a convenient way?

What will Terry think if he leaves Lester? And how will Ben communicate to Lester what he needs to do?

How on earth had Lester gotten where he was? Like Jonah and the whale, somehow the fickle currents had refused to hold him, had cast him up on the rocks. How unfair. Lester had wanted to die when he jumped and couldn't. Now Ben, who wanted in the worst way not to die would.

If he went after Lester.

If he didn't would Lester wait for the rescue team? Or would Lester think it over and decide to give the water one more chance?

What would Terry think of him, knowing Lester was alive, if ben didn't go after him?

What's the use, he heard her saying in his mind, of being strong if you let a friend die, all alone, because you won't try?

Yes, but what if I die? What then? Who'll stop Sand? Who'll keep you from marrying Dick Sand? (Who'll marry you? was an unspoken thought behind this.)

Who'll take revenge for my pain? Who'll stop the drugs? Ben was losing the conviction he'd gained when he vowed to expose Sand to the light. This was getting just too personal again.

Ben shut off his mind. He couldn't do the same to the queasy felling in his stomach.

He turned and looked at Terry, standing in the parking lot, arms folded, hugging herself. Like she was thinking the same thing he was.

Ben saw the flash of light far down the canyon. And then again. Sunlight reflecting from a vehicle. Even before he made it out he knew it was Sand's 4x4. Deputy Sheriff Dick Sand was in the saddle, riding to the rescue. Coming to save poor Lester. And to catch himself a murderer. Dead or alive?

Or dead at any cost.

Sand might or might not be able to cross the bridge below. Maybe not if the water was too high or the bridge was shaky from the pounding of water-swept debris and boulders that were being driven down the river by the flood. Sand could go around, over the old mining road, and only be delayed 20 minutes.

Tricky Dicky and his trusty .338 Winchester Magnum rifle with the nine power scope. If Ben ran away would he let Lester live? Or would he shoot down through the gap in the falls, where Ben now stood, and force Lester to choose between a painful wound or a peaceful death back in the water? Would Lester have enough guts to make Sand shoot him in hopes that his body would be found with bullet holes in it? Ben estimated that the chances of the body being found at all were slim. It could be held in the water till it decomposed or be washed so far out into the lake that it would become fish food.

Even Jonah had only made it once.

What effect would Terry have on Sand? Just what would he do? What should I do?

He felt the words as a moan in his throat.

Lester was a little fish, well hooked. Sand would not kill him with Terry around. Sand has his weaknesses too. Terry was one of them. But if Ben left Lester where he was he might be tempting Deputy Dick to kill him. While trying to save him. Or Lester might just give up again when he saw Sand and remembered everything that Sand had in store for him.

Ben could see Lester looking up toward him. His whole posture seemed to turn him into an eloquent, heart-hurting plea. Help me, Ben. Please help me.

Just like that night at Tibble Fork .

Ben saw his own hand go up again in the signs for wait and for friend. Part of him, he supposed it was the part that could drown and die, reacted in horror to what the message meant. At the same time Ben felt the old, overwhelming feeling of plain ordinary, simple everyday compassion sifting through him. What could he do. He was who he was. He didn't leave anyone alone to face the kind of danger Lester faced. Lester had cared enough about Ben to put himself in a position where the only way out for him was to kill himself. Could Ben be less of a friend?

No.

You're crazy! he screamed within himself. Absolutely nuts! Do you think that sympathetic feelings will keep that suckhole from scrubbing you like dirty rags in a washer? Yeah, that pool has a spin cycle. But it won't dry you out.

He saw REX's huge body contorted with vengeance, bloodlust and scorn. He felt the compassion begin to withdraw inside him.   You have to use others to get what you want, he heard REX saying. A great leader requires others to sacrifice themselves for his cause.

But it was too late for debate. Lester was looking up steadily at him like Daniel in the lion's den gazed toward heaven--expectantly, trustingly, faithfully.

Just jumping in won't get the job done. Too little chance that the currents will pull him to the center. Lester was a miracle of sorts. No swimmer could hope to go against the currents. Now he saw there was a new complication.

The tree was lodged at the outlet of the suckhole. It was a strainer, allowing the water to pass, but pinning and holding anything else, like a human body, with the pressure of the water flow.

He couldn't jump. He felt the throbbing of the pain in his head double and his cheeks burned. There had to be another way. A way where he didn't have to put his body into that churning hole below the falls. He felt beads of sweat start out on his upper lip.

Cold sweat.

He studied the outlet of the lake above the falls. It could be waded with the help of a rope during low water. How could it be done now?

If it could be done, if he could get to the rocks that divided the falls, he could rapel down the slab of rock, fish Lester out and get him back across the rope bridge without ever challenging the water monster that crouched below the falls.

Ben felt a little tingling hope stirring in him.

Ben turned and signed to Terry: Rope (question)

She signed: Yes

He made the sign for "bring" and pointed to the top of the falls. She turned and ran for the truck. Ben looked back down the road. There was no sign of Sand's van. That probably meant he was coming in on the other road. Ben had to hurry to get Lester up and still have time to slip away.

Terry brought him a one inch nylon, very strong. Ben ripped up a railroad tie from the edge of the parking lot, tied the rope around a sturdy aspen and around the tie.

The idea he had was to float the tie out into the current, over the far side of the falls. The tie might secure the rope well enough for him to use the rope to reach the rocks dividing the falls.

He waded out knee deep in the swift water above the falls, searching for footholds on the slippery rocks. Feeling the current trying to rip a foot out from under him. The tie was awkward to balance, but he knew if he set it on the water it would be jerked from his grasp and go over the wrong side. Sand wouldn't give him time to do it again.

Finally he dared go no further. Using all his strength he heaved the tie out far enough for it to get into the current going around the other side of the falls.

He saw the tie plunge over the far side, the line snapped tight but jerked and strained as the tie bounced in and out of the falling water.

The question is, will the line hold his weight? If not he'll be swept over the falls on this side as the line pulls up in a big looping bend and lowers him over. He won't be able to hold on after he slips over the falls and the tons of rushing water start to pummel his body. And the rope won't pull loose from the center of the falls to let him try to swing out of the way. The rope seemed to be wedged in the rocks sometimes. Then it snapped loose again, jerking and flopping about like a headless snake. He was not sure he could depend on it and he didn□t have much time.

What if another tree comes along and snags the rope?

The window of opportunity is closing fast. Sand will arrive before Ben can save Lester and fade back into the brush.

Ben decided he couldn't trust the rope to hold him as he waded across to the rocks. There had to be another way. He looked at Terry as he waded back to the bank.

"It's no good. The rope won't hold me."

"What will you do, Ben. Dick will be here soon." She looked anxiously down into the parking lot, as though Sand was already there.

"I'll have to try starting upstream with another tie and paddling out to the center and either grab the rocks or the rope out near the center." He stomach reminded him that that was exactly what he had done that day on the Colorado.

"Don't do it, Ben. Please." Terry put a hand on his arm. He felt the warmth as a little electric shock. The power seemed to be sapping his strength. His will. He pulled away. Turned away. But at least he bit off the words he was about to say: I have to go, Terry.

"You'd better get down to the parking lot. Make sure Sand doesn't get fancy with his rifle."

He turned back and looked at her and felt a lifetime of living in that look. If he died, he wanted to take that image with him. It was enough to break his heart. Seemed like he was always making her cry.

Ben grabbed another tie and ran upstream. He wadded out and shoved off with all his strength. Using the tie as a flotation device, he angled upstream and kicked hard to move across the current. He had fifty yards to get set up right and his target was no wider than a car parked sideways to the current.

He floated feet forward and bumped bottom a couple of times and nearly got a foot wedged in a crack. He managed to yank it out just as he was tipping over to go head down under the water.

But he lost his grip on the tie and watched it spurt on ahead of him. He saw the current suddenly push the tie strongly sideways just as it got to the rocks. As the water divided to go around the rocks the current actually flowed sideways. The tie suddenly jerked to one side two feet away from the rocks and pitched over the far side without it ever touching them. He would do the same unless he could grab the rocks or the rope.

The image of himself going over the falls into the maelstrom below flowed into his mind like liquid nitrogen and froze his thoughts rock hard. He saw himself approaching the rocks at an accelerating pace as the water began moving more swiftly. He was going over. There was nothing he could do. He felt his body going rigid, his mouth pulling open to scream.

He managed to swim a little and relocate himself to the left center so if he missed the rock he could try to grab at the rope. And then the water accelerated even more dramatically. Exactly the feeling of coming up over the crest on a roller coaster and starting down. Adrenaline blasts through him. He faces the real fear of death. It grabs at his guts and clutches at his head and stops his breath.

He can see the rope clearly now, but it has worked it way up on the rock because of the jerking of the tie as it bounces in and out of the waterfall down below. It may be out of reach of his clutching hands now.

The current starts to move him sideways and he is too far from the rock to make a grab for it. At the last moment his feet hit a buried rock ledge at the edge of the falls and he stands upright and he catches the rope with his left hand as he flies under it.

His sudden weight snags the rope in a crevice in the rock and he swings out over the abyss. He has a fleeting view of the boiling water far below. Then he pulls himself hand over hand and flips himself up onto the slippery rock. Just as he gets a grip by jamming his right hand into a crack in the rock the rope pops loose and goes slack again.

Shakily, Ben clambers up on the rock, heaves up some slack by lifting the tie, and wraps the rope tightly around the rock. As he pulls it taut it clears the water by about two feet. Ben would have liked about ten feet. To be far away from the currents. But the rocks just aren't that high. Time is so short and the rocks so slick that Ben has no time for debate. He makes his knots tight. Then he gazes back along the rope to the shore. He knows he could make that trip in under two minutes. It feels good to know that that part of the path is secure.

Unwittingly he looks upstream. Secure until the next tree comes along. Then gone forever.

There is no time to waste. He has to either go back now or move as fast as he can to find Lester. He spots Terry back in the parking lot, looking up at him. Strain in every line of her body.

Then he sees light glinting from the bodywork of a vehicle coming down through the trees on the old mining road. Ben feels the tension in him suddenly double. His stomach knots up and his hands feel weak. That can only be Dick Sand.

Time is running out much faster now.

Chapter 28
Ben Singer Takes A Fall

Looking back at Terry, Ben sees her running back down the hill to the parking lot. She must have started back up toward him when she saw Sand coming. Dick Sand's big four-by rig eased into the parking lot, Sand being cautious until he finds out what the situation is. Maybe he's calling for back up, calling in every lawman in the county to help him arrest a killer. And maybe he isn't. Perhaps he's just calculating his chances of handling all of this alone so that he can make it come out his way.

Where are his bloodhounds?

Ben pictured Sand's big magnum rifle. He remembered Sand boasting about the pinpoint accuracy of his hand loaded bullets. 338 caliber, 190 grain hollow points that mushroomed on impact. Small bullets compared to the size of the rifle. Bullets that could be speeded up dramatically by a large charge of powder so that they would shoot flat and hard and hit hard enough to bring down an elk or a moose. Ben had seen bucks that Sand had taken in season. Sand always paraded them around the campus on the fender of his van.

Big heavy deer, with a small hole little bigger than a dime on one side and a hole you could easily stick your fist into on the other. Sand bragging that the buck hadn't jumped twice after taking the bullet in the lungs at 250 yards. Ben isn't even 50 yards away from Sand's truck. He looks down at his hands and he sees them trembling.

Ben feels exposed and weak as he watches Terry talking animatedly through the truck window to Sand. She gestures to the falls and then again in his direction. Then she steps back as the door swings open and Sand emerges. He has the rifle in his hands and he is looking carefully all around the area. Wondering if there's any witnesses, or anyone out there to help me.

Will Sand shoot me with Terry watching? Ben wonders. If he murders Ben in cold blood he will kill Terry, too.

Or is he still trying to play Good Guy to Ben's Bad Guy? And can Terry play her part? Pretending to be Sand's fiance. A lot depends on the answers.

"And we find out right now" Ben said.

He sees Sand walk around to the off side of the truck, rest his elbows on the hood and swing the big rifle around till it is looking straight at Ben. He can't help feeling a tightness in

his chest, as though his flesh is trying to shrink away from the impact of a bullet that Ben would actually never feel, followed by the boom of the big rifle that Ben would never hear.

He sees Terry step up and shove Sand with all her strength. He actually sees the rifle move a little. Sand turns and looks at her, says something, and then swings the rifle back to aim again at Ben. Terry is now looking up at Ben, and out of Sand's view she signs: Shoot/No. Then she folds her arms and watches Ben while at the same time turning her head often to be sure Sandias keeping his word. Ben can't resist giving Sand his best grin.

I'm Robin Hood on the castle walls, it said. Stop me if you can.

Ben turns and rapells down the rope using his strength to make up for his inexperience. As he goest down he marvels again at how much can be done by simply being strong and fit. Much of a natural athlete's prowess lay simply in having a strong, well integrated muscle system in his body. Ben makes the forty foot drop in a matter of a minute or less, even without the standard rope climbing rigs. Only once, for just a second, did the rope swing him into the plummeting water. He was impressed at the power its falling weight gave it. If he allowed himself to swing out under the full force of it it would strip him off the rope. Nothing he could do, no amount of strength, could resist it. He just had to stay away from its power.

When he gets down Ben removes the railroad tie and snubs the rope around the rock. There is enough left for him to use it to climb along the rock and under the falls. He gets drenched, but is not hit by the mainstream force of the water fall.

In just moments he is beside Lester, who is sitting on the wet rocks, shivering, and looking like the Little Mermaid on a very bad day. He is gazing into the boil beneath the falls like he is waiting for a lost friend. His shoulders slumped, his elbows are braced on his knees with his hands dangling from loose wrists and his shoulders hunched up till his back looks like a vulture with folded wings. He shakes his head sadly and stands up.

Ben touches him lightly on the shoulder and Lester starts so violently that he almost falls in. Ben takes his arm and holds him firmly, securely.

"Hey, Les" Ben says. Almost nothing can be heard through the thunder of the falling water. Ben hopes his smile will help.

Lester looks at Ben and back to the seething water like a man being asked to choose between hanging and a firing squad. Lester has such a sick look about him, eyes so full of misery, Ben wonders if some of the water on his face is tears.

"You can always die, Les. Any day. Give living a chance, okay? If we stop Sand then it's all over. If we don't? Well if we don't, then we'll decide."

Ben has to put his mouth close to Lester's ear to make himself heard above the thunder of the water. He can smell the dampness and the musty smell a man got after time in the out of doors. And there was something else, sharp and tangy. Ben wonders if that is the smell of fear that people talk about.

"There was a hand," Lester said. "Reaching down to me in the water. Someone said: "Here, Lester. Let us help." In my mind. And a feeling, like someone really cared about what was happening to me."

"Axel," Ben says. Feeling the hair rise on his neck.

"What?"

"His name is Axel. He gave me a hand too." Too noisy. Too scary for a prolonged conversation.

"Let's get out of here, Lester. While we still can. Trust him, even if you can't trust

me. I'll explain later."

"Sand's got big trouble that he doesn't know about yet, Les. With the DEA. I've given them pictures, evidence, and the whole plan of operation in this area. I found people outside Sand's organization. He's done, Les. All we have to do is survive long enough for them to act."

Fat chance of that, Ben thinks. Lester will make it. But will I? Being dead's not all that bad, assuming Axel was dead, but it takes you off the playing field and leaves the work to others.

He sees a picture of Terry in his mind's eye and feels a deep breath expel itself as a sigh. And you missed out on so much living. So many days you'd never see. So many things you'd never do. So many pleasures you'd never have. All you can do is give it your best shot. Then leave it to your friends, like Axel, to make up the difference.

Lester looks openly skeptical. He glances repeatedly at the water. Lester seems to be choosing which devil to serve. Him or Dick Sand. Not realizing yet he would be climbing up out of this hole with Dick Sand out there with his rifle.

Ben ties an open loop seat in the end of the rope, puts it over Lester and has him set in it. Then Ben goes back up and out through the falls.

Ben turns to see Sand, 40 yards or so away, across the boiling maelstrom below the falls, looking steadily in his direction as he leans across the hood of his rig. Terry is still there, standing close and shading her eyes. Looking at the falls, then turning to look at Sand. Ben figures she is talking about a mile a minute to keep Sand from doing anything violent. It should be obvious that Ben's only way out is up the rope and over to the bank. Sand must know that no one would attempt to get away by jumping into the water below the falls. There was no excuse yet for shooting a wanted killer like Ben. If there was, Ben knew Sand would have pulled the trigger long ago.

Ben feels his insides draw up tight and his nose and ears and finger tips turn suddenly colder. In an almost leisurely motion Sand brings the rifle down and props it on his hand and rests

his elbow on the hood of the Suburban. Even at forty yards the rifle seemed big to Ben as he sees it swing and point directly at him again.

Terry moves closer to Sand and pushes him again. Ben also thinks he sees Sand's hand make a motion like it would take to jack a bullet into the firing chamber. Maybe Sand is going to shoot and say that Ben was moving to jump in and get away. He could claim it was an honest mistake and it would be just his word against Terry's because Lester wouldn't say anything bad about Dick Sand if Ben was dead.

Terry moves around and puts herself between the gun and Ben. She signs: Up/Rope Shoot/No.

He knows this is her word to him, not Sand's. If he tries to do anything but go back up the rope he knows Sand will shoot him. He sees her fold her arms firmly across her body. He also sees Dick Sand move quietly to one side so that he again has a clear shot at Ben.

How desperate would Sand be right now? Ben knew the first challenge was to live to surrender. What happened after that would be another problem. How long would he live in Sand's tender care?

He looks at the surging currents that torture the water around the rocks. The currents below the surface are wild and totally unpredictable. He feels sick again, and weak. He has to turn away an look up the rock face. Not at the pool.

Because now, at the foot of the pool, the tree is wedged tightly in the rocks, a big strainer ready to catch and hold underwater anything that comes to it.

It would love to cradle Ben in its spiky arms and croon to him a hissing, deadly lullaby while he struggled in vain to breathe, lungs burning, finally unable to stop himself from taking in a huge, sucking gasp of air. Only to feel his lungs fill with water. His mind blink out, as he went to sleep for the last time. He knew he should never have read about the act and process of drowning in the book The Perfect Storm . but of course, he had. He knew in lurid detail what drowning meant. It only focused his fear, sharpened it, and cut him in his heart.

The only trap on a river that some boaters truly feared. Once in its clutches you had only as long as you could hold your breath to break free.

Ben turns and looks up the rocks along the rope. It looks like the path to the pearly gates must look-golden and warm-compared to the cold, watery hell bubbling at his feet. He knows he can climb the rope, if Sand lets him. And he can haul Lester up without a hitch. If Sand lets him. What Lester will do when he sees Sand is another problem.

Let's find out. Ben grins in Sand's direction, for the sake of his nine-power scope that must be telling Sand when Ben last shaved. Evening was coming on, darkening the canyon. But Sand's scope would gather light for a long time yet. Knowing Sand the scope probably had a range finder on it and a sight point dot to boot. There is no help in the twilight for Ben. But also no excuse yet for Sand to pull the trigger on account of darkness.

Ben gives two hard yanks on the rope. He pulls hand over hand and Lester pops up out of the streaming water looking almost exactly like the prairie dogs Ben had seen bursting from their holes when a slashing summer storm flooded their town. Sodden, sorry, and terribly, terribly vulnerable to the lurking coyotes. Lester looks around, wiping the dripping water from his face and eyes. He looks at the water spewing and burbling at his feet almost the way Indiana Jones gazed into the pit of snakes. He moves carefully up the rocks, then stops dead when he sees Sand leaning across the hood of his Suburban. He looks at Ben and again lifts his arms and let them fall in little jerky motions that say `hopeless'.

Ben turns him around an points up the rope. He mimes himself climbing and then pulling Lester up to save his voice in the roar of the falling water. He is starting to feel cold, he'd been standing still too long. He can feel the ground trembling. His greatest fear, second only to the clinching feeling of one of Sand's high powered loads blasting through him from back to front as he goes up the rope, is that another tree would come over the falls and take their rope and with it their only hope of escape. Leaving them nothing but Dick Sand's mercy or the boiling river water to choose between. Some choice.

Really between the devil and the deep blue sea.

Ben starts up the rope, again using more muscle than skill. Wherever the rope hangs free of the rock he goes up hand over hand with his feet at right angles to his body like a circus performer climbing into the Big Top to do a triple somersault.

You watching, Sand? You remembering our fight? You feeling slightly sick knowing I beat you at your own game? You wondering how I changed so much so fast? Are you scared, Sand? Ben brings his thoughts back into line. He isn't competing with Sand or anyone else.

At the other places he plants his feet and walks up the wall pulling himself along with the power in his arms and shoulders. As he climbs he feels his body hunching a little against the possibility that Sand might shoot him at any moment. It helps him move faster.

When he reaches the top he immediately turns, bracing his legs wide on the slippery rock and trying to jam his feet well down into the rock at the edge of the drop off. He loops the rope over his shoulders and down along each arm. He starts lifting Lester before he is set or prepared to help But soon he faces the rock and kicks himself away to keep the drag off the rope. And he walks a little wherever he can.

Ben simply hauls up Lester's weight with his body, legs, and right arm. He bends, grabs the rope, straightens, lifting Lester by arm strength alone, and then repeats the process. Lester comes rapidly up the face of the rock and Ben begins to feel some of the strain of the physical efforts he's been making. He is breathing deep and he can feel his heart beat in his neck and chest.

He takes the rope near Lester and heaves him up over the ledge to the relative safety of the slippery rock that divides the rushing water. It is hard not to get dizzy or to jerk backwards as the water gives the sense that you are moving and it is standing still. Lester sits down immediately and refuses to look at anything but his feet. Maybe he feels Sand drawing a bead on him too. He pats Lester's shoulder and signs to Terry: Good/This Far.

She responded by unfolding her arms and moving back to stand alongside Sand. Standing slightly behind him she raised both hands high overhead and clasped her hand the way Rocky Balboa did in Rocky One when he finally managed to run to the top of the steps. Sand remained unmoving, but the rifle still pointed steadily at them.

Ben turned to Lester and guided him up over and around the rocks. As they move to the far side Ben searched the water upstream for any sign of floating debris. No trees coming that he could see. But it was getting dark, and his angle, so near the water surface, was bad. This was no place to hang around. Sand was waiting on the other side, but they had no choice but to move on before it got too dark to see what they had to do.

He made a quick, but effective loop sling for Lester so that all he really had to do was pull himself along the rope till he was over the bank and then free himself. The anchor tree stood back from the bank three or four feet so he needed no help if he was willing to make the effort needed.

"You can do this, Les. It can be real easy. Just don't think about anything but the rope. Don't look down. Just keep moving. Be sure and tug the rope over the buckle out there that joins the ropes, so it won't hang up. You won't have any trouble at all, and if you do, I'll come out and get you. But it will be better if the rope only has to hold one of us at a time."

And if a tree comes along, what then? Or if Dick Sand strolls up and slices the rope.

"It'll be dark soon, let's get this over with. Try living a little longer, okay? And watch the buckle link. Don't snag up on it. As soon as you're about over I'll come across. Don't hold me up, okay?" Ben grinned. "I don't want to keep Dick Tracy waiting."

Lester gave Ben a sick, doubting look, like a man who had just been assured that an amateur could walk the Grand Canyon on a tight rope if he held an eagle feather between his teeth.

"I don't know, Ben. I went under once."

He was shaking now. Not just his teeth chattering in the cool, misty wind coming up from the falls, but all over like a man with malaria. Hypothermia and fear. What a combination. But he had to go and he was still in good enough shape to make it. He just didn't think he was. Time for a little psychology, Ben thought.

"Of course, if you want, I can go first and pull you across, but the sag of the rope might put us into the water out in the middle there."

Lester glanced at the rope and the rushing water. He was thinking about being left behind. About touching the water again. Ben felt relief when Lester shook his head, like a man resigned to climbing in the barrel at Niagara Falls.

"No, I'd rather have you behind me."

Lester took a deep breath that came out in a shuddering sigh. He looked longingly at the part of the pool visible below the falls. This should have all been over, the look said. Why am I still here, still alive, still afraid?

You died, didn't you, Ben thought. It took courage of a sort even in your despair to step off into that. Courage of a sort to take charge in a way and say that there was one kind of life, a life of humiliation and shame that you would not live. And so you died. But you aren't a warrior reborn. You still fear death.

"Do it your way, Les. When you get across buy me some time in you can, if you feel like it."

After all, I just saved your life. I wonder if you are happy about that.

They both looked over to the bank. Sand wasn't there standing by the tree to arrest Ben. They couldn't see the parking lot around the rock pile they stood on. He was on his way up, then. Ben needed only a small break to make it into the brush. Sand can follow if he wants, and bring a machine gun too, if he wants, Ben thought. Ben knew right where his buried equipment was. He wasn't as helpless as Sand might hope he was. Where's Sands wolves?

Trying not to appear anxious, Ben rigged Lester up in the sling. He expected Sand to appear over the slope, up from the parking lot, at any moment. The adrenaline pumped in him and he

felt that he was gathering himself for the effort ahead. He was ready for the challenge. He was also getting tired and cold from the constant soaking mist and the breeze that blew up the canyon.

He sent Lester on his way. The rope sagged and swayed as Lester pulled himself along. Half way over Lester's nerve failed him and he stopped and wrapped his arms around the rope. He looked past his feet at Ben, agony on his face.

Ben started to move out along the rope, getting ready to swing out and wrap his legs over the top of it so he could pull himself along hand over hand to get to Lester. The vibration and the increased swaying of the rope goaded Lester. He began hauling himself along in huge jerks, ignoring the swaying, his mouth moving. Ben could hear nothing above the roar of the waterfall. In two minutes he was over the bank and began to free himself from the sling.

Ben peered over the rock and couldn't believe his luck. Sand had made a major mistake. He was still leaning across the hood of the truck with Terry close to him. Ben watched the rifle in his hands move back and forth in a small arc as though he were keeping track of both Ben and Lester.

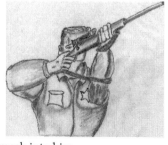

Tough luck, Sand, Ben said to himself. He saw himself crossing the rope and ducking into the brush before Sand could get up the hill. He grasped the rope, arched his back over the rushing water, checked his grip on the damp nylon and then hooked his legs up over the top. He began pulling himself rapidly along, ignoring the swaying and the sagging of the rope that brought him down too close to the water. The smallest snag going over at this point would smash into him.

A third of the way across he heard a booming, cracking sound and felt a distinct tug on the rope. He twisted and had an almost upside down view of the parking lot. Terry was jumping up and down near Sand, trying to punch him in the face, trying to hit the rifle. Ben could also see rifle smoke drifting away from them.

Sand had fired. The question was, at what? Ben couldn't believe Sand would miss it, whatever it was.

Ben suddenly felt like he'd been dipped in ice water. His breath caught in his throat, his grip weakened and he felt his legs starting to release their grip on the rope. He lost his isometric systems for a moment and became the old, weak Ben Singer. He almost fell into the cold stream of water rushing over the falls.

Sand swept his left arm out and down in a impatient motion that caught Terry with her feet off the ground. His lower arm or hand caught her in the stomach and she collapsed to the asphalt like a rag doll dropped by a careless child. Sand hadn't even glanced in her direction. He was looking at Ben. Ben felt like a buck deer on opening day who'd been caught out in a meadow at daylight. Ben saw the rifle coming up again, swinging toward him.

He'd been wrong.

Horribly , fatally wrong.

He felt his body shrinking and pulling again as he drew himself in against the expected impact of a jacketed hollow point hunting bullet that traveled with supersonic speed and with enough force to expand in him, ripping through muscle, organs, sinew, even bone. The impact would shock him so badly that he'd go numb and drop from the rope like a poisoned insect falling from a fruit vine.

He was three feet from the buckle, one third of the way across. He had to keep moving. Be a moving target, and he had to act now. He couldn't just hang here like a bull's eye target, swinging gently in the wind.

He reached out to move on and as he did he felt another hard tug on the rope. He heard a metallic clink and then the distant crack of the rifle. His eyes were drawn to the buckle that joined the ropes as a dawning horror swept over him. Sand was not missing. Sand was hitting exactly what he aimed at. He just wasn't aiming at Ben. Shards and sharp spikes of metal stuck out from the buckle in all directions. Almost nothing was left of the part that bound the ropes together.

Cold fear froze Ben in place, one hand on the rope, the other reaching out for the next handhold, his mind trapped in the awful visions and sensations of his ride through the Colorado River rapids. Of his view of the boiling, deadly water pulsing below him If he could just make it to the other piece of rope, on the other side of the buckle

In that instant the rope parted.

Chapter 29
A Family Reunion

In that instant the rope parted. Ben crashed down into the rushing water, fear screaming through him, clutching the rope with all his strength.

Then, with a wrenching emotional effort, he let go. Found himself falling, his stomach coming up into his throat. Fear squeezing the breath from his lungs, raking his throat raw with the harshness of his scream. His brain, clicking like lightening, was telling him that the rope would only hang him upside down over the falls and swing him over the rocks where the water would jerk his body off the rope and plunge him to the boulders below. To have any chance at all he had to do the thing he feared most--force himself to drop into the heaving, seething pool beneath him.

Ben released the red hot, sullen anger that boiled inside him. He felt it shoot through him, burning out the paralyzing fear that had locked up his body and mind.

Dick Sand. He focused his outrage.

Sand would not get away with this! Getting rid of Ben Singer would not be this easy. Ben sucked in a massive breath.

To have a chance he had to hit the center of the plunge pool below the falls, to absorb the shock of falling three stories without hitting the rocks at the side or on the bottom of the pool. If he traveled with the falling column of water it would carry him right down into the pool and slap him against the bottom.

Fatal.

He also had to cut through the powerful reverse currents that would suck him back into the falls where he would be recycled through the suckhole until there was nothing left of him. He had to avoid being pounded along the bottom by the tons of falling water, only to be bashed and battered against the rocks at the bottom of the pool as he was pushed outward toward the tree.

If he was sucked under and behind the falls it would likely be a death trap.

He could only try what the survival experts had said might be possible in a three dimensional eddy like this one. The idea was to dive deep, get down into the layer of water that was moving downstream near the bottom of the pool and get away from the powerful currents of the suckhole. Some water was flowing out of the pool. He had to find a way to go with it. But he was certain if flowed through the tree ..

A desperate chance. At best he could hope to make it to the outlet of the pool. But there the pinon tree waited like the final guardian between him and life.

If he became entangled in it's branches, if they even snagged his clothes, he would never get another breath of air. He would finally, in desperation, inhale, fill his burning lungs with water, and suffocate.

Ben flipped and hit the water feet first, expecting to break a leg hitting the water, or worse yet, to straddle a drifting log or the railroad tie he's used as a flotation device. He hit the water with a force that almost buckled his knees. He'd hoped to stay upright and penetrate the water like a spear, to use the momentum to go as deep as he could. But he felt the effect of the powerful surface current surging toward the falls the moment he hit. It was like jumping onto a moving escalator. Before the water swallowed him he felt himself being pulled at an angle, aimed toward the falls.

Then, like a mouse in a washing machine, he lost all sense of balance and direction. He felt himself being pulled and pushed from what seemed like all directions at once. He tried to keep his eyes open. He had to know which way was up. It looked like the lighter water was off to his right, then he realized that no matter what his sense of balance told him, he was on his back and looking up. Swirling debris, leaves, twigs, moss and more distracted him. But he felt something hard and sharp hit him in the back.

He turned over and grasped the rocks, felt the current, and for a moment feared that it was tugging him toward the falls. Then he saw a large brown trout holding in the current near him. With a flick of it's tail it disdainfully moved off, to get away from this strange intruder.

Ben hoped he was in the current that led away from the falls and he moved with the current as fast as he could pull himself along the rough bottom. Then he saw the dark mass of the rock that divided the falls on his left. He was headed in the right direction. He saw debris above him being sucked upward as the current reversed itself to go back to the falls. He felt a tugging suction trying to lift him from the bottom.

Certain death.

He fought with all his strength to stay against the bottom. To pull himself downstream.

He glimpsed the broad tail of the big trout as it disappeared into the murky water, moving to his right, to avoid the tortured currents in front of the rocks where the twin streams from both falls met and combined. The haystack and the spewing, arcing, frantic, fountaining of water. The hydraulic pressures would be tremendous, and the currents totally unpredictable. The wise old trout was survivor. He knew where the safe water lay. He was showing Ben the way.

His lungs were beginning to burn already. He didn't have the air to go around even once in the currents below the falls.

His time sense said he'd been under about five minutes. Part of his mind knew that was a lie. He couldn't hold his breath even half that long. He was fighting a spasmodic jerking of his chest as his body tried to inhale. He could hear a terrible, hollow ringing in his ears.

He knew that he had to find his way out of the pool quickly. About then the bottom angled up sharply and he hit his head on the hard wooden trunk of the tree that was wedged in the rocks at the outlet of the pool. Ben felt the current strength that was trying to suck him under or into the tree. There was no room to go under, no time to try to climb over. The disadvantage of the pinion was that there was no bare trunk he could slide up and over. The branches started at the base and went to the top. They were thick, green, limber and seemed determined to snag him. The current was pushing so hard at him that he feared being wrapped around the tree, to be held dangling and helpless until he died.

The spasmodic jerking of his chest was getting worse and a red border was framing everything in his eyesight.

Ben felt the current strength increase in pressure and velocity as his strength began to fail.

He wouldn't be able to overcome this final death trap. Ben was being pinned to the tree while the water tried to wrap him around it just like the current could wrap a rubber raft around a rock.

As his eyesight dimmed and his chest heaved almost uncontrollably, he began to think longingly about just letting go and sinking into the growing blackness around him.

Then he saw a lightening of the water to the left and to the right of him. Two men stood there, one on either side. They were not shadowy like REX. Ben recognized his father and the warrior from the hillside battle. They were looking at him expectantly.

What do you want? he thought. Have you come to take me with you?

Apparently not.

They both appeared to be lifting on the tree. Ben reached into himself. Found there a determination to prevail or die.

He saw Terry and Lester and TJ.

Dick Sand winning.

Ben felt a final surge of raw emotion, anger, frustration, hope, fear, one or all, but it exploded in him like a bomb. He twisted against the power of the water, planted his feet, put his back against and partly under the tree near the root section and then straightened his legs with all that was left in him, determined to burst his heart or to move that tree, or both.

The natural buoyancy of the tree helped him somewhat, at least at first, and he was able to overcome the power of the root that was pressing the tree against the outlet rocks. As he moved the root section upward the water pressure against the tree pushed it down stream. This broke the base loose from the rocks it was jammed into.

Ben heaved again till he felt his neck veins bulge with the effort. He fed into his muscles every desire he had to live, to do good, to fight for what was right. To endure. In the murky water it seemed that the men at his side lifted with him.

With a sudden sodden snapping sound a root broke. The tree shuddered in the current, rolled, and the base of the tree began moving downstream, pulling the rest of the tree along behind it. As the root section popped to the surface Ben went with it. His head broke out into the air and he sucked in a deep, sweet lungfull of air.

A breath of life.

But Ben still faced real danger. Below, the standing waves of the rapids boiled over and around the rocks in the stream bed and fifty yards below the stream made a sharp, nearly right angle turn. Ben knew from his reading that there would be a massive log jam there.

That if he stayed with the tree it would pin him under that pile of debris. But swimming to the bank could be hard, if not impossible, he knew, because of the helical circulation that tended to keep everything afloat in the center of the main current. That surface current would tend to pin him in the center of the river along with the tree until he got to the curve.

Ben rested through the first few waves, breathing deeply, staying on the side of the tree away from Sand's position. He was riding free, feet forward, with a bull-dogging grip on some of the roots. The waves were steep, but the water was deep and he rode the roller coaster thinking ahead.

Where were Sand's people right now?

       *   *   *

"I warned him to stay where he was" Sand said. "He was trying to escape. I could arrest you for trying to help him."

"You could have walked up the hill and stopped him!"

Terry felt the blood heating up her face and felt the nails of her balled up fists digging into her palms. She also felt the real agony that was still in her stomach where Sand had hit her.

"Then he would have jumped down the falls and escaped."

"Escaped through that?" She gestured at the boiling pool. "You've killed Lester too."

Her throat caught on the word because it meant Ben was dead. Drowned somewhere in the falls, drifting with the current, all the life gone from him. He didn't deserve that kind of death.

Sand smiled the infuriating way he had, slow, smug, so sure of himself. He was pointing up the hill. She turned to see Lester coming toward them, hunched over, the picture of pure physical and mental misery. But he was alive, looking over the edge of the falls, into the pool below.

Terry felt Sand come to attention beside her with a start. She turned and saw that the tree that had been trapped at the outlet of the pool had broken free and was moving ponderously through the standing waves below the falls.

Sand brought the rifle around and, jacking another round into the chamber, sighted through it at the tree. He took his time, seeming to examine every square inch of the tree. Lester shuffled the last few yards to join them. Sand ignored him.

To Terry he looked like a wet and woebegone kitten. His expression and his body posture never lost its sad, morose, defeated articulation. But the eye on the side away from Sand winked at her in a grotesque exaggerated, unmistakable way that said Ben was still alive.   The message staggered her. She hugged Lester to hide her surging emotions. Then fear hit her again. Was Ben near the tree? Would Sand see him? She turned on him and pushed him hard, even moving him a little, enough to spoil his view through the scope.   Then she stepped back, her sore stomach reminding her of Sand's strength and his cruelty.

"Get some help," she let herself scream. "Maybe he made it under the falls, like Lester. He could be trapped under there and it's getting dark. If you don't get on that radio right now I'll turn you in for dereliction of duty. You can see under the falls from up there."

She pointed to the spot where Ben had stood when he saw Lester. She didn't mention that you could also see under there from the place in the parking lot where she's first spotted him.

"I'll go and see if he's there".

There was no change in Lester to indicate this was a bad move. And she prayed that Lester hadn't seen Ben under the falls. If he was there Dick Sand could give the phrase "shooting fish in a barrel" a whole new meaning.

Sand had calculating look in his eyes. They narrowed to slits as he worked his way to some decision, as he turned to look up the hill. Looking past him down stream Terry saw Ben pull himself up the far bank and lay for a long few seconds half in and half out of the water. Plenty of time for Sand to spot him and draw a bead on him with his fancy rifle.

Terry lashed out with a foot and nearly broke her toes kicking Sand below the knee.

"Don't you dare go up there. Call for help. Get Search and Rescue started up here this minute. Dick ..Dick come back here!"

This was said to his back as he began moving up the hill. But she let him go and was careful to do nothing to cause him to turn around. And she wouldn't allow herself to turn and try to see Ben. She was afraid Sand would see it in her and guess the truth.

She let her heart sing instead.

Chapter 30
Sand Takes Control

Terry watched as Sand climbed the hill and peered under the falls. She noticed that he kept himself in sight, turning often to be sure Terry and Lester hadn't moved. She couldn't trust herself to look at the place where Ben climbed out of the river. But she could see it in her mind and her heart felt light and easy.

Until she saw Sand coming back down the hill, looking all over now. Pausing to gaze into the forest through the big rifle's scope. Uneasily, she watched him approach across the parking lot.

Terry saw a change in Dick Sand's eyes. He looked to Terry, to the Falls, at Lester, at the spot where Ben disappeared, back to Terry again. In the moments that took something seemed to switch off inside him. A stillness gathered around him.

Lester searched his face, seemed to read his future there, then dropped his chin to his chest. Shuffled his feet a little, and began rocking back and forth ever so slightly like a small, terrified child afraid to run, afraid to stay.

Sand was looking into the water again. Maybe thinking that since it solved his problem with Ben Singer so well that it could solve his problems with Terry and Lester. Sand looked down the canyon, checking to be sure they were alone.

When Terry saw his eyes again she saw why Lester was afraid. She felt a trickle of raw terror starting along her nerves. There was nothing there. It must be the way a swimmer saw the eyes of the shark that was about to sunder him. A cold, remorseless, irresistible, empty, inhuman machine.

Ben had been right. Terry could see that now.

Sand was a monster.

Ben had proved himself. Helping Lester the way he had. A floating sensation of profound relief warred with the worry in her mind. Her original feeling about Ben had not been wrong. He was, or at least, he had been, a moral man, good. Dedicated. But he was so different now. The anger she saw when he fought with Sand. Was he still the man she had loved? Dick Sand had done so much to him. How could he still be the same person inside?

Was he still so out of control that Axel would not be able to save him? Had anything actually been solved? Ben might be good, but he wasn☐t good enough. Not against a man like Dick Sand.

A thought froze her in place.

Sand thought Ben might be dead. That he probably was dead. Where did that leave her. And Lester . Expendable? Useless? A threat to Dick Sand?

She now knew Sand for what he was. And he knew she knew. The pretending was all over. Was there any reason why he should keep her and Lester alive? None that she could think of

She looked around, a breathless feeling making her pant a little. They were still all alone. He could easily kill them, dump them in the water, let the water cover his tracks. The perfect alibi. Assuming the bodies were ever found. Terry took a half step back.   Sand turned his dead eyes on her and froze her to the bone. She couldn't move. But she had to do something to help her and Lester to go on living just a little longer.

"He got away, you know," she said. Feeling her hands clench and unclench as she spoke. Choosing her words oh so carefully. She'd told Ben she would handle

Dick Sand. Could she?

"We both saw him come out of the water over there."

She pointed to the place where Ben had rested on the bank before disappearing into the brush.

Sand just looked at her, not at the place. But there was a light now in the back of his eyes. Calculating. Something had stirred down inside him somewhere, in that mind that was black as moonless midnight. He produced a small cylinder-shaped object and spoke into it.

"He may be on your side, headed your way. He just came out from under the falls. He can't be armed. We'll wait a minute. See what you can find."

He looked at Terry and then at Lester. His eyes said: Don't move.

Terry kept looking down the road. Hoping against hope someone would pull into the parking lot. Then the ripping sound of automatic rifle fire came from the woods above where Ben had disappeared into the brush. Sand's face widened into a grin. Lester began to rock back and forth again.

Sand spoke into the cylinder.

"You get him, Herschel? Is old Ben a gonner?"

Silence.

"Herschel. Herschel, you there? Answer me!"

Just then a man plunged out of the brush and fell on the bank, holding his knee in both hands. Behind him, in the declining light, Terry saw Ben appear, another man in front of him. The man's hands were tied out in front of him. A rope around his throat was clutched in Ben's hand. The man looked very worried. Ben spoke into the little black cylinder in his other hand.

"You can have this one." Ben's voice emerged from a small speaker/microphone clipped to Sand's shirt.

Ben motioned to the man on the ground.

"He can't run so he's no good to me. But this man, Herschel, he and I are going on an Apache picnic. He stops running or slows me down, I jerk the rope tight. The knot won't ever loosen up." He tugged the rope and Herschel reacted immediately, pulling his head up, stepping forward a little. "You'll find him tied to a tree somewhere. Most of him anyway. When I'm done. In the meantime I hold you responsible for their lives.

"We got TJ's photo album, Sand. You're all done. My grandfather sent copies to my cousin in the FBI in Phoenix and to a local TV station. My cousin Dexter works for the FBI down there. They're going after someone named Monterro. That was about a week ago."

Sand raised the rifle. His hands shook, hard. His face was alight with burning hate. Ben turned and was gone, running into the brush, Herschel struggling to keep up and not tighten the knot. Sand brought the rifle up and fired at random into the hillside.

The man holding his leg rolled out of sight. Then Terry heard a voice coming out of a little speaker on Sand's handset.

"Monterro has canceled your line of credit, Sand."

"What?!" Sand looked like he was going to bite the little machine in two. "How do you know? Who told you?"

Terry heard a raw anger and menace in his voice. He'd never spoken that way around her. She took another half-step back and suddenly found the black eye of the rifle staring straight into hers. Sand gave a little shake of his head. It was enough.

She stopped moving, stood very still, almost hypnotized by the snake-black eye of the big rifle. Her stomach cramped. She knew how Ben felt when Sand shot at him.

When she had shot him.

That thought caused her to flinch, to hug herself. What if she had killed Ben!

"The word came down on the net while you were target shooting at Singer. Somebody sent pictures to the Phoenix Sun Times and they called Mr. Monterro. To ask him for an interview."

"Oh, he's not a happy camper, Dicky. I guess you could say Singer saved your life. We were settin' up on you when he popped up behind us. Shot me in the knee with a steel ball from a wrist rocket and just took hold of Herschel and tied him up. Never saw any man handle old Herschel that way."

"Anyway, he smashed the guns. That gives you kind of a head start. But the word's out. Come daylight everybody'll be out to collect what's on your head. They even sprung old Orville out of Yuma to come help

"Too bad." The voice sounded easy-going, warmly conversational. "Thought you were a comer. You woulda been, too, Dicky. Except you took on the wrong man. Shoulda left Singer alone. Yessir, that's what did you in all right."

"Oh, and Dick? Now it's gettin' dark. You might like to know that Singer didn't run Herschel off at all. He's right here with me. Being guarded by a kill-trained Scotty dog.

"You hear that Sand? Singer said `this here dog is kill- trained. Don't move.' Herschel looks at this little dinky dog and then at Singer like he thinks it's a joke, you know?

"Singer just looked at him and tugged on that Injun knot, to get old Hersh's attention. Then he looked him real slow in the eye and said. `He barks, and I come back and kill you.' Just like that. Then he's gone. Off into the dark.

"You know, Dicky, I figure, he does you in, he won't want nothing for it. Thought if I gave him a little hand, sorta hold you in place, as it were, while he gets around behind you, I could claim that reward myself. Hope you enjoyed our little visit. Hasta lavista, componero."

The voice stopped. Dick Sand stared about him. trying to peel back the darkness that had descended on the canyon. The sound of the falls masked all the normal night noises. And Ben was out there somewhere.

Stalking Dick Sand.

Sand turned abruptly and motioned Lester and Terry to move together. He handcuffed them roughly. Pulling the bars down much too tight. Terry winced and felt her hand begin to go numb. He was careful to keep himself behind them as he moved them around the van and slid in first.

Roughly he pulled Lester and Terry in beside him and started the engine. Just then the rear window disintegrated in a shower of glass shards and they all jumped at the sharp slapping sound of the steel ball hitting the window. Sand whipped the wheel, did a fast turn, keeping Lester and Terry's side of the van toward the direction the projectile had come from. He drove out of the campground and up the canyon road that led to his place.

Terry massaged her hand, seeing the hate and rage in Sand's face, knowing it would be useless to ask for so little a human kindness as loosening a handcuff when she knew he was going to kill her. As soon as he was safe.

Just because she was Ben Singer's friend.

Because it would hurt him.

Ben ran for the bike. A coldness was filtering into his body. It was the coldness of the cave shelter. When Dick Sand was the only one left. When the darkness gathered and the Wolf rose to kill Ben Singer. When all Ben could do was watch.

Now the Wolf had Terry. If he lost sight of him Terry would die. Sand would hurt her first. Just to torture Ben. That's how Sand was. Now Sand had nothing left to lose. He would be sure and punish everyone he could.

Bud arrived in time to join Ben on the bike. Ben nestled him in snugly for the ride.

Ben started the bike and broke from the brush, down a steep embankment. Leaping the ditch next to the road, and gunning the bike up the road after the fading lights of Sand's van.

What would Sand do? Did he have an escape plan?

Without a doubt.

Dick Sand was a detail man. He would have everything in place. One slip and Ben would lose him. He would crawl into a hole somewhere and be gone. Terry and Lester would live only as long as he thought Ben was breathing down his neck. As long as he thought they could protect him from Ben.

Ben strained his eyes to see the road. He couldn't turn on his lights. He strained to see Sand's van, to be sure it went up over the top, to Sand's place and not up the Tibble Fork road, which also led over the top and down into the valley.

As soon as he saw Sand take the right hand fork, heading home, Ben gunned the bike and roared up the left hand toward Tibble Fork. At the reservoir he drove the bike hard down a fifty foot gravel embankment, crossed two branches of the river, bouncing and sliding on the gravel bottom, spraying water above his head in the channels, fighting the bike, risking everything to a fall. The bike slithered up the far bank into the trees and Ben started horsing it up a game trail that led from the water to the crest of the hill.

In the dark he risked spearing himself on dead tree branches, falling into arroyos. Breaking the bike on a rock. But he could use the lights. Sand couldn't see him from this side of the mountain and if he could reach to top he could meet Sand coming up the endless hairpin turns of the canyon road.

Ben topped out, cut left along a game trail that ran just inside the trees above the road. Down the canyon he could see headlights coming up around the last turn. Ben cut the lights and motor and leaped from the bike, pulling the wrist rocket from the back of his belt as he ran through the screening brush and slid to a stop, panting, as Sand came over the hill.

As the van passed he drew back his arm and shattered the side window next to Sand. He was rewarded with a violent, tire screaming swerve as Dick Sand fought to keep the vehicle on the road.

I'm still right here, Sand. Don't go down the hill thinking you've lost me. Don't do anything foolish, like hurt Terry or Lester. You need them. To protect you from me. Do you remember me, Sand? From that day at Derky's Lake?

Ben brought the bike out onto the road and stayed a hundred yards behind Sand as he went down the grade. He had to be sure Sand pulled in at his place. He could go on down the canyon and at the intersection go anywhere. Lose Ben completely. But if he did he'd be driving a Warren County Sheriff's patrol van that would stand out anywhere he went.

Sand would have planned better than that. He had another vehicle somewhere. Along with everything he needed to start over again. Or to hide out in comfort for a long, long time.

The coldness wouldn't leave Ben. It seemed to grow stronger as he followed along in the quiet night. He couldn't let Sand win. But he had little to stop him with and Sand had Lester and Terry. Their lives were in Ben's hands.

On impulse he cut up into the trees when he came near his campsite and paused less than a minute to recover the ancient sword and slip the scabbard into its place, hilt within easy reach, like old time cowboys used to carry their rifle. He settled his bow into its clamps on the back of the bike, checking the quiver to be sure it was full of arrows.

Ben regretted not having a gun. He had no idea how to get Terry away from Sand, short of killing him. If he saw the end coming Sand would kill them both anyway. Just out of pure meanness, knowing even as he was dying that he was killing Ben too by taking away everything he loved. Winning even in dying. Sand would do it. There was no question of that.

Ben racked his brain, trying to force a plan to form. But nothing emerged. He was tired. His emotions in shreds. His inner voice screaming at him that he had to save Terry from Sand.

He pulled up closer to Sand's vehicle when they got within a quarter mile of the turn off to his alpine cabin. He saw the gate open automatically as he approached. At he last moment Ben decided not to follow Sand through the gate. He slid the bike into the brush along the road, grabbed up some branches, and jammed the latch so the gate could not lock. As he did he could hear the thrum of high voltage electricity singing its deadly song in the fence.

He had to assume that Sand could not stay in one place. Not a place as obvious as his own home. Not with his own people hunting him.

As long as Ben was free, alive, out there in the dark somewhere close, Sand would have to leave Terry and Lester alive. To use them as hostages. As a shield to protect him from Ben. There would be no doubt in Sand's mind about what Ben would do to him if he harmed them and then tried to leave alone.

That was the only weapon Ben had at the moment. He doubted Sand would give him time to develop anything else.

No, Sand would be back out and he would not hurt Terry yet. Ben pulled out the night vision glasses he had taken from Herschel. He could see through the trees, down into the opening at the front of Sand's cabin. He saw the garage door go up and the inside light go on. He could see an older model Ford pickup truck with a camper shell sitting in the garage. Facing out, ready to go.

Terry and Lester came out of the van with Sand crouching behind them, the rifle in his hands. He jerked them roughly backward until he could step out of sight, into the garage. Apparently on command, Terry and Lester took two steps back out into the open. Easy targets from the garage, which was suddenly plunged into darkness as the lights went out. At the same time floodlights set around the grounds lit up, bathing the surrounding area in overlapping circles of eye burning white light. Ben jerked off the night goggles before his eyes were hurt or the lenses blanked out, leaving him blind.

Sand's message was plain. Any threat from Ben and Sand's rifle would light up the dark garage and blast Lester or Terry. Sand only needed Terry to keep Ben at bay. Lester was excess baggage. Ben hoped Sand wasn't thinking that too.

In the meantime Sand could move anywhere in the darkened house. Ben was glad he hadn't trapped himself in the compound. He moved back a little into the brush in case Sand was using night goggles to search for him. He kept his eyes roving through the darkness in case Sand tried to slip up on him. In case Hershcel found out how to untie the knot on his throat. Because he and his partner would be as eager to kill Ben as they were to get Sand. Clean up all the loose ends at once. Ben motioned to Bud to keep an eye out up the road, just in case.

*   *   *

Dick Sand moved smoothly through the dark cabin. He knew exactly what he wanted to take and he knew where each item was. Paperwork, names, phone numbers, computer files. Monterro wasn't the only `importer' in the business. He'd planned to leave him and set up on his own anyway. It would just happen sooner, that was all. He had enough dirt on Monterro to make him mind his own business. Sand felt his grin stretching his face as he hurried through the living room.

"You got all the cards, Dick ole boy," he heard his voice echo softly in the dark, caught the note of merriment in his voice. Planning will do it every time.

He picked up a set of phone numbers as he passed his desk. Mercenaries who would do anything if the price was right. Men who wanted in to his organization. Ready at a moment's notice. An instant army if he needed one.

"Just reach out and touch someone," he couldn't say it without laughing out loud. Money was power. You could buy anything in the world if you had enough money. "And I got plenty. Before I go I'll have five times as much more. Singer will be dead. All the loose ends tied up. A phone call will get Monterro straight. Yeah. The good times just never stop."

He'd just swing past Monterro's "warehouse" on his way out and take a pick-up load of his best stuff. The street value of a pickup load was .. Sand felt himself grin again. A lot. That all. A lot. Translated into power it made Sand invincible. Absolutely unstoppable. Guaranteed. Singer had dug himself a hole that his character wouldn't let him climb out of. He was dead and didn't know it.

Everybody was one step behind him, and one step was all Dick Sand ever needed. Except for Ben Singer. The dummy. He wasn't even in the game. He laughed a little at the idea of Ben Singer out there in the dark somewhere armed with a wrist rocket. He was just thrashing around. Bumbling like always. Desperate to save his girl. Tied to her hand and foot by his feelings for her. Feelings were a weakness Sand never indulged in with good reason.

Sand felt his lip curl in contempt. That was Singer's basic weakness. The big flaw in his character. He cared. It would kill him in the end.

"The end is near," Sand sang tunelessly. "It's almost here."

A flash of burning hatred escaped into his mind from where he kept his emotions, bottled, controlled, mostly unused. He'd reward Ben Singer for his interference. Leave him dead. Or wishing he was dead. Blast everything he cared about. Splatter that little farm girl all over the mountainside. Let him die trying to save her. Or stand there and suffer and shake while she died. Either way, Ben would learn again who was the Man.

"Either way, Singer," he said softly, in the dark. "It don't matter to me. But it's going to happen. Count on it."

He punched in a number on his phone. In just moments it was picked up. He heard a deep male voice on the other end.

"I'll be in Rock Springs before daylight, Mel," he said. "I'll need maximum security for at least two days.

"You used to being rich? Can you handle large amounts of money? Oh, and I'll need to meet with some people right away to set up a security net." Sand listened.

"No, I'll take care of that in a day or so. We don't need a permanent place yet. A few phone calls and everything will be peaceful. Then we can make our plans and find us a real good place.

"Good security for 72 hours is all I need ..

"No, no need for you to know what I'm driving. I'll call when I get there. If I like what I see you'll have a permanent position in my company. It goes with your own money tree."

If I don't you'll be dead.

"Yeah, well, gotta go. Got to tie up a couple of loose ends." Sand laughed. Three loose ends.

He hurried through the house now, picking up boxes of computer disks, gym bags and duffel bags filled with gear. He punched in a special code that wiped his computer hard disk clean, then activated a mechanical device to douse the entire disk with acid. No one would extract data from that mess. Especially not after the fire. He set a special timer, gave himself twenty minutes, and went back out to the garage.

Dynamite and gasoline would burn the cabin to the ground. If some of Monterro's monkeys were around by then, well that would be okay too. Remind them that Dick Sand was not a man to mess with. No sir. Not a man to mess with.

He opened a locker and pulled out what looked like two fly fishing vests. He checked battery levels on each transmitter/receiver in each vest. Then he loaded the truck with his gear.

He called Terry and Lester into the garage, put a vest awkwardly on each one and tied them snugly with cotton cord. He didn't undo the handcuffs so the jackets hung badly them.

But with a pound of plastique explosive in each one, they didn't have to fit well to do the job.

He forced them roughly back out into the circle of light, then flipped a switch and spoke into a microphone that he took down from a wall bracket by the door. He used his softest, most friendly voice. The one he'd used on Ben the night he drove him out of Warren Valley.

"Listen good, Ben. I won't say it twice. The vests have enough explosive to level this house." He stepped out into the light, carrying his rifle. He help up what looked like a garage door opener.

"You see this, Singer? A deadman switch. If I let go, for any reason, the bombs go off.. Just that simple. I lose, you lose, big. So back off, Singer. When I get what I want I'll leave these two along the road somewhere. If you come after me, I'll kill them sure."

"Give up, Sand." The voice came out of the dark, from everywhere. From nowhere. "Now, while you still can."

"Get in the truck" Sand snarled. "Now. Or I leave you and trigger this from up the road. Move!"

Terry and Lester made an ungainly bundle as they struggled to get into the truck. Sand forgot them and went to the other door, got in, and started the engine. They made it in as he clashed the gears and the truck spurted out of the garage. Sand had to slow down to allow the gates to open, then the truck roared out of the gate, spun gravel digging its way up onto the pavement, and went back up over the hill. Back to the junction with Tibble Fork.

****

Desperation driving him, fatigue slowing him, Ben ran for the bike. Wondering why Sand hadn't made a run for the Sundance junction, down the hill the other way. In a few short miles he could have turned left up Deer Creek to Heber, Park City, the freeway to anywhere. Right would take him down to Warren Valley and to the freeway there.

Ben loaded Bud onto the bike and then struggled to get it up on the road, headed back over the mountain. Puzzling. Why was Sand headed back into the mountains? Why wasn't he running like a scared rabbit?

When had Sand ever done that? Ben thought. When was the last time he ever ran from anything? Ben had to give him that. He always met you head on. Kept coming. Always had an ace-in-the-hole.

Determined that if he lost, you would lose too.

The cold fear in Ben grew as he wearily struggled to get the bike up to speed and headed back over the pass. The night was soft and warm, the air full of the summer smells of the mountains. Bugs clacked against the small windshield and made him duck his head. Thinking of Sand's big rifle. Feeling himself reaching for the rope.

Falling.

He shut off the images and tried to override the surging tide of emotion. Fight down the sense of impending loss. To put out of his mind the image of Terry with a bomb tied to her riding through the night with Dick Sand.

He didn't have to take the trail this time. Sand would know he was there, behind him in the dark.

What scared Ben was that Dick Sand didn't care anymore.

Chapter 31
The Old Lobo Runs For The Hills

Down to the junction, back up Tibble Fork road. Ben had been there once already tonight. He ran the area through his mental map. Why would Sand head this way? The road turned to gravel just beyond the reservoir, then ambled up the mountain to old lumber mill sites, ghost towns back in the trees. Some old mining camps. Then the road crossed the flank of the mountain, became a set of dirt track trails that worked back down the mountain. One into Warren Valley, the other down into Salt Lake Valley. Either would lead eventually to the freeway. But why go the long way around?

To avoid pursuit? It didn't make sense. Ben was sure the truck wasn't known to anyone Sand wanted to avoid. He'd had the jump on everyone when he left Derkey's Lake. Why was he messing around on the backside of a mountain the middle of the night?

He was after something. That had to be it. Something too important to leave behind.

Drugs

Hidden somewhere on this mountain.

Smooth, Ben thought. So smooth. Old mines lay scattered all along the flank of the mountain. An old mine could be cool, dark, even-temperatured, dry. A place known only to Sand where the mule loads of drugs where stored, waiting for transshipment across the country. Far below, in the valley, was Salt Lake City. The "crossroads of the West." Roads, highways, and interstates led in all direction from there.

Sand's plans became clearer in Ben's mind. He had a storage warehouse here somewhere. Filled with drugs. He was going to fill his pickup with them before he left the state.

Ben's tired mind churned over. Where was the mine. Could he get there first? What would Sand do to Terry and Lester? He wouldn't take them any further than the mine. Ben was sure of that. He'd read enough survival literature to have some idea of how many ways a bomb could be detonated. Sand, with time and unlimited money at his disposal, must know everything Ben knew and more.

He knew something Ben didn't. Something that made him not care one way or another if Ben followed him. It meant he believed he could kill Terry and Lester, maybe Ben too, and get away clean. He was going about his business. Carrying out his plans as though Ben didn't exist. Ben felt his courage slipping. Sand didn't consider him a threat at all. As far as Sand was concerned Ben was already dead.

The coldness in Ben began to make him shiver. A steady shaking, a cold sweat trickled down his back despite the warmth of the summer night.

No plan.

No solution.

Time was running out.

Ben's mind was a blank.

Maybe all he could do was die with Terry. While Sand stole quietly away to take up his evil work some place else. Ruined other lives.

Ben shook harder as he saw himself pulling his bow to full draw, sending a razor head ripping through Sand's body. Watching him fall. Seeing the explosives go off, ending all their lives. Three good lives for one bad one. But at least Sand would be stopped.

Unless he was wearing body armor.

I wouldn't put it past him.

Doubt took a deeper hold on him as he wearily fought the bike over a very rough mountain track that seemed to be angling back up into the woods.

Or Ben could hang back, stay alive. Watch Terry and Lester die. Then take up Sand's trail. Spend a lifetime if necessary on a trail of vengeance. To bring Sand to justice. An empty lifetime. Lonely. Guilt-ridden. Twisted and deformed. A creation of Dick Sand.

Better to die now than live that life.

Ben saw himself again, a nightmare memory, floating ahead of him through the dark woods.

Shouting!

"You can't do that, Sand! Stop it!"

Leaping across the fire.

Smashing into a rock solid Dick Sand. Hearing him laugh at Ben's puny efforts.

The beating, the humiliation, the pleasure in Sand's face when he was hurting them.

Only this was now. Ben was strong. But Sand was still too much for him. Beyond his strength, his cunning, his scheming plans. Laughing, his face fading away into the darkness. Leaving Ben with terrible pain. With the loss of everything he loved. Leaving him an empty life where every desire was burned to ashes by the shame, the frustration.

The unmanliness.

Sand was the better man.

Sand was the only man.

Sand was The Man

Ben was only a moldering bundle of failures, frustration, rage, remorse, loneliness and a soul-deep thirst for vengeance.

"Dick Sand owns you." Grandpa's voice. Speaking in his mind. "He's your evil twin and he's making you just like him."

Ben saw himself punching empty air as Sand's visage melted into the night. Ben felt the white-hot rage that seemed always to be banked, smoldering, deep inside him break out. Begin to burn through his veins. He felt again as he felt when he had fought Sand on the beach at Derkey's Lake. Almost berserk. Ready to howl and bite the trees.

His muscles knotted, his systems set in so hard it cramped his breathing, made his whole body shake.

He had to do something. Standing by and letting Sand win was not an option.

Bud whined and looked back anxiously at him. Bud was never comfortable around him when he gave way to rage.

Ben saw again the huge warriors on the ancient hillside. Saw the women and children armed for battle. All of them destined to follow their unbridled rage and thirst for vengeance into a battle they could not win. Follow to certain destruction.

Ben knew this. Was sure he was on the same road. But he could find no other solution for himself except to follow after them.

Ben jerked his mind back. Cold adrenaline pumped ice water through his veins. Sand had left the dirt track road. He almost seemed to be traveling over open ground, weaving through the trees. But when he got to the place where he'd turned Ben could see a very faint two track trail heading off at an angle along the shoulder of the mountain. Angling upward into the towering stand of old growth Douglas Fir and new growth lodge pole pine.

Headed for some obscure mining camp or ghost town, Ben was sure. Forgotten. Unvisited. Except by Dick Sand. And maybe the ghost of Indians the Spanish had worked to death as slaves in the mine.

Ben felt the hair crawl up on the back of his neck.

He forced himself to concentrate carefully on the sounds of Sand's truck and on the course of the flickering lights moving through the trees. Sand would be stopping soon. Ben couldn't afford to over run him.

Just then Bud leaped from the bike and then paused a moment until Ben stopped. He trotted out of sight, into the dark spaces between the trees.

Scouting?

Running away? Leaving Ben to his fate?

Ben heard Sand's engine shut down. The silence of the mountain closed around Ben like a smothering black velvet blanket. Quickly he killed the bike engine so Sand couldn't locate his position.

He felt like he wanted to throw up, to try and release some of the tension that screamed up and down his nerves. It was only a matter of minutes now before Sand would load his truck and leave. Precious moments that meant life or death for Terry and Lester.

And for Ben Singer.

No plan.

No solutions.

Ben pulled the bike back into the shadows, where Sand wouldn't see it if he went back out the way he'd come in. Ben wondered, as he crept away from it if he'd ever see it again. Ever ride again. See another sunrise.

No plan.

No solutions.

Sand was winning.

That meant Terry was only moments away from dying.

Ben took his bow, slung the sword over his back, tied the tip of the scabbard tightly to his belt so he could draw the sword smoothly and quickly. So it wouldn't rattle as he moved through the brush.

Ben selected an arrow. He couldn't bring himself to choose a razor tipped broadhead. The more he thought about it the more he knew that Sand was wearing light body armor.

Sand was Sand.

He wouldn't leave out such a critical detail. Ben could see Sand laughing as the arrow bounced harmlessly off his chest. As he pushed the button that would end two precious lives.

Hands shaking, he selected a blunt-headed shock arrow. Sand's head was a small target. But the arrow would put him down if Ben got a clear shot. That's all he could hope for. That was all Sand had to defend himself against. If he held the deadman switch in his hand he didn't even have to worry about that.

So much for the great Benjamin Franklin Singer.

Superchief.

Superchump.

It would have been easier, far easier, to have simply died in the cave in Whitehouse Canyon. Maybe Terry and Lester could have lived then. Maybe someone else would have stopped Sand.

Maybe.

Ben felt what little strength and confidence and anger he had salvaged slipping away. Like water draining from a bucket full of holes.

"You're not alone, Ben." Axel's voice. In his mind? In his memory?

"Don't be Sand's twin, Ben. Triumph because it's your duty to struggle against evil. Not because you personally hate Dick Sand. Remember what your Grandfather told you."

Light and Truth

Not pride and vengeance and blood.

Ben shook free of all feeling. It was time to do something. This was life and death, not a debating society. He felt the body zones re-energizing strongly. Drawing power in the face of death from reserves Ben didn't know the human body possessed. The strength of desperation. No reason for holding back anything in reserve. Leave it all on the field of battle tonight.

It was prevail or die.

No middle ground.

Ben fought down the senseless rage that was bubbling inside him, banked it, forced it out of his mind with an effort of will. He tried to fill the emptiness it left in him with light and truth. To live the last moments of his life by values and principles. Not by pride and rage and thirst for vengeance.

Sand needed to be stopped. It was Ben's duty to try. To do all he could to resist the evil Sand represented. Even if he died in the attempt, Ben needed to keep Sand from getting away.

His mind settled into an emotionless, icy clarity.

Stop thinking of death.

Time to think of what he could do with the remaining life he had.

Ben scurried through the trees. Soon he saw Sand's truck, out in the open, in a clearing against the mountainside. He was backed up to a dark opening in the cliff face.

Sand's gold mine.

Where he kept the wealth his slaves earned for him. While he scorned them in life and paid them with death.

He couldn't see anyone. Lester and Terry must be with Sand, inside the mine.

Ben jumped when he heard a heavy weight hit the back of the truck and slide forward. Hitting the forward wall of the truck bed with a soft THUNK!

In a moment the sound was repeated. Sand was loading the truck.

Silence.

He'd gone back for another load.

"Give him something to think about," Ben heard Grandfather's voice. The old Apache trick. Give your pursuers something to think about. Show your fangs. Ride over the first hill, dismount and shoot the first rider that shows up. Make everyone else very cautious.

Ben took out his hunting knife and, using rocks as supports, propped the blade against the front tire. He moved carefully back into the trees, listening, trying to see into the dark maw of the mine. He could see the metal gate that normally covered the mine opening. It was swung back out of the way. It was made of metal straps welded or bolted to form an iron grid with spaces too small for a person to crawl through. But large enough to let the resident bats in and out. An ecologically designed solution designed to save lives.

The gate was designed to keep people from getting lost in the mine. Most of the old mines had been covered this way. A perfect cover for Dick Sand. He'd done his homework well. No one could get into the mine. Few would even know it existed.

THUNK! THUNK!

Sand was back. Ben couldn't see him. He was humming a little to himself as he worked. Ben crept back into the dark and circled to the left to bring himself into a better shooting position. Moving ever so slowly he stood up, using a tree for cover.

THUNK! THUNK!

The truck springs creaked a little as the truck settled under its load. Sand must be nearly done.

No plan.

No solution.

Time running out.

Ben's heart began pounding in his chest. His breathing got hard, raspy sounding in his ears. Panic started creeping into the cold, settled center of his mind.

Nibbling away.

Sweat started trickling down his back and sides, tickling him.

Distracting him.

Ben heard the gate hinges squeak.

Startled, he moved a little. A dry branch popped under his foot.

He heard Sand's voice, full of good humor. Almost gleeful.

"You got to choose now, Ben." The voice was gentle, conversational, relaxed. Like it was when he was beating Ben and kicking Lester.

"Run and live. Stay with them and die.

"We both know what you're going to do. You're weak, Singer. Like I showed you all along. Do gooders always get mixed up. Too emotional. All tangled up in other people's lives.

"That's you, Singer. That's why you lost."

Ben heard the gate close with a rusty CLICK!

He saw a red light blinking steadily back inside the mine, somewhere close to the entrance. The blood red light showed him the outline of Terry and Lester. They were inside the gate, fastened to it somehow. The vests were gone.

Then it hit Ben. Like a sledgehammer. Timer on the vests. Blinking in the darkness. Counting the last moments of their lives.

Sand came around the truck, the control dangling from his hand. His thumb still tightly pressed down on it.

Now was the time to kill them all. To take Sand along. Ben started to draw. He hurt so bad it was like a physical pain.

Sand moved to the door of the truck and opened it. Ben came to full draw. Caught Sand's head in his bowsight. He couldn't miss.

Should he fire?

Sand looked into the darkness.

"Don't worry, Singer. Two minutes and it will all be over. It was fun, Singer. Watching you bumble around.

"Now you get what anybody gets who's in my way A whole world of hurt.

261

Enjoy."

A small grey shape hurtled out of the darkness, growling fiercely. Bud leaped and nipped Sand's hand, startling him. Making him drop the control.

Ben flinched, lost his draw, felt his nerves burn red hot.

No explosion.

Bluffing?

Afraid Ben might kill them all?

Or so confident that Ben was a bumbler that he was beneath Sand's contempt?

Ben came to full draw and released as Sand dove into the truck and slammed the door. Bud grabbed the control and ran into the dark.

The blunt arrow slammed into the side of the truck, inches from the door.

Sand starts the truck as Ben grabs another arrow and watches in dismay as it bounces harmlessly off the bullet proof glass in Sand's side window.

In moments the truck is gone. Sand is gone.

Only Ben and Terry and Lester are left.

The lights blink, twinkle in the dark cave like the eyes of a dragon getting ready to erupt an awesome fireball of unquenchable flame.

Out of the cave.

Engulfing Lester and Terry. Blasting into atoms everything Ben cared about.

The thought slams into him. There is still time to run for the safety of the rocks.

To survive.

Like he almost left Lester at the falls.

Then he feels warmth against his back.

LIGHT AND TRUTH

Without thought, Ben whips the blade from its scabbard even as he leaps toward the gate.

Toward the dragon waiting to consume him.

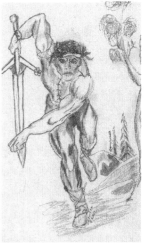

He raises the sword high above his head as he nears the gate. He sees Terry and Lester try to pull away. There is a chain linking them to the gate.

Skidding to a stop in front of them Ben brings the heavy bladed sword swinging down with every ounce of desperate strength behind it.

No holding back.

No time for a second try.

The blade, forged of folded, hammered steel that sold in its day for the same price as gold whistles through the air, sunders a line of strap iron a foot above to a foot below, and right alongside the chain. Easier and faster that hacking at the hardened steel in the chain and lock. Pivoting, whirling the blade in a glittering arc,, Ben brings the sword horizontally, swinging it like a big league batter aiming for the home run bleachers.

Ben grabs one side of the opening and with a wrenching jerk he opens it wide, bending the iron straps back and to the side.

Terry squirted from the hole and would have run straight away. Ben caught her arm and swung her feet off the ground, propelling her along the rock face. Lester followed.

The red eyes stopped blinking.

Ben ran.

The cave erupted with a roar, the gate was flung across the clearing, shattering a tree and wiping out huge chunks of brush.

But the hard walls of the mine contained the blast, channeled it straight head. Like a gigantic cannon. The force of the blast missed them as they sprinted behind the nearest boulders.

Ben immediately looked up to see if rocks had been shaken loose above them.

Shaken, Terry clings to him weeping, Lester gazes in awe at the destruction wreaked by the blast. They moved out into the trees. Away from any possible rock fall.

Into the dark in case Dick Sand came back.

Ben quickly unloaded the bike, leaving Terry his emergency camp gear and food and a woolen army blanket to fight off the cool night air. Told them to wait in the woods till daylight if he didn't come back. Then to work their way back down to Tibble Fork. There were always people there. But watch out for Herschel and the others.

He checked and found the broken haft of his hunting knife glinting in Sand☐s tire tracks. The blade was gone.

Good.

He hugged Terry, holding her tenderly so as not to hurt her. Leaving most of his heart with her as he pulled away and jerked the bike around to go after Dick Sand. Ignoring Terry's plea to let the law handle it.

No time for that if Ben could stop him now. Lives to be saved. Suffering to be stopped. Ben's mind was full of the TJ's who had slaved to make Sand rich. Who had given their lives to feed his ego.

The monster needed to be stopped. At any cost, now that Terry was safe.

Ben brought the motor to life and rode off, pausing just long enough to allow Bud to leap into his lap. He couldn't resist hugging the little dog close against his belly for a moment. Prince he wasn't. He was better. His heart bigger. His courage greater. Ben owed him more than he could ever pay.

Then he focused on sending the bike hurtling through the dark along the trail Dick Sand had taken. Sand was taking a back way down off the mountain, headed for either Warren Valley or Salt Lake Valley. Either way, to disappear back into the human jungle of the drug world.

Ben wanted to be sure and say goodbye.

Chapter Thirty-Two
Ben Singer Says Goodbye

Driving around the shoulder of the mountain, Sand heard the rumble of the explosion, saw the landscape behind him outlined briefly in blazing white light, felt the ground vibration up through the truck. Sand felt his grin stretch his face. Wider than it had for a while. It was always fun to win, especially the close ones. He had to admit, that this had been closer than anything he'd ever had to survive.

Sand shook his head, the grin still in place, the old merriment flooding through him.

Ole Benny. That boy was just like cow manure. Every time you turned around you were steppin' in it and the smell followed you everywhere.

A feeling of relaxation was filtering through him. He would go on. Life would proceed according to plan. Dick Sand would stay at least one jump ahead of every coyote that came after him. And if he couldn't, it wouldn't take them long to realize that they weren't chasing a prairie dog. They were dealing with The Man ..

His mind refocused sharply as he rounded a bend to see the road narrowing and angling across the lower part of a steep shale rock slide that disappeared above him in the dark, extending halfway up the mountain. The road seemed to cling to the loose rock like snow to a steep slope, ready to slide away into the dark abyss below at the slightest sound or vibration. He wondered if the blast had shaken anything lose up above.

He geared down to approach cautiously. As he did he suddenly realized that one side of the truck sloped too much. The truck was bumping and jerking so badly along the track that he hadn't noticed it earlier. A heated flash of anger incinerated the good humor he'd felt. He got out to check the tire.

He cursed when he saw that it not only was flat, but that there was a broken knife blade imbedded in the rubber. Then he just had to laugh, a big booming laugh that echoed away into the dark. A final act of frustration. Ben was dead, lying around the woods in many small pieces. But old Benny just had to keep trying. Sand chuckled softly, shaking his head in wonder. What a wimp he was after all.

He moved to the back of the truck. No problem. He could change the tire and still be in Rock Springs before sunup. He set about getting the jack from behind the front seat, lowering the spare from underneath the truck bed. Whistling quietly to himself. Trying not to think of Ben, not dead, so committed to vengeance that he'd let Lester and Terry die alone so he could come after Sand. Nope. Singer just wasn't made that way. He would have died trying to save them. Still, the silence of the night was deep and spooky and he felt the hair rise a little on the back of his neck.

Best get this done and move on.

*   *   *

Ben glided through the trees, his body heavy with fatigue. He had recovered only a little from his exertions at the falls. He felt a great weariness tugging at his courage. Then he recognized it for what it was ..fear. A great reluctance to pursue Sand. The shame and fear he'd felt when Sand had beaten him started to seep back into him, to make his hands sweat and shake a little, to gnaw away at his confidence. Sand loomed larger and larger out there in the dark. Big and dangerous, vicious and deadly. Ben had done nothing to him since beating him at the picnic. Sand was absolutely untouched by anything Ben had done. While Ben had been scrabbling around, getting by on luck and little else.

He felt the old Ben Singer re-emerging. Trying to take charge. To tell him all he really had to do was step back into the dark forest ..let Sand go. Let the law take its course.

Let Sand get away.

Terry and Lester were safe now. There was nothing to be lost if he let Sand go.

He saw TJ's face, floating in the dark sky, out over the lights of the beautiful Salt Lake Valley.

Except his self-respect. Except the lives of the people like TJ that Sand would destroy before he was stopped. He thought of Sand disappearing into the valley below .like a wolf among sheep. Maybe changing trucks again, getting away completely, to go on killing innocent people until someone finally ran him to earth.

Ben felt a massive sigh shudder through him. If he could he had to finish it now. Stop Sand even if Sand also stopped him. Hoka Hey, as the Sioux would say, it's a good day to die. Ben's Navajo mind rejected that idea. But not the thought that Sand's evil must be removed from the land. That was a thing worth doing, no matter what the cost.

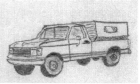

Ben took a game trail that topped out on the shoulder of the mountain about 300 yards above the road. He stopped well below the top so the sound of the bike motor wouldn☐t carry through the night air. He could see the winding track where it crossed a large rockslide and he could see two miles of road beyond where it angled steeply down into the valley. There were no headlights showing anywhere. He opened his mouth slightly so he could hear better in case Sand was driving without lights.

Then he heard the sound of metal on metal and his eyes were drawn back to the rockslide. A flash of coldness made him shiver when he saw the truck, and then the figure of Dick Sand working to remove the spare tire.

Ben pulled his bow and quiver off the bike, checked them quickly, wished again he had a gun, and then moved quietly down through the brush toward the road and Dick Sand. Not like hunting a deer. This animal was more dangerous bare handed than any wild beast. And he was armed to boot. For a moment Ben was grateful that Prince was gone. This would be difficult and very very dangerous at best. With Prince in the game it would have been impossible. Ben saw Bud off in the brush, keeping pace, looking at Ben and grinning.

Sure, Ben thought, keep my spirits up. Maybe in ten minutes I'll be like you, off in some other world, getting acquainted with Axel's other friends.

But I won't mind too much as long as I'm sure that Dick Sand is in Hell, where he belongs.

A twig popped under his foot. Cold fear flushed through his mind. He wasn't concentrating. Another false step and Sand would

Warrior's Way

bring out the big rifle and brush Ben off the mountainside and into eternity before he could ever get close enough to use the bow. He moved on, not thinking anymore, just using his Indian mind to become one with his surroundings, to judge what he should do.

Would he just shoot Sand in the back from ambush? Would he step out and challenge him to a fight? Let him go for his gun and try to beat him with an arrow? Ben was weary enough to doubt if he could beat Sand again in a fight. How was he going to stand up to Sand with arrows when Sand had bullets. And the will to use them. Sand had killed many times. Human life meant nothing to him.

But could Ben take a life, execute even a vicious, evil man such as Sand? Or would he freeze in the final milliseconds of the confrontation and allow Sand to go free, and to have the satisfaction of killing Ben in the bargain. The books said most people die trying to solve the moral riddle and come to the conclusion that if I don't kill him he will kill me. Survivors mostly killed first and debated second. Ben wasn't certain which kind he was, but a sinking feeling in his gut was telling him that he was about to find out once and for all.

There was no more time for thought. Sand was at the front of the truck, preparing to lift the spare into place. Ben had to either act now or to fade back into the dark and just let Sand go.

Gazing at Sand's broad back Ben was tempted simply to loose an arrow at him. From fifteen yards he would not miss. It would slice through Sand's armpit, bypassing his armor. He pulled up the bow, brought it to full draw, fixed Sand's upper back, his heart and lungs, squarely in the bow sight. Then angled slightly for the area of his arm.

He felt the raging lava begin to seethe and roil in him. The whole world narrowed down in his vision till only his target was left. For TJ, for Terry, for Lester, for the numberless host of those Dick Sand had ruined, Ben felt his hand begin the automatic movement that would loose the bowstring and send the razor sharp broadhead cutting clear through Sand's body. To cut the evil out of him once and for all.

Then Ben was amazed to see himself shifting his aim! Unwilled, his bow arm lowered, the sight shifted. The hand on the bowstring released its grip and the arrow sang, straight and true, squarely between Dick Sand's legs, burying itself in the spare tire.

Almost in slow motion Ben saw Sand jerk, start to jump up, fall backward as his boots slipped in the loose gravel on the road, even as he heard the explosive pop of the tire and saw Sand's lower body disappear behind a cloud of dust and as he heard Sand's shout of surprise, exasperation ..and fear.

"Lose the gun, Sand," Ben said. He heard the murderous throb of his voice. Part of him was very sorry Sand was not skewered on one of his arrows, coughing out his life in the dirt. That part of him wanted badly for Sand to do something, anything, that would justify killing him.

Ben had automatically notched another arrow. Sand lay on his back, looking upside down at Ben, his mouth open, slack with surprise. But his eyes already were focused clearly, watchful, intense, calculating. Watching for his chance. He never quit. Never stopped looking for an opening. Ben recognized once again that he was facing one of the most dangerous creatures on earth. He felt the hair rise on his neck and goose pimples ran down his back and arms as the vision of the wolf man in the rock shelter came back to fill his mind.

Ben took a step back and stumbled a little in the dark. He saw Sand gather himself to draw and fire. At fifteen yards he wouldn't miss any more than Ben would. Ben stiffened and aimed squarely at Sand's face. He felt as much as saw a stillness move through Sand. A caution, perhaps a trickle of fear, after all, Ben had beaten him once. Few men could say that, all of them far back in Sand's past. Maybe that doubt was enough.

"I like you just where you are, Sand. Now lose the gun. Easy, with your left hand, you know how I like it done. Do it."

Sand reached over carefully, removed the big magnum from its holster and tossed it gently up alongside the truck. Not out of reach far enough to satisfy Ben. But there was little he could do about it. He realized that at best, if he wasn't willing to execute Sand outright, that he was in a stand off.

Sand seemed to know it too. He suddenly grinned, sat up, and leaned against the flattened truck tire that sat against the truck. He rubbed his hands on his pant legs like he was dusting them off, not like they were sweaty with fear. Ben couldn't read his face in the dark. Couldn't tell how much of what he said was bluff.

Sand chuckled softly, almost to himself, shook his head, an spoke in the friendly tone that Ben hated so much.

"You're still a wimp ain't you Benny? You have to be mad the kill someone. You can't do it cold. So you're hoping I'll just give up and peacefully go to jail. Kind of make you a hero.

"Won't work, Ben. You and I both know you won't shoot me with that thing. You'll just have to come down here and put the cuffs on me." Ben went cold inside as he saw Sand slowly raise his hands and then begin working himself into a standing position, using his great strength to move his body effortlessly upward.

"You man enough to do that after all the exercise you had today, Benny?" The razor edge was back in his voice, the challenge open in his face, the deadness back in his eyes. He was back in command of the situation.

"Nope. You still don't have no backbone, Singer. You know who the Man is don't you. Well, I got to be on my way."

Sand turned and started along the truck, toward the pistol lying on the ground. Ben's arrow struck the pistol and carried it under the truck, out into the dark abyss beyond. As he quickly notched another arrow he opened his mouth to tell Sand he would shoot him through the legs if he had to but the words came out as a growl as he saw Sand had reacted instantly, spun on his heel and launched himself across the hood and was disappearing into the dark on the far side of the truck. Ben's hurried shot cut the air above his head and arched harmlessly out into the dark.

Ben heard as much as saw the far side door open and then slam shut. He heard the near side door lock even as he dropped the bow and leaped for the truck.

Ben pressed his face into the glass and saw a huge, shadowy Dick Sand rummaging in the glove compartment, hands searching frantically. Looking for a hideout gun that wasn't there. Ben went cold as he saw Sand slide forward and jerk the back of the seat forward. Even in the dark Ben could see his grin as he began to work the big rifle out from behind the seat.

Ben's mind shut down under a shocking, icy flood of fear. Compounded of his feelings when Sand shot the rope and dropped him over the falls and the vision of himself riding on Sand's truck like a four-point buck after being shot at long range.

Ben couldn't run. Too far to cover. In moments, Sand would blast him right through the side of the truck. There was nothing to be done. Sand had won. Sand had won ..Ben felt the bitterness start to well up inside him again, for the last time. How lonely death would be knowing Sand was still loose in the world.

Into Ben's mind leaped the small boy's image of a huge man tipping over a car in the parking lot of the Navajo Mountain trading post. Not me. I can't do that, Ben felt despair ripping through him. Draining the last of his strength. Even as he saw that Sand almost had the rifle free.

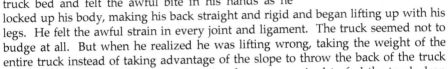

I'll die trying, he remembered himself saying in Whitehouse canyon. Not like a rabbit run to the ground. If he shoots me don't let it be while I'm standing around like a fool's hen in the brush.

Ben bent at the knees, hooked his hands under the truck bed and felt the awful bite in his hands as he locked up his body, making his back straight and rigid and began lifting up with his legs. He felt the awful strain in every joint and ligament. The truck seemed not to budge at all. But when he realized he was lifting wrong, taking the weight of the entire truck instead of taking advantage of the slope to throw the back of the truck

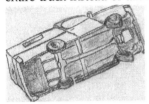 over the edge, he was surprised to feel the truck drop sharply and rock on the springs. It must have surprised Sand too. Ben saw his face peering out the window, trying to locate Ben. He saw real fear on Sand's face for the first time.

He shifted along the truck bed, set himself again, and felt Sand's weight hit the far side of the truck as he heaved again. He wondered if Sand was trying to jump out. That question was answered when the interior of the truck lit up like noon day and a smothered roar accompanied the blasting of a magnum hollow point bullet out through the truck door where Ben had been a moment before.

Fear shot adrenaline into his body. Anger heated up inside him. The raw, red hot magma broke free. The warrior's rage surged through him. Sand would not win. Ben felt the strength of desperation and hope that had filled him at the falls as he struggled to move the tree. He reached down inside himself to free up and focus every ounce of strength and of outrage that was in him.

And in the next moment he staggered forward a half-step and almost fell down the slope. Helpless, exhausted, he sank to his knees, fell forward and caught himself on his hands. He was amazed to see Sands truck tipping on over, in a ponderous, almost leisurely movement that smashed the door shut on the far side, cutting off the sharp sound of Sand's scream as he was trying to escape.

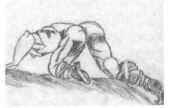

On the first roll the camper shell shattered and bales of drugs scattered down the slope, tumbling and sliding alongside the truck. On the second roll, picking up speed and momentum, the truck fetched up sharply against a massive pine, breaking its back, wrapping partway around the tree, but not smashing the cab.

Chest heaving, body aching, Ben got unsteadily to his feet in time to see Bud bounding down the hill toward the truck, skipping lightly over the loose shale. Then the truck door screeched open and Dick Sand flopped out on the ground like a spent fish flopping feebly in the bottom of a boat.

Ben moved down the slope, careful not to start a rockslide, finding the going easier than it looked. Wondering if he would have the strength to climb back up.

He found Bud sitting, grinning, beside Sand, who looked like he had gone ten rounds inside a washing machine set on the spin cycle. He was battered, his nose was bleeding, one arm at a crazy angle that must mean it was dislocated or broken. He moaned, seemed almost to be crying softly to himself.

Ben found a length of rope, knotted it around Sand's neck, sat him up against the truck and tied the rope out of Sand's reach in the tree. He checked his pockets to be sure he didn't have a knife to cut the rope.

Sand's eyes were open. Intelligence still burned there. But somehow the old Dick Sand was gone. For the moment. Ben saw the eyes following him, knew Sand could understand.

"You know the knot, don't you Sand", Ben said. "Don't let it get pulled tight whatever you do, unless you have some great desire to see what Hell is like a little early."

Ben climbed the side of the truck, watching Sand's feeble attempts to be sure he didn't get tangled in the rope. He pulled out the big rifle, being careful not to let Sand see that the scope was smashed and broken.

"You know about my kill trained Scotty dog too, don't you? He'll stay with you while I go up the road aways and bring help back. But if I hear him bark "

Ben watched as Sand transferred a part of his worry from the rope to the dog.

"Don't be long, Ben," Sand said weakly. "Please. My arm "

"Yeah. I won't do to you what you'd have done to me in the same circumstance. You can count on that, Sand. Because like you said, I'm not anything like you. And I wouldn't want to start now. Terry and Lester started ."

He saw the shock hit Sand like a physical blow.

"Yes, they're both alive. They went for help when I started up here. I expect help anytime now."

"How .". Sand swallowed. "How'd you do it, Ben? There was no way you could save them and yourself, too. I just figured you wanted revenge more than you wanted to save them."

"You figured I did what you would have done, you mean."

"How'd you do it?" There was a hint of awe in Sand's voice.

"I used Light and Truth, Sand. Light and Truth."

Ben left Sand shaking his head, turned, and climbed up the slope. From the road he could see headlights shining through the treetops back over the ridge. Wearily he started back for the bike. When he glanced back he saw Dick Sand, huge, but misshapen somehow in the dark, leaning against the truck, cradling his arm, clutching the rope, staring fixedly at the little dog sitting off to the side

Chapter Thirty-Three
Ben Singer Comes Home

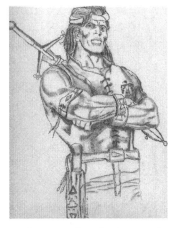

Dr. Hartman intoned: " ..And so we are met here today to honor a young hero, a fine scholar, a brave man, an honest citizen who, by personal sacrifice and by great personal effort, even at the risk of his own life, has helped eliminate from our society a group of very evil people who were preying on weak and innocent members of our community ."

Ben felt Terry squeeze his hand. He glanced down at the ring that sparkled on her finger. He looked up to see an even brighter sparkle glowing deep in her eyes. Looking out over the crowd in the WWCC Ballroom he spotted Grandpa and his mother, Tony and uncle Charlie .he suddenly realized that nearly every male member of his extended family was somewhere in the room. He felt a warm glow. They had supported him. Even knowing him as he was, they had moved quietly to surround him with a safety net.

Further back he saw Terry's parents. He was looking forward to introducing them to Grandpa. That would be quite an experience for both sides of the family ..Ben smiled at Terry again. Life was just beginning now, not ending under Dick Sand's unholy influence.

Ben thought of Sand, in prison. Awaiting trial on so many charges, but being tried first on capital murder charges in TJ's death. Utah still had the death penalty. He'd seen Sand in court. Cradling his arm, which had shrunk dramatically from atrophy and disuse. Sand was almost a cripple now. And he seemed even more crippled emotionally, burned out, grey, listless, pathetic. Ben shuddered despite the warm sunlight when he remembered how badly he'd wanted to be like Sand. Use his methods .feel his anger and contempt. The only "friend" Sand had left was Rhetta.

Ben shook his head, wondering.

Well, at least Sand could look forward to Rhetta's letters. He grinned inwardly as he remembered Terry's exasperation with her when she flip-flopped   and suddenly announced to everyone who would listen that she was taking on a new "charitable project". She would work, she said, for the humane and ethical treatment of felons....

Ben came back to reality with a jolt when he realized that Alex had just walked in, taking a seat modestly, in the back. His business suit was a little out of style, his bearing still erect and enduring. His smile was cheery, full of friendship, compassion and understanding. A true friend. Ben owed him .oh so much ..He felt his eyes sting. A mist turned the sunlight into rainbow colors. That rainbow of joy at the end of a great storm. The beginning of a peaceful summer day.

Ben realized clearly now that Alex was someone he wanted to be like. He'd have to look into this whole Whitehouse Society deal now ..see what it was all about ..see if he could learn to live by more if its ideals.

" ..We are happy to announce this day that Ben Singer has been restored to his place in this school as the recipient of the Thornton Scholarship in pre-law studies. In addition, Mr. Ted Nielsen, mayor of Warrenville, is here to make a special presentation to Ben at this time .Mr. Nielsen.

The mayor stood up to scattered. mild applause and stepped to the podium.

"Dr. Hartman, Board of Counselors, and directors, Chief Hensley, my fellow citizens .I'm pleased to be able today to make a special Citizen's Citation award for meritorious community service to Mr. Benjamin Franklin Singer."

He turned and motioned to Ben. "If you'll join me here, sir."

Ben stood easily, moved quietly and smoothly across the podium to stand by the mayor. He was an inch shorter, but broader, vastly more powerful, making the mayor look small by comparison. The mayor seemed to react to this, to the impact of Ben's presence. His hands shook a little as he placed the ribbon and the attached gold medal around Ben's neck. Turning back to his audience he said:

"This award comes with a $10,000 cash award, which I am pleased to present, at Ben's request, to the city drug rehabilitation program to help begin an outreach program for teen and preteen drug abusers in the community. Mr. Singer is not only brave and able. He is also a dedicated civic-minded young man. This plaque, Ben, is in recognition of the great service you have rendered your fellowmen. I understand you were instrumental, at the risk of your own life, in breaking up a vicious drug cartel extending clear into Mexico. This resulted in nearly 100 arrests, several of them apparently top drug dealers in the Phoenix area. This happened because you directly, single handedly saved the lives of two people and captured the man who was directing the drug ring in this area, along with a quantity of drugs and a set of records that exposed the entire operation.

"We want to acknowledge at this time the help your family gave in locating drug routes, identifying people carrying drugs, and in bringing several of them, including two very dangerous men who were known killers."

Ben smiled at his family. They had been behind him all along. Trying hard to help him. He felt a stirring in him. A healing, a closing of wounds, deep down inside. The banking of the angry fires that had burned so strongly in him. In the Navajo way, a restoration to the Beauty Way, the Pollen Path of Hozho that his people valued so deeply. He glanced at Alex. In a flash of sudden insight he understood what Alex had been trying to teach him all along.

Ben had wanted to do good, to be good. He had wanted the right things all along. Sand had knocked him off center so badly that without Alex's mentoring Ben would surely have gone the wrong way. Used Sand's and REX's methods. Destroyed himself, murdered his character, forever lost sight of his goals and dreams. Become as venal and miserable as Dick Sand.

But I was right in the beginning, Ben thought. I lost faith in myself and in my values for a while, but I had made a lot of good choices up till then. Maybe Alex was right. Maybe I deserved a helping hand. It was touch and go there for a while. But in the end I served my values and it turned out well in the end. Ben felt a little shudder pass through him. How close he'd come to murdering Dick Sand. How glad he was now that he hadn't. Even if no one else had blamed him, he would have felt it was a basic betrayal of all he stood for, all he valued in life.

Ben vowed to learn this lesson well. Now, when he wanted to do good, as he went through life pursuing his goals, seeking to live by his values, he would watch for others like himself. People who wanted to do well, but had temporarily lost their way. He'd know what to do. That was the marvelous reward of a bitter, bitter experience. Now he knew he had walked the way himself he wished that society could be changed so that good men didn't have to suffer at the hands of people like Sand. That would be something to live for, to work for.

He saw Lester, coming in late, but with a young girl that had to be his sister. Ben knew the FBI had set up protection for her and had arrested some of Sand's people when they came after her. He heard the mayor droning on

" ..a special research scholarship in juvenile law in the memory of TJ Davis. This will enable Mr. Singer to expand his service to his people by becoming an expert in those laws and programs aimed at preventing the beginning of drug abuse patterns in the young.

Mr. Singer, we are proud today to congratulate, to openly applaud the efforts that you made, singly, alone under great duress, to end in a great public service."

Ben felt himself shifting nervously, he knew just how little he had done. How much he owed to others, how completely he had failed, almost to the last moment.

He smiled at Alex, who gave him a thumbs up sign and a dazzling grin. Alex rose and walked up the aisle, heading out. No one seemed to notice him, nor the small, perky dog that tagged along behind. Bud looked back over his shoulder, then did his famous circus back flip, grinned at Ben and then followed Alex.

Alex turned and looked at Ben and Ben realized Alex had been reading his thoughts again. Alex signed: Peace Go With You My Friend. He smiled then he and Bud passed from Ben's sight, out the pavilion, headed back to where? Ben saw in his mind's eye the book. He would find Alex in the book. That's where he would start his search for Alex and his people.

Alone? Ben thought. Are any of us ever alone in what we do? Good or evil, it seems there are other who are concerned, taking part when they can. Ben wondered who REX would find to take Sand's place. He shivered as he thought what that would be like.

The sun broke through the clouds again and bathed the audience and Ben in warm, glowing light. He motioned Terry to join him and he stood with his arm around his good friend. His sweetheart, as he listened to the sound of sustained applause. There were, after all, it seemed, a lot of good people who appreciated those who tried to do what was right. He had no need to ever feel alone in doing good, ever again.

Since the events of 9/11 this seems more important then ever. Good people are emerging from their backgrounds, taking part, taking a stand for the best of our values. May you join them....along the Warrior's Way.

Jon H. Hansen, M.Ed.

AUTHOR'S NOTE: There are many events in history that describe the desperate plight of societies locked in wars of extermination. The events in this book were chosen because hey happened here in America around 400 A.D. according to the Book Of Mormon. This book is published by the Church of Jesus Christ of Latter Day Saints (Mormon) in Salt Lake City, Utah. You may get a copy from them or send me an E-mail for a copy with an index referring to these battle scenes and other aspects of a true Warrior's mentality that you may find interesting. No Mormon Missionaries will call on you if you get the book from me. Check the Webiste occasionally for updates on this and for the location of a discussion group if one springs up around the principles in this book.

J Hansen

Email: writerjonhansen@comcast.net Mail: Jon H. Hansen, M.Ed., P.O. Box 970022, Orem, Ut 84097

APPENDIX A

Student feedback indicates that more is needed than the explanations woven into the story. This Appendix seems to fill that need very well. It is introduced here so that you can study the entire subject and then return to the story for the polishing and refinement it can give. This material enhances the work of Covert Bailey, a famous exercise guru, found on the internet and in the bookstore. He tells you what needs to happen, and the Warrior's Way information shows you how to do it the best, most efficient and natural way. It's a combination that is hard to beat. There will be a link from my website to Bailey's website soon.

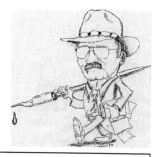

Jon H. Hansen, M.Ed.
Wordwright
Illustrator

Email: writerjonhansen@comcast.net   Mail: Jon Hansen, M.Ed., P.O. Box 970022, Orem, Utah 84097

AGAIN REMEMBER THAT YOU MAY BE UNDERTAKING A MAJOR REORGANIZATION IN THE WAY YOU HANDLE YOUR BODY. SEE A DOCTOR BEFORE YOU BEGIN AND CONSULT A DOCTOR AS YOU GO ALONG SO YOU CAN MONITOR MUSCLE AND JOINTS, BUT JUST AS IMPORTANTLY, THE FUNCTIONS OF HEART, BLOOD, CIRCULATION AND ALL YOUR BODILY FUNCTIONS. REMEMBER THERE ARE NO SHORTCUTS OR MAGICAL ELEMENTS INVOLVED. THIS IS A MASSIVE CHALLENGE TO YOUR BODY THAT CAN DEVELOP GREAT PHYSICAL POWER IN YOU. IT MAY BE STRENUOUS AND DEMANDING AT FIRST.

TAKE HEART FROM THE FACT THAT SOME "NATURALLY" STRONG PEOPLE ARE ACTUALLY LAZY. THEY DO LITTLE BEYOND ENERGIZING THESE SYSTEMS. AFTER A WHILE IT WILL SEEM EASIER TO DO IT RIGHT THAN TO PUT UP WITH THE STRAIN OF DOING IT WRONG. GIVE YOURSELF A BREAK AT FIRST AND YOUR EFFORT WILL YIELD RESULTS. THE EFFORTS WILL BE JUST SUFFICIENT TO EQUAL THE THRILLING SENSE OF SUCCESS THAT ACCOMPANIES IT.

TAKE THE TIME TO DO IT RIGHT! YOU SPENT YOUR WHOLE LIFE GETTING INTO THE SHAPE YOU'RE IN. USE THESE IDEAS TO DO A COMPLETE MAKEOVER, BUT REMEMBER THAT MUCH OF THIS DEPENDS ON THE STRENGTH OF THE LIGAMENT ATTATCHMENTS THAT CONNECT BONE AND MUSCLE.

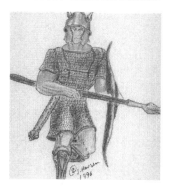

THINK ABOUT HOW MANY ATHLETES SUSTAIN INJURY NOT TO THE MUSCLE, BUT TO

THE LIGAMENTS. LIGAMENTS THICKEN AND STRENGTHEN MORE SLOWLY, OVER TIME. GIVE THEM TIME TO COME ON LINE BEFORE YOU BEGIN EXUBERANTLY DISPLAYING YOUR NEWFOUND STRENGTH AND ENERGY….. BUT MOST OF ALL… ENJOY!

The First Great Key To Super-Strength—The Body's Middle Zone

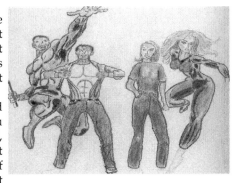

What actually is, and how we perceive what is are usually two different things. Our mental image of what happens when we push down on the gas pedal in a car hardly describes what really happens. This subject is the same. I'm using many examples and illustrations and ideas to help you visualize how the really powerful, natural strong men get that way without special exercises. But they don't think of it this way at all, and Nature hasn't written an "owner's manual" for the body detailing it.

So….. We have to start somewhere. Among the illustrations I devised to help you understand what's going on, I've found the idea of the body being roughly divided into "zones" to be helpful to readers.

Definition:

In the late 19th century physical culture was all the rage, like it is today. Today we just call it the fitness craze. Well…..anyway, some famous physical culturists began to study a very peculiar phenomenon. While most people were hitting the gyms and turning themselves inside out in pursuit of fitness…..(sound familiar?) some guy would show up who didn't know a dumbell from a jump rope but was so strong that he pulverized and out-performed the best weight lifters and exercise enthusiasts hands down.

A little research revealed that such men had always been around. They were often the kings, generals, bandit kings of the ancient world.

How come they're that way, the pundits and gurus of fitness wondered.

Edwin Checkly, for one, after a massive study involving thousands of interviews and photographs, concluded that everyone of them, whether a Chinaman, a Turk, an Irishman, whatever race, lifestyle, diet, and activity pattern, all had some things in common.

Habitual ways of managing their bodies. In a marvelous leap of insight he concluded, and then proceeded to demonstrate, that the habits created the strength. As opposed to the normal, intuitive idea that they had the habits because they were strong.

So…… What we have in this book is a description of those habits. I'm coming at this from Checkley's viewpoint, but the illustration devices are all my invention. I use Checkly so I don't get certain people mad at me who sort of inculcated me into a modern Native American warrior society that also treasures and passes on a lot of this knowledge.

The French Army around World War One was teaching some of this to recruits. So why isn't it well known?

Jon H. Hansen, M.Ed.   274

Why isn't everybody doing it?

You'll draw your own conclusions. But I and some of my readers who have tried hard to share this knowledge have concluded that it's because this isn't a magic bullet. Not some glitzy sugar pill. It's real, and it's hard to do at first. Most people can't get beyond the "at first" part......

Will you?

Some satisfy themselves to do some of it, or all of it sometimes and thus stay slim and shapely and vital. Others opt for the power mode. I did. I went from 6'5" and 190 pounds to 6'5" and 260 pounds. In police work, in school teaching (junior high) and in a thousand physical confrontations in life, I went for the power.

Sounds cool, huh? Well calm down. Because I lived my life more like the 'warriors' described in the book I never had to use it. Well, maybe a few times in answering domestic disturbance calls involving three or more men. Or when I stopped a potential riot outside a basketball game in a small town one Friday night........

The point is, dear reader, that this is not about me. It's not about how I chose to make use of the knowledge.

It's about you. It's about each of us, in our marvelous variety. Male, Female, old, young, handicapped, and so on. It's best that you quickly transfer your study to yourself and to the people around you. If these principles exist and truly describe the human condition you'll be able to see it as soon as you know what to look for.

My job now, as it was in the classroom for many years is to help you "perceive the referent". Meaning that you form a working mental image of your own of the things I'm attempting to describe in words and pictures. We each have to re-invent for ourselves a model of how the world works. You need to make this knowledge your own and find your own best way to use it.

That's easy. All you have to do is "energize" the muscle systems and you'll immediately "feel" it. From there practice, observation, and self-monitoring will do the rest.

Because it isn't rocket science. Lots of people who could never pass my history courses are still stupendously strong. Because they have the body management habits that create that strength.

So lets get to it.

We have to start somewhere. Among the illustrations I devised to help you understand what's going on, I've found the idea of the body being roughly divided into "zones" to be helpful to readers.

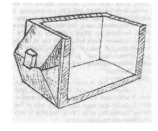

The central aspect of the habits of 'natural' strong man that sets him apart from everyone else is the way he manages his pelvis.

The bones of the pelvis contain points of attachment for muscles that form the foundation of human erectness. The body management habits of very strong people center there in peculiar ways.

The box represents the box of the pelvis in the

Warrior's Way

human body. The open part is the front.   You will see this box inside some of the other illustration too.   The assembly on the side represents where the hip bone attaches. The pelvis and the muscles attached to it are the keys to natural strength and athletic power.

The spine is balanced on the pelvis, literally sitting on the lower vertebra that are fused to the pelvic bones.

Muscles attaching to the front of the pelvis and other muscles along the sides plus the gluteus muscles (your behind) attaching to the back of the pelvis, can be used to determine the position of the pelvis and the lower back (and the spine). In the illustrations these muscles groups are cross-hatched and darkened.

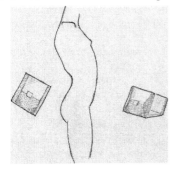

The thing to focus on is not tipping the pelvis from side to side but from front to back. Most people slouch along with the front of the pelvis tipped down spilling its contents (your guts) over the front. This is the first thing we have to deal with and one of the toughest because a deep forward curve in the lower spine and a drooping front of the pelvis are so common that illustrators and artists and even coroners have accepted it as "normal"

Normal it may be in terms of the fact that it's found almost universally in humans.   But "natural" it ain't, in terms of our naturally strong people.

If you aspire to liberating athletic power in yourself (to become a "natural" athlete) you'll study kinesiology in some detail on your own or with a coach. (that's the science of human movement, etc. Lots of athletic coaches study it. Google can tell you more.) For most of us, a basic understanding is plenty. You can learn so much from just watching people and paying attention to what you feel in your own body that great detail isn't necessary.

For our purposes it's enough to know that if you pull up the front of your pelvis you flatten out the curve in your lower back. That's all you really need to know.

WHAT'S GOING ON HERE?

In managing (mismanaging) the middle zone there are two main categories of failure. They are as different in their results as day and night. The poorer way leaves a person very weak, usually fat in their middle years, always physically undeveloped.

The other comes from partially energizing the mid-zone muscle groups, but

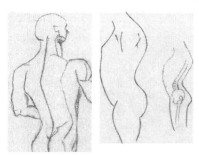

failing to finish the job and do it right. Many athletes display this second type of body handling, and they are precisely the ones who later in life can develop the "beer belly" and degenerate easily into the worst (weakest) type.

Mark it down for future reference that the dividing line between these two groups lies in whether or not you energize enough of the mid-zone to force yourself to breathe

correctly. Watch carefully for that discussion a little later on.

Notice that in every example I've given except one (I sure hope you can spot which one it is!) that it's the mid-section (belly) that sags. Lets take a look at the illustrations while I try to describe to you what's happening here.

Plate two shows two views of the pelvis, both tipped forward, and between them, a human body, also with the pelvis tipped forward. This, however, is a diagram of a person who breathes more or less correctly and thus is not a worst case example. Picture the forward curve the spine must have in this person.

The way you tell in real life is that the person's upper body, shoulders, neck, and arms, will be well developed and strong and the head will set better on the shoulders, rather than hanging forward over a collapsed chest.

The back view gives some hint of this deep curve in the lower spine. It exists in infinite variety in people. Some have a sagging belly out front and some do not, but the tilt of the pelvis is easy to spot once you know what to look for.

Picture the weight of a car pressing down on that curve. NO WAY!

Allowing the pelvis to tip forward is a major source of weakness. The question is, how do you get the tip out of it?

Plate 3 shows a front and a back view of a standing man. Certain muscle groups are shaded in. These groups, the abdominals, the laterals and the glutes, can contract to pull up the front of the pelvis and hold it isometrically in place. These muscles (especially the glutes) are described as being "unusually coarse". This may hint at why they can endure being energized day and night. Because they can. And when they are, the lower back, the mid zone, is held in bands of muscle that lock the spine into place.

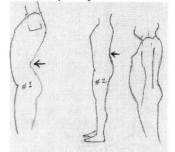

Take time to study the pictures, the front view and the back view, to get a sense of what's being said here, but **don't try it yet. You'll need to read the story to see how Axelron shows Ben how to start gently doing this so you don't do yourself an injury.**

Focus on these three profiles in the area where the arrows point. Number one shows a deep curve, with the pelvis tipped far forward. But the upper body and neck are robust mainly because the breathing is done in the upper chest. Many athletes that later go to pot will present this physique when young. Number two shows much less curve. This is more like what you want to achieve. Except the view has the figure standing on his heels.......WRONG!....but we'll come back to standing later. The third figure represents those who slump, allowing the chest to collapse down into the body. The breathing is mostly done with the belly muscles that should be holding the back flat. This is the type that fights to stay in shape, is generally very weak and often very fat. There are such a large variety of bodies and genetic inheritance plays such an important role that much has to be said about "morphotypes".

TIME TO TRY IT OUT

To energize these groups stand with your feet pressing down firmly on the ground. Eventually you should find that you naturally place your feet about shoulder width apart, indeed that you begin to stand much like the comic book superheroes. (Can there be a connection here? There can indeed!) You will also find a slight forward lean to your body, the weight resting more on your toes, less on your heels. Energize your behind muscles (glutes) strongly and feel them at once pulling down and pulling in under your pelvis region. At the same time, use the abdominal and lateral muscles to push your spine, and the entire lower back, backwards. Straightening out the curve in your spine.

Quick! Observe. Did you have to change your breathing, did you start breathing in your upper chest, almost panting, because the muscles you normally breathe with are suddenly otherwise occupied? Like you breathe when you have to bend over and heave on a heavy weight?

If you did, sorrow and rejoice at once. Sorrow because you probably have the poorer management habits, rejoice because you have the most to gain from learning to handle your body correctly!

Now you got it. 24 hours a day, forever. Yeah, right. Maybe thirty seconds or a minute for you at first. Then those atrophied muscles start screeching for oxygen and punishing you with pain like you were being crucified .

But that's your goal. Since those muscles were designed to do this job you will be utterly amazed at how much progress (how much stronger you can be) in just a couple of weeks of effort. As you may have learned from being fit once, it's nice to live in a body where the muscles have tone and energy. A big part of our sense of well being resides in the muscle/ligament/joint systems of our body. As well as the cardiovascular system, which you may notice is getting a pretty good workout by now.

WANT TO SIT DOWN?

You'll lose it if you do. Sitting is a special case if you're going to do it right. We tend not to get the buttocks muscles tucked under us right. And we stop pressing back with the laterals and abdominals.

The way I do it is I sit down, put my feet far out in front of me, then raise myself on my feet and elbows and strongly energize the glutes. Then I sit down, push down hard, and force myself to sit very erect, with the abdominals and laterals doing their job. When

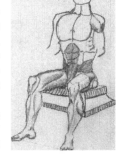

you read a little further on about the diaphragm and the key role it plays, I'll explain how, when sitting, you can use this key muscle to force yourself to rotate the pelvis in under you and then to lock these muscles into their static, isometric, holding positions. If you're a number one, who normally sits poorly you'll amaze yourself at how much energy you burn just sitting!

Poor sitting, and too much of it, is what turns a lot of twos into middle-aged number ones. If you can sit right, as you'll soon discover, you are working all the upper body muscles as well as forcing yourself to breathe correctly. (You probably aren't, but you are much closer and in a while you'll know how to get it right.)

You can work up a major sweat just sitting there. That's why the "naturally" strong are strong. They are exercising their bodies constantly. Not in big, exhausting exercises. But in small, incremental ways that use muscle nature designed to do the job, and that total up to stupendous power sometimes. Even lithe and erect women, whom you would not describe as "powerful" are nevertheless very strong and muscular in a feminine way. Much of their slimness and their unconcern for diet can be traced to the fact that they have these systems energized day and night and are burning calories that you simply store as fat. And remember, those feminine curves we so admire or envy (depending on our point of view) are created by muscle not sculpted out of fat and cellulite.

This exercise (essentially a static or holding exercise) uses what is called "slow twitch" muscle that has a bigger blood supply and can build up amazing endurance. When you try to hold yourself up with other than slow twitch muscle you just get tired.

Plus, both men and women, have and maintain large amounts of very fit muscle, which is the latest thing for fat burning. (As if they didn't know about it in ancient Babylon)

When you sit, sit. Don't slump. Be sure you use your slow twitch muscles. Google's getting a workout today, huh? Visit Covert Bailey or catch him on public television. He's made this clear for me and he can for you, too.

THE DEADLY ERROR

The big mistake is in sitting round shouldered, letting the abs and laterals relax while the back of the chair takes up their work, and then allowing the breathing to settle out of the chest. In proper sitting the body leans forward, not backward. The weight falls somewhere between the glutes and the knees. Find someone who sits well and observe. Also look at the body that goes with it.

Since we sit so much now days it is very difficult to maintain natural strength. It was easier when we spent the day standing and walking. I now stand often at my work, using a tall file cabinet to work on.

Remember, the instant you aren't doing it right atrophy sets in. Do it right! Gain the incremental rewards of strength and stamina that these things give you. Study those around you until your are convinced that it really is the "natural" way that was designed into your body. Then do it day and night, arrange yourself, persevere. Enjoy the rewards.

LET'S DEAL WITH BREATHING

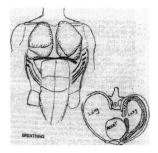

As you look at the plate on breathing, and assuming you've been to the doctor and are sitting or standing with you middle zone properly energized (those pitiful overworked muscles screaming at you yet?), consider the following:

Note where the lungs lie in the body. They are high up, looked at from the top down, they fill all the upper chest. Is there, therefore, any real physiological need for you to breathe with the muscles that you have locked up in holding your lower spine and pelvis in place? (Belly breathing?)

Viola! As though nature had anticipated us, the lungs are clear up above these muscles. Moreover, they have their own group of muscles to aerate them. Breathing costally, that is "rib breathing" has been around a long time as a health aid.

Costal breathing can be seen in dogs and lions when they pant to cool themselves. It involves whole groups of muscles in the chest that a number one physique only uses in the direst straits, the biggest emergencies, and therefore poorly. Once you energize the mid zone and keep it there, you have to develop these systems, again adding to endurance, muscle tone, and strength in shoulders and chest. This exercise is like weightlifting in the gym. You lift the weight of your chest and shoulder with each breath. Try it awhile and you'll begin to see why natural strong men are so strong in the chest, shoulders, and back.

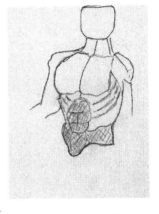

Next time you see the build of a "natural" athlete look for all this, mid zone and glutes strongly energized, and watch the breathing when they have run a race. Or watch any person like this and you will see the shoulders rise as they breathe. Then find a sloucher. Especially someone whose body seems layered with fat that hangs from them almost in folds. Watch. No shoulder movement. They have lost or never had, this physical benefit of using this whole muscle system. No wonder they get blown away in a physical confrontation.

Look at the person sitting in front of you. If you see the shoulders and chest gently rising and falling you'll begin to see what I mean....This is real. Some people do it and some don't.

I was recently in a reverse arm wrestling contest with a 78 year old man... don't ask we were deciding who got to do something.....I said the loser gets to do it. Then, when we started, I started pulling his arm down, to make him make my wrist touch so I would "lose". It's a hoot when you do it with grandkids. But he decided not to win. He's 78, I'm 64. He's been naturally fit all his life, but not super-powerful. He weighs maybe 175 pounds to my 260. It took me almost three minutes to "lose" the contest. And my elbow is still sore.

He's a natural "costal" (rib) breather. I know, I've watched him for years. I only hope when I'm 78 I'm in as good a shape has he is.

You can learn more about this at the website if you read the article on costal breathing. It was a big deal back in the days of Edwin Checkley...

Well, back to work.

Breathing "properly" means that you use the upper chest muscles to lift the chest, then expand the sides of the chest, then push down the diaphragm if you can (or need to). Looking at the drawing, this fills and empties the lungs very effectively. You can "pant" when you need to and amaze yourself at how long you can maintain physical effort because you are quickly filling and emptying the lungs.

BE CAREFUL NOT TO CONSCIOUSLY BREATHE IN A WAY THAT CAUSES HYPERVENTILATION, WHICH IS TAKING IN TOO MUCH OXYGEN AND UPSETTING THE GASEOUS BALANCE THE IN THE BLOOD. IF YOU WORK CAREFULLY YOUR NATURAL SYSTEMS WILL QUICKLY GET USED

TO TRIGGERING THIS "NEW" SET OF BREATHING MUSCLES. AND YOU WON'T GET DIZZY AND LIGHTHEADED FROM "OVER-BREATHING.

Down under Walking I inform you that these principles have been taught in the French army for a long time. I hope by now you are prepared to understand that nothing I'm telling you is new. It's just sort of secret, that's all. You'll get more of that back in the story of Ben Singer. But let me quote you something from a book published in 1923: (He started his work around 1890)

Edwin Checkly, Checkley's Natural Method Of Physical Training, Phila., PA, The Checkley Bureau, 1923, Illus. by H.D. Eggleston. Copyright 1921 by Edwin Checkley, Jr.

"necessarily he had to perform a certain number of movements while instructing his pupils; outside of that he never took exercise, depending entirely on his method of standing and walking, and the ordinary exertions of the day to keep him in his perfect state of health and vigor." p. viii

(Elderly gentleman speaking) "I heard Checkley lecture once, and I was so convinced by his argument regarding breathing, that never since that time have I gone a day without practicing his methods of breathing. It took me some time before I mastered his "costal breathing", but in the 25 years since then I have enjoyed the best of health, and old as I am, I can walk for miles without fatigue and can skip up three flights of stairs with the best of them. I think that as a general rule, there is no crank like a physical culture crank, but Checkley was different. Probably I liked him because he proved to me that I could attain vigorous health without the laborous calisthenics that I so despise."

IBID p. ix

Reportedly he died in an accident at age 75. The doctor remarked that he was young and vigorous as a man of 50. Still as strong as he was from 30 years before, looked like his picture at age 45.

Now if you're young that may not seem so great. Go to a rest home. See what awaits you someday. Avoid it. And enjoy these benefits early in life.

THE GREAT KEY

I don't know how many muscles are involved in all this. As one of my seventh grade students might say, there's bunches and bunches.

I do know if we had to control each one separately with our minds we couldn't think about a whole lot else. So nature has given us some help. And the key to locking up the middle zone properly and to breathing correctly all lies in controlling just one muscle.

The diaphragm.

Yeah, I know that's a toughie. We've all got one, we just aren't used to controlling it all that much.

If you look again at the diagram showing the lungs you will see a dark, thick band just below them. That represents the diaphragm. You might as well know there are lots of specialized activities out there, like karate for instance, that have a lot to say about how you breathe and about how to use this muscle. What I'm going to say goes against some of it. But that's no big deal. What we're talking about here is just every day, run of the mill, routine body management stuff. When you get exotic, like in yoga, you may learn more and it will be useful to you.

In the meantime, this is important because using the diaphragm right forces the abdominal muscles, the lateral muscles, and even the glutes that form your bottom, to lock down tight, rotate your pelvis into position, and to stay put while your breathe.

So what you say? Well, there's one little complication. Your body loves to breathe in its old, lazy way. You can lock things up, and the minute you divert your mind to anything else, your mid-zone will start to deprogram, let go eccentrically, instantly. Irritatingly, constantly.

Your diaphragm is the villain here. You've used it for breathing so long that it's hard to just push it down as low as it will go and t hen keep it there. You get

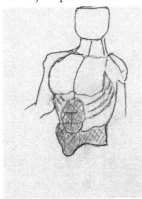

distracted and the diaphragm goes back to participating in the breathing process and the mid zone lets down on you and before you know it you're a number one again.

But if you push the diaphragm down strongly How can I describe the process without getting gross? I guess I can't. When you grunt you use the diaphragm. When you're constipated you push down strongly with it. Maybe also when you're having a baby. I was around for the birth of seven of my ten kids and that pushing was coming from somewhere!

Anyway, the key to this is that when you are energizing the mid-zone, tightening the abs, laterals, and gutes, and rotating the pelvis, if you push down as hard and as far as you can with the diaphragm you'll feel it force the other muscles to lock up completely, the pelvis rotation goes further. You feel the power. But you also feel that you're holding your breath.

But you have to keep the diaphragm down there to maintain the lock up. You have to breathe in short, almost panting breaths using the upper chest and the sides of the chest and not involving the diaphragm at all for normal, `resting' posture. (As when you are sitting or standing without any further physical effort.)

A thing I've noticed might be useful to you. A characteristic of people who do this is that the veins in their arms stand out all the time. Mine only used to do that after I "worked out". Watch for it in yourself, recognize it in others. That other might be a person worth studying a little even if they haven't gone the whole distance and created great raw physical power in their bodies.

Hey, if it was easy we'd all do it. As it is, the "natural" strong man with real power is rare today. Because people rarely get into these habits anymore. It can be done, you can breathe costally, not using the diaphragm much. This is hard at first if you are a slouching couch potato. It is, in fact, the major barrier to you overcoming your weaknesses. Because the newly energized muscles are screaming for oxygen and your new breathing pattern may not be effective until the chest muscles build up and the chest expands somewhat. That means, bottom line, that you will probably only be able to do this for short periods of time at first.

But do it 100 times a day. When resting and laying in bed do it all night. Lying down will take most of the strain and demand off your muscles and the breathing system can keep up and can build itself up. Don't launch into some crazy exercise program that only adds to the strain on your system and only exercises some muscle groups. Lay this foundation first.

Then start walking. Done properly, the walk will strengthen you tremendously. But only after the breathing system catches up to the new demands on it.

Remember, you're laying a foundation. Be wise and do it right. Build from the bottom up. (There's a pun there somewhere. Notice how full and strong the `bottoms' of naturally strong people are.)

One of my favorite examples of correct breathing is the actor Jack Palance. (Urban Cowboys-he was the old cowhand that died. He also does after shave commercials and you can catch him on the old movie channel.) One of my friends said of him years ago that he moves like a panther. He was on the Oscar awards a year or so ago (age 72 or so) doing one arm push ups to show that he was still fit, able, and ready for acting roles. If you spot him, watch him breathe. And watch some of his old movies where you can see him in action. Another good example is Woody Strode. A black actor, who even late life, showed amazing natural strength and poise.

Clint Eastwood, if you follow him from his days as Rowdy Yates on Wagon Train up to the present shows much of this also.

All these men and others may also exercise. But they do so in addition to having a fine physical foundation of natural strength and fitness.

WHAT ABOUT WEIGHT LIFTERS, ATHLETES, AND OTHERS WHO EXERCISE REGULARLY?

There are two major types. Those who energize the zones and breathe correctly and exercise on top of that and those who don't, who simply occasionally exercise some of their muscle groups. Guess what atrophy does to them the moment they quit? Yup. And often you can see it. They are covered with a soft layer of fat, they have poor "posture" and don't have the dynamic movements and muscle definition of the "natural" athlete.

Boxing is a good place to see this. Evander Holyfield shows many of these traits and when you see him in the ring, his body muscles are sharply defined. He's basically strong and "well built" even when he's not in the ring. Other boxers, even though skillful, and perhaps winners, lack that and have great difficulty "staying in shape".

As Alex is trying to help Ben see, these habits create a basic foundation upon which you can build athletically if you wish. If you don't, you still are basically strong and fit.

To lift weights or not, or do any other particular type of exercise is strictly a matter of personal choice and has nothing to do with whether or not you choose to do what Ben is learning from Alex.

MOVEMENT

After all the isometric strain of holding my middle-zone right and breathing correctly, you want me to move?

Yup.

Like a superhero.

Take a look at the panel marked "Superhero". All you see are pelvises, upper legs and lower backs.

What don't you see?

The slightest hint that that area of the back is de-programming, de-energizing, relaxing in any way, in spite of the obvious physical activity. That's what.

That's what it means to release "athletic" power. A classic example is the side view of a fullback, seen from the side, streaking for the goal line. The back is held flat, the bottom tucked under, legs seem to extend strangely ahead of the body.

You will see this all around you in various sports activities now that I've heightened your awareness of it.

We don't usually run the 75 yard dash every day, nor take on the physical challenges of the superhero. But before we leave them, pause for a sober reflection on the fact that they do these things. And doing them helps make them what they are.

If you aspire to join them, lay this foundation well, then use it in your sport. You'll learn how much "natural" ability simply comes from holding the body correctly isometrically so the isotonic muscles can perform athletically!

Moving, average, every day moving, comes down to keeping the mid-zone energized constantly, breathing correctly, and then doing what you do. You'll find that bending over has to be done differently. You may bend the upper body, but the lower back remains flat. All movements seem to start from or to be controlled by the powerful mid-zone foundation. Turning, twisting, rising, setting. Practice on your own, watch others. Think: graceful, powerful, each movement cushioned by the alternate contracting and relaxing of muscle. Don't be clownish in this. Don't become a swaggering buffoon. Watch the men of quiet, confident power. As your body develops endurance and form and strength, be like them. Remember most of this is simple, quiet isometric holding. **That's why it escaped your notice before. But all that is at an end now. And remember, the quiet isometric holding is what develops for you a powerful body that can unleash amazing isotonic power at will. Have you ever been intimidated just by the physical presence of a powerful man? Then you know what I mean.**

Join their ranks. Slowly, patiently. But stop today being what you are and become the best you can be. Now, stop dreaming and lets get the last of this done. So that you and I can get on with the rest of our lives.

WALKING

Much has been written on this subject. Is not so mysterious as what we've been discussing. It's just .and I hope you can understand all this now it's just that if you don't take into account first whether or not you use the isometric systems in your body correctly, all the stuff about diet and exercise miss their mark. Walking, done with the balanced hips and flat back, is the secret to a truly powerful physique. So explore all this in detail, as you walk. You'll feel it as you get it right so don't let the detailed directions throw you. Read them and then TAKE A HIKE! :)

Example: if you're a slumping, lazy couch potato your body doesn't burn as many calories. More is stored as fat. Starvation diets put you into the gain, lose cycle. Exercise lasts only as long as you do it and the only muscles you benefit are those engaged in the exercise. Moreover, if you try to exercise without the isometric foundation of mid-zone energizing and proper breathing, you may be putting terrible strain on your lower back and on other parts of your anatomy. Exercise may be very distasteful to you.

How can any diet or exercise system work the same for you as id does for the "naturally" strong person who goes around 24 hours a day with the isometric system energized? You don't even live in the same universe with those people. The terms and conditions of you life are radically different than theirs.

Only when you close the gap do other things like diet and exercise start to make sense. What I'm saying is, I guess, that you violate the natural way. How then can you expect the natural way to work for you? Does it? See what I mean? You can't blame yourself for not knowing. But now that you know, I expect you to apply your new insight, and your basic intelligence, and the driving desire we all have to be our best, and to do our best, to every aspect of your physical life.

So ..what does that have to do with walking?

Walking was the thing all ancient warriors did lots of. Done from the isometric foundation it is all you need to build stupendous strength into your body. Done in a lazy. sloppy way, without energizing the mid-zone, etc., it is no better than any other exercise, does not burn many calories, and the benefits stop when you do.

Walking, then, is additional exercise. Used on top of these other things it can:

Exercise muscles from your toes to your head, especially the back muscles that lend so much to power and formliness.

Exercise and strengthen the muscles engaged in isometrically holding the mid-zone and others, including the breathing system.

Build powerful legs and buttocks.

Stir up and aerate a body that is tired and stagnant from too much isometric holding (as when you sit for long periods of time).

Increase blood flow to feed and cleanse hard working muscles.

The neat thing about this is, that to get these benefits you don't have to "go for a walk". It's something that you will do countless times a day, every time you have to get from one spot to another. However, you may find it restful and helpful to stroll several times a day during the buildup period to stir things up and to ease tiring muscles. And you may want to explore some of the writings on correct walking, "power walking" and so on if you decide to get serious about building physical power and plan to take long walks.

But, like breathing, we'll just deal with the normal, every day, nuts and bolts stuff. You can add the bells and whistles later if you want to.

POWER WALKING MEANS "HIP-STRIDING"

Alfred Hitchcock and Perry Mason walk from the hips down. No movement of the pelvis region. They have a weight problem. John Candy is a more recent example that might be familiar to you.

There are infinite varieties of walk, just as there are infinite varieties of ways to energize and hold the mid-zone. We aren't going to waste time describing what you can see by simply observing those around you. Because, again, you never

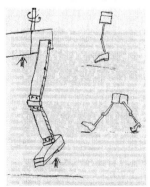

learn to do it right by seeing examples of people doing it wrong. Once you know what the process is meant to be, then you will recognize it when it's being done right. (You'll seldom see it being done right by men. Women are much more likely to do it correctly. (Unfortunately, different physical make-up limits what a man can learn from a woman on this subject. I leave you to explore it further on your own. But let me warn you in advance, if it isn't already obvious, you won't help your case for manliness any by walking around like a woman. You'll need to watch the hip stride of powerful men and learn from them. You'll see it often in massive linemen strolling to the sidelines together after turning some poor ball carrier's upper body around backwards during a play. Heaven help you if you see it striding toward you on some dark side street.)

Rodeo cowboys, with the big silver buckles, can often be seen, when walking toward you, to be hip striding. The buckle turns from side to side as the hips rotate. Most babies walk with a hip stride too so you should be able to observe this.

Refer to the plates that illustrate walking. I've used "boxies" to help you see the internal pelvic box and what it does when we walk. Your task will be to figure out what muscles accomplish this and how to use them without deprogramming your mid-zone isometric systems.

What are you complaining about? I told you once already. If it was easy every one would be doing it. As it is, if you get it even part way right you're going to be able to join that rare group of "beautiful people" that walk off with so many of the rewards of life. Can't you find in yourself a willingness to pay a reasonable price for that great gift, knowing as you do now, that there are no gimmicks, short cuts or magic pills? The application of reason, intelligence, knowledge and will are what are needed here. Maybe you ought to go back to the story a while and share in Ben's struggles.

Well, anyhow .my kid's and my student's eyes glaze over when I get up on my soapbox, too. So un-glaze and lets get back to work.

This is the last thing I need to tell you.

To understand what the boxies show, you need to realize that one reason the mid-zone is so poorly handled is that there are no bones in it to hold anything up. The spine runs up the back, and that's it. What we gain from this arrangement is the marvelous flexibility of the human body.

Okay so remember what I said about muscles being able to be both isometrically and isotonically energized depending on the need? And that they can hold, move a joint, or gradually let down against the resistance of gravity?

Some of those mid-zone muscles do double duty when you walk. **(Where do you think the strength comes from? By now you know it has to be developed by exercise. Where do those natural "hunks" get those great looking abdominals from, anyhow? They are working on them with each step they take, while you lumber along like Perry Mason on his way to court.)**

You can understand this several different ways, but let me start by having you think of the knee and the ankle as hinges. When you throw your leg and foot forward the hinges open and lock. Your foot can come down at the heel with the toes pointing up at pretty good angle. (Look at the illustration.) What you do is lift your hip up a little and literally use the hip (the pelvis, to throw that leg forward. And I mean throw it. That means that the hip goes forward first and stops and then the leg continues forward and the knee opens up and the foot is turned up.

Okay .now, what's the rest of you doing? Looking weird, I'm afraid. Lets add some more to the picture. Focus on the back leg. The knee is open, the foot is pushing off with the toes. PUSHING OFF! I say, not just passively rolling around back there, actively doing something.

Notice what the hips are doing, or what the pelvis box is doing, it's being rotated around the spine and is traveling back with the rear leg just as the other hip is traveling forward with the front leg, and remember, the hip going forward has been raised a little so the foot clears the ground. Have you seen somebody exercising by holding the hips steady and turning the upper body back and forth? This is the way the naturally strong do that exercise. Constantly, with every step they take. Imagine what this does for the waist muscles after a while.

Why am I smiling? I'm seeing you trying all of this for the first time. Teetering, awkward, embarrassed. I hope you're not out in public somewhere. Like I said, if it was easy, everybody would be doing it.

How's your mid-zone? Still with you? Sometimes it helps to stop, stand and assume the correct standing "posture" and then to start walking again.

Now, back to the "throwing" part. Not a sloppy, lose-limbed movement like a puppet on strings. You have muscles. Use them!

Tighten the thigh muscles so that leg you "slung" forward is gradually stopped by the pure contraction of muscle. Turn that foot up using lower leg muscle. On the leg and hip going backwards, do the same. Feel like you are rolling on ball bearings made of muscle. Especially in your feet, literally lift yourself up on a rolling cushion of muscle as you walk.

Watch the top of the head of a good walker, from a distance. The head does not bounce up and down! All the movement takes place elsewhere. That is what is known as a regal gait (the walk of kings)

Learn to cushion every physical movement you make with the gradual contraction and release of muscle. That, my friend, is where the cats get their "cat-like" grace. They don't move around with their bodies hung loosely on their joints, suspended from their ligaments like dirty wash on a clothesline. They walk, move, with MUSCLE! Try it. You might like it.

Watch the French Foreign Legion march sometime. These principles have been taught in the French Army for a long, long time. (But they didn't tell you, did they) The Legion's march was outlawed once in France. It's insolent. It's about half-speed, almost an insolent stroll. But it's a hip-striding walk that you could well learn to emulate (mimic, imitate).

<table>
<tr><td>

This plate shows the body from above. The dotted lines represent the torso or upper body and the square box represents the pelvis. It shows that the pelvis rotates forward with it's attached hip and leg. Remember also, the advancing hip lifts up slightly to help the foot clear the ground

</td><td>

It's a marching step that the Legion has used to cover miles and miles in the hot desert sands. Learn a little about them. How they have vowed never to leave their

</td><td>

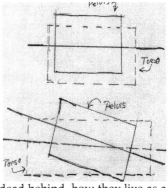

</td></tr>
</table>

wounded or their dead behind, how they live as a brotherhood, answerable only to themselves. It will give you clues about the ancient warrior societies from which they have grown. There are many things about them I don't like, but this part of their mystique is admirable. I use their stroll, and the

Warrior's Way

principles I've explained to you, all the time.

Now for the "feeling part"--what you may experience when you are doing it right. If you maintain the mid-zone, fully energized, and the breathing forced high into the chest, the rotation of the hips has some peculiar effects on the stomach and back muscles that you have probably never felt before.

In front, for example, the muscles all across the front of your abdominals, will contract alternately, with each step. When you feel that you'll at last begin to understand why the "naturally" strong don't have to do sit ups or other abdominal exercises. They do them all the time, more gently, longer lasting, building ENDURANCE. And the strength of a Russian weight lifter. A weight lifting book I have has exercises broken down into two separate routines, one done one day, the other the next, to exercise two different groups of isotonic muscles. But on both days they require you to do sit ups.

That's how important the mid-zone is. It also means the mid-zone can take exercise every day! Day after day. Without need for rest. Remember the "coarseness" I spoke of?

So when you walk, when you sit, stand, sleep, you should be building strength and power and ligament thickness in that zone of your body. Then those muscles can support the spine, add twisting power to your movements, permit you to do acts of real strength and power.

Now, do you begin to see the whole picture?

One last thing, when you walk correctly, you will also feel your back muscles contracting and relaxing right up to your shoulder blades. Above that, the muscles are involved in breathing, getting their own exercise, building their own power.

When you see a true hip-stride you will see a powerful man or woman. They go together. Hopefully now you see that he doesn't walk that way because he's strong. It's the walk that helps to make the strength.

Get up. Take a walk. Follow him, and Ben Singer, along the trail to a warrior's strength. And I hope, to find the honor of a true warrior.

THE END, AND THE BEGINNING

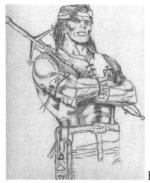

BEN SINGER

In **WARRIOR'S WAY** you can learn to energize and manage the three key muscle zones that all "natural" athletes use to give their bodies gentle, steady, muscle-toning, fat-burning exercise that can, if done correctly, build the stupendous physical power that we sometimes see in natural strong men.

Nature has not made these people your "natural" superiors. You have deliberately made yourself inferior to them by not using this gift nature has given all of us.

Then join those "naturally" fit and vital people yourself by learning, along with Ben Singer, how to energize the muscle control system that lies dormant and unused in so many of us. That is so poorly energized in many others.

Do this before you diet, before you exercise, before you take up athletic training. Learn first to unleash the power of the "system" to help you grow powerful and fit even as you sleep! Then, everything else you do will double its benefits to you.

Follow Ben in a headlong race to stop Dick Sand from killing his sweetheart. Join Ben in the fight of his life as he uses his new-found strength and learns from bitter experience, perhaps too late, to choose the WARRIOR'S WAY.

DON'T BE WIMPY ANOTHER DAY! JOIN BEN SINGER ALONG THE WARRIOR'S WAY!

For more information and to read an article that will teach your some things you can use right away:

Visit the author's Website at:

http://home.comcast.net/~jonhansen44

Jon H.
Hansen,M.Ed.
Wordwright
Illustrator

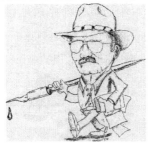

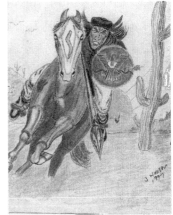

ISBN 142512781-9

31806324R00163

Made in the USA
Middletown, DE
12 May 2016